D1823344

Recent Advances in Cancer Management

Recent Advances in Cancer Management

Edited by Jasmine Johnson

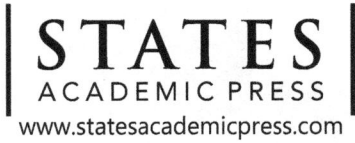

STATES
ACADEMIC PRESS
www.statesacademicpress.com

States Academic Press,
109 South 5th Street,
Brooklyn, NY 11249, USA

Visit us on the World Wide Web at:
www.statesacademicpress.com

ISBN: 978-1-63989-461-1

Cataloging-in-Publication Data

Recent advances in cancer management / edited by Jasmine Johnson.
    p. cm.
Includes bibliographical references and index.
ISBN 978-1-63989-461-1
1. Cancer--Treatment. 2. Cancer--Prevention.
3. Cancer--Treatment--Technological innovations. I. Johnson, Jasmine.
RC270.8 .R43 2022
616.994 06--dc23

Table of Contents

Preface

I am honored to present to you this unique book which encompasses the most up-to-date data in the field. I was extremely pleased to get this opportunity of editing the work of experts from across the globe. I have also written papers in this field and researched the various aspects revolving around the progress of the discipline. I have tried to unify my knowledge along with that of stalwarts from every corner of the world, to produce a text which not only benefits the readers but also facilitates the growth of the field.

Cancer refers to a collection of diseases wherein there is an abnormal growth observed in the cells, and this could spread to other parts of the body. The management and treatment of cancer depends on the type of cancer and the stage. A few of the therapies and treatments used for the management of cancer are chemotherapy, bone marrow transplant, surgery, immunotherapy and targeted drug therapy. Chemotherapy involves killing cancer cells through the usage of drugs. A bone marrow transplant helps in the treatment of a damaged or diseased bone marrow. It also allows for the administration of higher dosages of chemotherapy. This book attempts to understand the multiple branches that fall under the discipline of cancer management and therapy. It strives to provide a fair idea about this discipline and to help develop a better understanding of the latest advances within this field. This book will serve as a reference to a broad spectrum of readers.

Finally, I would like to thank all the contributing authors for their valuable time and contributions. This book would not have been possible without their efforts. I would also like to thank my friends and family for their constant support.

Editor

Role of an Atomic-Level-Based Approach for Improving Cancer Therapy

Santi Tofani

Abstract

Looking at the atomic level of biological activity, the electron spin may be considered a key parameter, governing fundamental biological processes. Spin states have a major role in defining the structure, reactivity, magnetic and spectroscopic properties of a molecule. In the last decades, there has been a growing interest in the use of magnetic fields (MF) to study their influence on different biological systems, considering their effect on electron spin energy levels and consequently on redox-related cellular changes. Different authors have studied the use of magnetic fields as potential antitumor agent as well as an adjuvant agent to chemotherapy and radiotherapy with promising results. Overall, the published data support the presence, in laboratory animals, of antitumor efficacy in many types of cancer including adenocarcinoma, breast cancer, melanoma and neuroblastoma. Those antitumor effects seem to be associated with no observable side effects or toxicity in animals or in humans. More studies are necessary, mainly at the clinical level, to understand the real potential of this atomic approach in improving availability of cancer therapy. In addition, this approach may contribute to fulfill a knowledge gap facing biomedical science today, the one between the atomic level and the cellular level.

Keywords: magnetic fields, quantum biology, free radicals, cancer treatment, apoptosis, atomic biology, spin state in biological systems, antitumor effects, electromagnetic fields, biological effects, electron spin, p53

1. Introduction

Only 25 years ago, at the beginning of the 1990s, chemical biology was just an idea. Since then, that idea evolved into a global community of scientists, dedicated to understanding science at the interactions of chemistry and biology. The work of this community has greatly contributed to the development of medical science.

Among these studies, the molecular studies (molecular biology branch) have traditionally played a very important role in chemical biology research. From a panel of experts, the Nature Chemical Biology editors [1], the need for covering the remaining greatest knowledge gap facing biology today has been underlined: the one between the atomic level and the cellular level.

In fact, since molecules are made of atoms, the new frontier should be to study the influence of atomic structure on biological activity. This may be considered a natural evolution of medical science development. This development has made impressive progresses through centuries, moving from considering humans as an entire entity to considering organ system, organ, cell, cell components and, nowadays, molecules (molecular biology). In this trend, the missing additional part is the atom, and as a consequence, this new branch of medicine should be based on what we could call "atomic biology" (**Figure 1**).

This opens a fascinating scientific adventure: we strongly believe that Physics has to play an important role for the reasons better explained below. The development of a new branch of medical science that, in analogy with Chemical Biology, we can call Physical Biology, can have the main objective to study the influence of atomic structure on the characteristics of the biochemical reactions influencing cell life. A most important contribution is requested to elucidate phenomena at the base of biomolecular activity, influencing the genetic pathways that regulate cell life in genetically based illnesses, like cancer.

For this typology of illnesses, in fact, Chemical Biology and its branch Molecular Biology have been unable to help Medicine to obtain completely satisfactory therapeutic results. More selective treatments to avoid important adverse effects are needed.

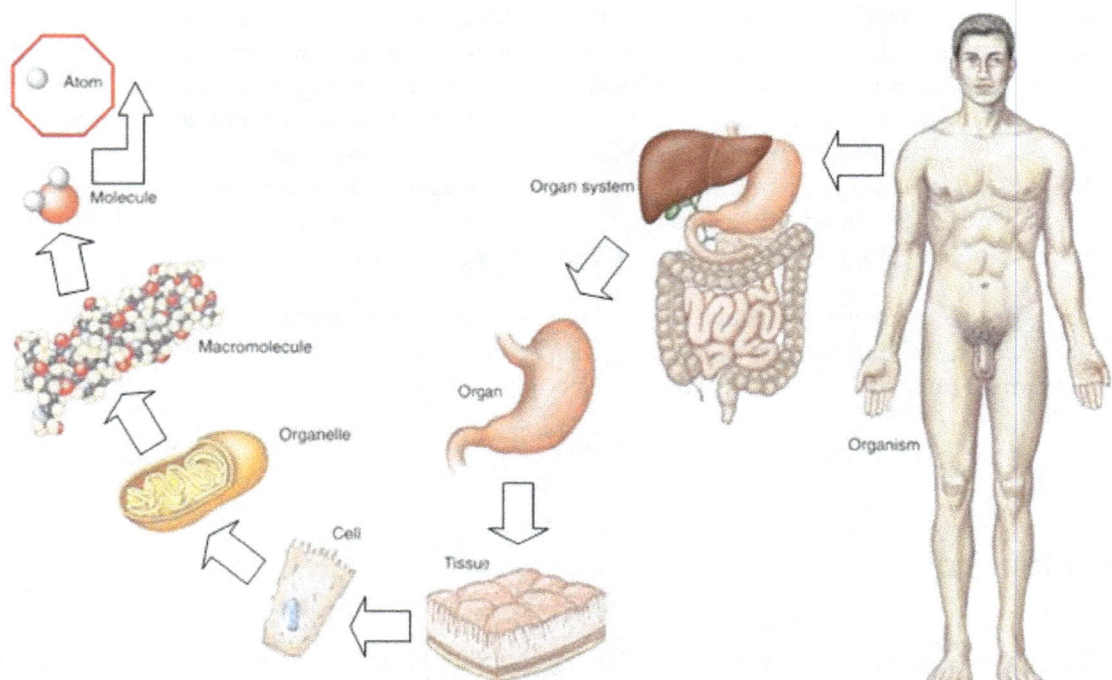

Figure 1. Trend of medical science from its beginning to now. With time (see from right to left), medicine has been developing considering first humans as unity and then made by organs, tissues, cells, until arriving to the present time of molecular biology. Since molecules are made of atoms, the next frontier should be the connection between atomic and biological levels.

The fundamental laws of physics have the capability of describing the very tiny processes that are at the core of life in matter. Because of this, we know for example that using magnetic fields with specific characteristics we can influence spin energy levels. This, for example, gives the possibility to medical doctors to use magnetic resonance imaging to have a very powerful clue of what happens at molecular/atomic levels of the biological structure and function, having consequently the possibility of making diagnosis with an accuracy not possible before.

We know from chemistry that electron spin state has a pivotal role in all the reduction-oxidation reactions that are at the core of the cellular metabolic pathway, governing the behavior of the biological system, influencing genetic stability. The synthesis of many complex molecules often requires the oxidation of their precursor, via the use of molecular oxygen. Availability of electrons to transfer changes when electron spins assume specific energy levels. These energy levels are known from quantum physics to be easily influenced by magnetic fields. Physics allows the use of specific static magnetic fields like those used in magnetic resonance imaging, but almost two/three order of magnitude (100–1000 times) less intense, not thermal, to influence electron spin state.

Aim of this chapter is to analyze the scientific reasons why a more physics standpoint approach to biological processes, or in other words an atomic-level-based approach to biological processes, may contribute to cancer therapy. We will consider biological processes from an atomic-level prospective, analyzing first the correlation between the atomic structure, its influence on availability of electrons, and key biological functions connected to cancer genetics and consequently the available literature reporting results obtained in different laboratories on the use of magnetic fields to influence cancer biology.

2. Atomic structure and fundamental role played by electron spin in key biological processes

Considering the three particles (electron, proton and neutron) constituting the atomic structure, the electron is the only elementary particle and it plays a pivotal role in chemical/biochemical reactions. Electron exchange allows chemical reactions to take place and electron transfer reactions are critical steps in diverse arrays of biological transformations, ranging from photosynthesis to aerobic respiration. Electrons are classified inside all the elementary particles according to their spin value that, being half integer, collocate them inside one of the two families of elementary particles, the fermions [2]. So, the spin has a fundamental role in the nature of matter's structure. Spin is an intrinsic property (form of angular momentum) of particles connected to their behavior in the presence of magnetic fields, where they seem to act as small magnets. In classical physics, a charged spinning object has magnetic properties that are very much like those exhibited by these elementary particles (**Figure 2**). Similarly, physics describes elementary particles in terms of their "spin." Despite this, spin is a purely quantum-mechanical phenomenon; it does not have a counterpart in classical mechanics and obeys quantum physics laws.

Fermions and then electrons obey the Pauli exclusion principle, which states that two identical electrons cannot exist in the same state, that is, electrons paired in the atomic structure in a way to have opposite spin value. Without Pauli exclusion principle, chemistry would not

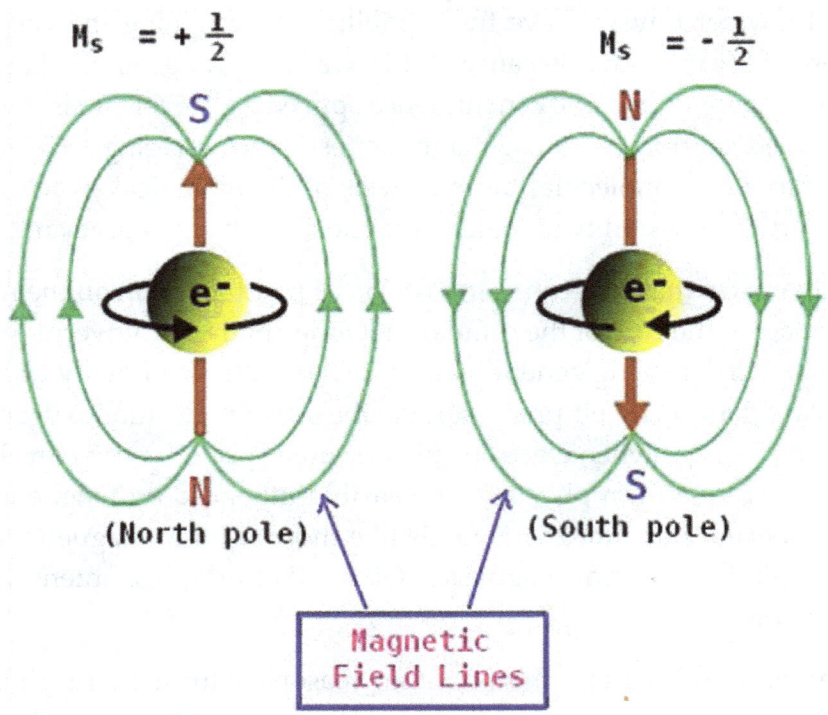

Figure 2. Electron while traveling around nuclei or between atoms/molecule rotates about its axis producing a magnetic field (from physics in fact we know that any moving charge produces a magnetic field) called angular momentum or spin. The electron spin value is ±½ depending on the direction of its rotation.

have the Periodic Table. For these reasons, spin is an essential property influencing the order of electrons and nuclei in atoms and molecules, thus having great physical significance in chemistry. Therefore, we may consider the spin a very important physical entity when studying biomolecular processes. The spin, although being purely quantum-physical, has profound implications for real-world, large-scale systems like, for example, living tissue. In most cases, according to Pauli principle, electrons need to pair up to allow the system, to which they belong, to reach a lower level of energy. This process of electron pairing up facilitates stability in the system (i.e., chemical stability in a biological environment), but it is possible only when, as above states, electron spins have opposite values. This favorable situation depends on the electron origin as well as on the conditions of the chemical environment. When the electron pairing up is not possible, the system accumulates an excess of unpaired electrons. This process leads to the formation of different spin states of individual electrons as well as of molecular species containing unpaired electrons.

Chemically, any molecule containing a single, unpaired electron is defined as free radical. Free radicals are often highly unstable elements which in fact are chemically highly reactive (**Figure 3**). In many cases, the spin state has been found to be a key factor governing the behavior of the biological system since their influence in chemistry and bioinorganic chemistry [3].

The spin state has a pivotal role in all the reduction-oxidation (or redox) reactions that are at the core of our metabolic machinery. Redox reactions involve the transfer of electrons from one reactant to another. This kind of reactions is so important that our life depends on them. The synthesis of many complex molecules often requires the oxidation of their precursor, via the use of molecular oxygen. The utilization of molecular oxygen is vital in many biological

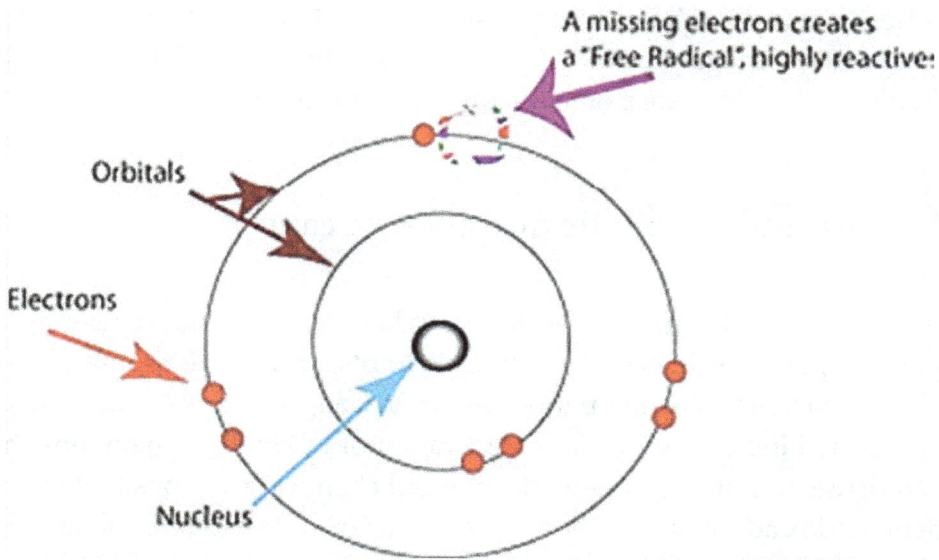

Figure 3. Atoms that do have an unpaired electron, like the atom here presented with atomic number of 7 (nitrogen), are called free radical. Because of their uncoupled spin, they have a not nulled magnetic moment and, in agreement with Pauli principle, they look for a counterpart to reach physical/chemical stability. For these reasons, free radicals are highly chemically reactive.

pathways. The ability of aerobic organisms to harness the power of molecular oxygen as a terminal electron acceptor in their respiratory cycles has revolutionized the evolution of life. Oxygen itself is a diradical: Oxygen-based radicals are also often referred to as radical reactive oxygen species (ROS), such as superoxide anion (O2−) and hydroxyl radical (OH.). Electrons constituting molecules generally have opposite spins. These electrons stay in different orbitals and may take part to the bond formation. A peculiar characteristic of the oxygen structure is that it has two electrons that are not spin-paired, lying in different orbitals, and each of them is looking for an additional electron to pair up. In this case, the process of electron pairing-up, making two pair per atoms or four pairs per molecule, is oriented to produce water molecules to reach a state of lower free energy. Redox reactions are facilitated by enzymes since they have binding sites that can keep oxygen in contact with oxidizable substrates for a long time. This contact time, longer than that made possible only by collision, substantially improves the chance of spin reversal and allows the two electrons to pair up, process that otherwise would be not possible due to limited energy, below the kinetic barrier that would be provided by only collisions. Another important aspect is that enzymes may have such characteristics to catch and withhold available energy from oxidation processes, activity very useful and important in ATP high-energy-related compounds. In addition to this, we know that redox reactions affect signaling between molecules bound to DNA with potentially key effect on cell cycle. It has been shown that oxidative stress conditions may control the very important tumor suppressor protein p53 activity on different promoters using DNA-mediated electron transport [4–6]. One of the most challenging endeavors from both experimental and theoretical point-of-view is to elucidate the role and effect of different spin states on the properties of a biological system, even deciding which spin-state occurs naturally. There is in fact a growing interest in spin states in biochemistry from a chemical standpoint [3]. It can be supposed that a more physics-dependent approach may contribute significantly to this elucidation. In fact, being the spin a purely physical entity (localized magnetic moment/field), its energy states can be theoretically better influenced by physical means than by chemical reactions. In fact, starting from the 1980s, magnetic fields have been widely used to influence the free radical chemistry, thanks to their influence on electron spin state energy levels [7].

3. Redox balance and metabolic processes in cancer

The maintenance of redox balance is considered a key factor for the cancer cell metabolism [8–11]. Adaption requires for these cells to be able to respond to the proliferative signals that are delivered by oncogenic signaling pathways. After malignant transformation, many cancer cells show a sustained increase in intrinsic generation of ROS which maintains the oncogenic phenotype and drives tumor progression throughout chemical reactions that are electron spin state dependent. Redox adaption through upregulation of antiapoptotic and antioxidant molecules allows cancer cells to promote survival and to develop resistance to anticancer drugs [12].

The dependence of tumor cells and cancer stem cells on their antioxidant capacity makes them vulnerable to agents that dampen antioxidant systems. There is a realistic prospect for treatments aimed to dramatically increase intracellular ROS to kill cancer cells by decreasing their antioxidant capacity. This may be obtained using compounds that inhibit antioxidant systems or through inhibition of specific signaling pathways that upregulate antioxidants in cancer cells. The resulting increase in reactive oxygen species may then induce tumor cell death either through random damaging functions of ROS or by specific induction of apoptosis via death signaling pathways. The advantage of such a strategy is that normal cells are not significantly affected since they have lower basal ROS levels and therefore are less dependent on up–/downregulation of oxidative stress [13]. A supposedly more simpler strategy would be to selectively influence the ROS concentration and then redox activity in cancer cell by directly influencing the spin state energy levels by using appropriate magnetic fields.

It is important to note that dealing with ROS concentration we have to consider the double-edge sword of ROS action. In fact, for example, a chemopreventive and an antitumor action have been reported by the use of nutraceuticals derived from fruits, vegetables, spices, and other natural products used in traditional medicine that show antioxidant efficacy. This lasts in agreement with observations [14, 15], suggesting that antioxidant enzymes like the mitochondrial antioxidant manganese superoxide dismutase (MnSOD) may function as new type of tumor-suppressor gene. The above suggest both "upside" (cancer-suppressing) and "downside" (cancer-promoting) actions of the ROS. Thus, similar to tumor necrosis factor-α, inflammation, and NF-κB, ROS act as a double-edged sword.

4. How magnetic fields can influence biological chemistry through spin state

The fascinating aspect of spin states is that the formation of spin-correlated radical pair states between enzyme and oxygen radicals is magnetic field sensitive. In fact, the use of appropriate magnetic fields is capable of changing the spin states of radical pairs modifying the rate of conversion between singlet (S) and triplet (T) and consequently influencing the free radical recombination rate and finally their concentration with downstream biological consequences [16].

Let us now see more in detail the mechanism through which magnetic fields influence spin states and consequently free radical chemistry. Radical pairs are typically formed by electron transfer or photolytic bond cleavage from a molecular precursor. The radical characteristics and then their chemical reactivity depend on their spin states of their unpaired electrons that, like all electrons, present an intrinsic spin angular momentum (quantum number $s = \frac{1}{2}$) characterized by two states, known as spin up and spin down. These two states are labeled by the magnetic quantum numbers $ms = \pm\frac{1}{2}$ (ms specifies the projection of the spin angular momentum on a fixed axis). Spin-correlated radical pairs are generated according to the physical law that implies the conservation of total spin angular momentum, a singlet molecular precursor leads to a singlet born radical pair, while a triplet precursor leads to a triplet born radical pair. The correspondent two spins of the born radicals will be aligned antiparallel and parallel for the singled and triplet born, respectively. S_0 is generally used for the singlet state, its total spin quantum number S is zero as well as its overall spin angular momentum, so their energy is independent of any applied magnetic fields. Vice versa, the three triplet states T_0, T_+ and T_- are defined by a total spin $S = 1$ and spin projection numbers equal to 0, +1 and −1, respectively. In the presence of an applied static magnetic field, the energy of the T_0 state is therefore also field independent, whereas how the energies of the T_+ and T_- states are shifted by the Zeeman interaction is proportional to the strength of the external applied static magnetic field (**Figure 4**). In the absence of an external static magnetic field, interconversion between the singlet and triplet states of the radical pair is driven by internal electron-nuclear hyperfine interactions.

The use of an external static magnetic field influences the interconversion between singlet and triplet states (see circle in **Figure 4**), influencing the rate of recombination of radical pair and consequently influencing free radical concentration. Even if the energy released by the magnetic field to the electron spin is significantly less than the thermal energy, the interesting aspect is that the spin-correlated radical pair, being in a nonequilibrium state, allows a kinetic effect if subsequent radical reactions are spin selective.

The frequency, amplitude and orientation of the magnetic field that perturbs the radical pair dynamics depend significantly on the local enzymatic chemical environment [17]. Specifically, the use of magnetic fields of moderate intensity (milli Tesla, or mT, range), static and/or at extremely low frequency, (frequency up to 300 Hz, down to 3.3 milliseconds) acts through the Zeeman effect removing the degenerative triplet energy levels. Considering the very short life span of a free radical (from microseconds to nanoseconds), it sees the extremely low-frequency magnetic fields as static, which intensity is time dependent.

It results, as discussed above, in the splitting of three levels of different energies, decreasing the probability of transaction from triplet to singlet spin states. The rate of free radical recombination, at a frequency from low to zero, depends on the intensity of magnetic fields that regulates the conversion from triplet to singlet state (**Figure 4** crossing between T_- and S_0).

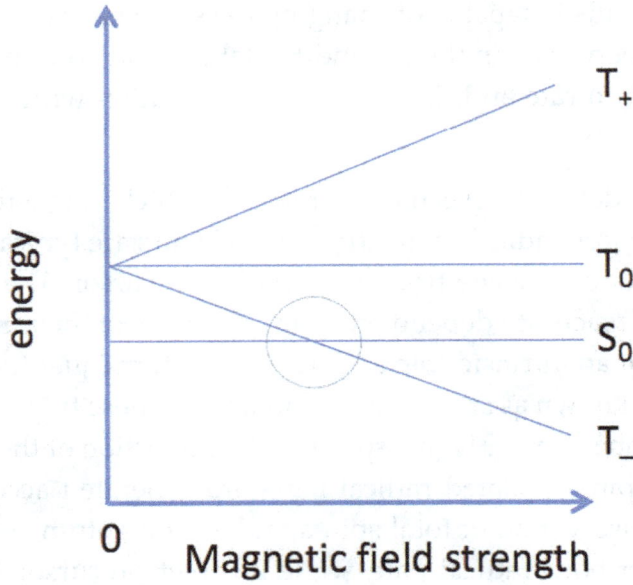

Figure 4. Effect of the Zeeman splitting on the singlet (S_0) and triplet (T_0, T_+ and T_-) states. As we can see, increasing magnetic field intensity, the degenerative energy levels of triplet separate to reach a value (circle) at which we observe the crossing between T_- and S_0.

Magnetic fields at much higher frequency (a mega Hz, or MHz, order of magnitude) used in combination with static magnetic fields can also have importance in influencing the spin states and then the correspondent chemical reactions. There are in fact multiple interactions in which weak magnetic fields (intensity on the order micro Tesla, or µT) at higher frequency can change the population distribution in the various spin states, among them the electron-nuclear hyperfine interaction. External static in combination with high frequency magnetic fields can alter radical pair spin dynamics by Zeeman and HFI resonance effects and thereby change the relative yields of reaction products that derive, alternatively, from singlet and triplet radical pair states [18–20]. Many biological molecules exhibit hyperfine splitting constant that ranges from 0.1 to 35 MHz [20–22], so fields of this frequency may be used to influence hyperfine coupling resonance. Magnetic fields at this higher frequency and very low intensity have been used, together with static magnetic fields, to influence hyperfine resonance, decreasing the intracellular superoxide concentration to selectively increase rat pulmonary arterial smooth muscle cell proliferation [23].

One can then suppose that appropriate magnetic fields may be used to perturb spin energy levels influencing the singlet-triplet and vice versa transaction probability and therefore controlling specific biochemical reactions and metabolic pathways. Different experimental data support the above hypothesis that magnetic fields, mainly static and extremely low-frequency fields, influence the ROS chemistry. This hypothesis is in agreement with the conclusion of a survey conducted, considering 41 scientific original publications showing that the use of this type of fields is capable of influencing the ROS chemistry in biology [24].

In addition, data coming from one multiannual, multicenter, multidisciplinary cancer research project have been reviewed [25]. In this project, static and extremely low-frequency magnetic fields having intensity on the mT range were used to influence electron spin energy levels and consequently ROS chemistry and related redox cellular signals showing promising results. In fact, important anticancer effects have been reported in vitro as well as in vivo through an influence on the genetic pathway that increases apoptosis via the p53 protein with no adverse effects in different human cancer models.

5. Magnetic fields as a new potential effective antitumor agent acting through the electron spin

In the last decades, there has been a growing interest in the use of magnetic fields, in studying their influence on different biological systems, considering their effect on electron spin energy levels and consequently on redox-related cellular changes and on genetic instability [25].

Different authors have studied the use of static and extremely low-frequency magnetic fields as a potential antitumor agent as well as an adjuvant agent to chemotherapy and radiotherapy with promising results. Overall, the published data support the presence of antitumor efficacy in many types of cancers including adenocarcinoma, breast cancer, melanoma and neuroblastoma.

Different Italian Health Institutions and Universities have realized the importance of this potential new approach to cancer treatment by starting, years ago, a multiannual, multidisciplinary, multicenter research project, conducted, for the laboratory part, mainly in a GLP-certified laboratory. The project aim was to validate the hypothesis that an atomic-level-based approach to biological processes may help to improve cancer therapy. The project has produced a variety of results published in different Journals. Later, the research activity, which can be considered a continuation of the project, restarted in the Medical School of a Chinese University.

Different from other projects, the considered one provides an entire set of data obtained from a series of multiple in vitro and in vivo laboratory trials, as well as a pilot study conducted on humans. Project carried out with this logic have yielded a corpus of data, organized and linked together in a logical fashion to allow organic and more complete, articulated analysis than with those coming from a single study. These characteristics are even more important in the fields of bioelectromagnetisms, where different authors have been using different magnetic fields and different biological means, providing a huge set of data difficult to correlate and then to interpret. These are the reasons why in analyzing the published data, supporting the efficacy of magnetic fields to induce antitumor effects, in agreement with the hypothesis that an atomic-level-based approach to biological processes may contribute to improve cancer therapy, we start with those coming from the above-cited project. Analysis of data coming from other project will follow (see the paragraph "Scientific consensus on the anticancer efficacy of magnetic fields").

5.1. Connecting atomic structure to biological activity

The multicenter project first objective was to find a connection between the fundamental law regulating the structure of matter and key biological function(s) regulating the stability of genetic machinery and the conservation of the species. First the atomic structure was analyzed, realizing that the key parameter governing the formation of matter as well as its stability is the (electron) spin state as above reported.

In fact, let us consider the biological processes at the base of our life. The human body is constituted by almost 37,000 billion cells, and as an average, billion cells replicate every day; for each replica, almost a thousand billion of DNA bases replicate for every cell division. These incredible numbers tell us how complex and at the same time fascinating is the biological life as we know it. Which incredible organization Nature has set up to avoid as much as possible diseases due to the inevitable mistake during such huge number of copies of DNA basis. This organization allows that most of these errors will remain silent, but also minor errors can have a serious impact. In addition, despite its essential role in storing genetic information, the DNA molecule has limited chemical stability and is subject to spontaneous decay [26].

Processes such as hydrolysis and oxidation occur at significant levels *in vivo*, in part due to reactive metabolites continuously generated in various physiological processes. In addition, external factors like radiation and genotoxic chemicals will further stimulate DNA damage formation. The inherent instability of DNA constitutes both an opportunity and a threat. DNA lesions can block important cellular processes such as DNA replication and transcription, cause genome instability and impair gene expression. Lesions can also be mutagenic and change the coding capacity of the genome, which can lead to devastating diseases and conditions associated with genome instability, including cancer, neurodegenerative disorders and biological aging. At the same time, without mutations, Darwinian evolution would not be possible.

Cells use different biological processes like DNA repair, apoptosis and others like autophagy working in a well-defined and coordinated manner to contrast genome instability and prevent much as possible the onset of serious diseases.

Analyzing these processes, apoptosis appeared the most interesting one to be connected with the key physical parameter governing the stability of matter, that is, electron spin. In fact, apoptosis is the process set by cells to control genetic machinery in order to avoid replication of cell having an altered DNA. Thousands of proteins take part in a well-organized manner into this process that will send to death the cell with altered DNA before replication. In case of cancer, among thousands of proteins, the p53 protein, called the "DNA guardian," seems to have a key role since, in mutated form, it is present in most cases of human cancers. This protein is considered so important that its encoding genes taken together are the most studied protein and genes in literature, with a total of more than 80,000 entries in PubMed [27].

5.2. Magnetic field characteristics, cell culture results and tumor growth inhibition

As seen before, different papers relate to p53 activity with redox machinery and ROS formation [4–6]. Accordingly, an intriguing hypothesis is to consider the possibility of selectively affected tumor cell growth using appropriate magnetic fields such as to influence redox signaling via an effect on electron spin state energy levels of ROS/enzymes that are connected with p53 activity/status (scheme of **Figure 5**) [28].

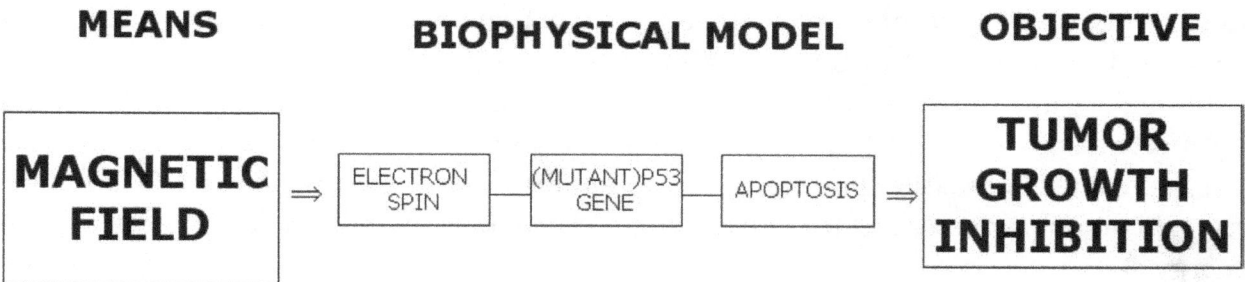

Figure 5. Biophysical model used to produce antitumor effects. Magnetic fields' effect on free radical recombination rate, activating redox signaling that influence mutant p53 activity and inhibit tumor growth via apoptosis.

According to the above-reported effect on the influence of magnetic fields on electron spin state, characteristics of the fields that are more suitable to influence cancer cell redox activity and p53-dependent apoptosis should result in agreement with known theory [7, 16, 28–30]. A series of about 100 in vitro trials exposing three different cell lines (MCF-7 human breast adeno-carcinoma, WiDr human colon adenocarcinoma and MRC-5 human embryonal lung fibroblast) have been performed and apoptosis as a function of magnetic field exposure characteristics (intensity and frequency) has been assessed [31]. The magnetic field characteristics that gave best results were constituted by a combination of static and extremely low frequency, to form an extremely low-frequency modulated static magnetic field with intensity varying between 1 and 8 mT, as shown in **Figure 6**. The total time average intensity of this magnetic field was 5.5 mT. The characteristics of this field, experimentally selected, were in agreement with what was predicted by theory. The efficacy of this field has been confirmed in an animal trial exposing different group of nude mice bearing a WiDr human colon adenocarcinoma, each group with different magnetic field exposure regime, assessing tumor growth inhibition and apoptosis [31].

The in vitro results, obtained using different magnetic field frequency as well as intensity, show that magnetic fields are able to induce apoptosis like death, only in the considered

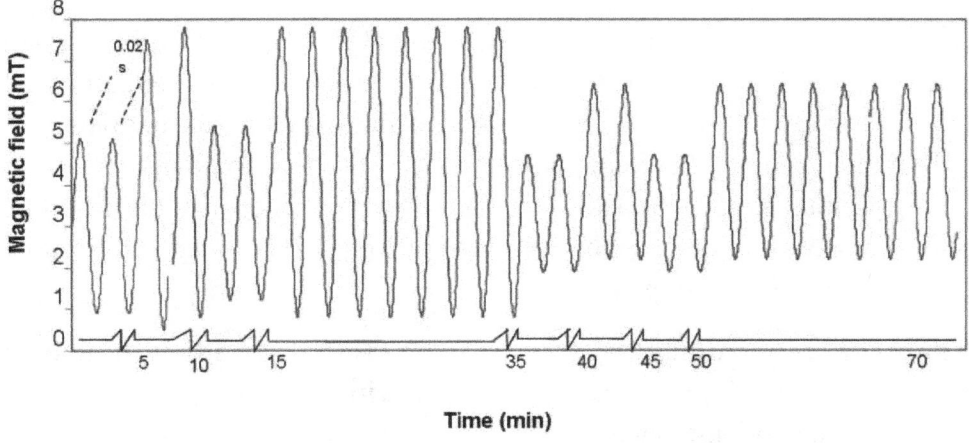

Time (min)

Figure 6. Magnetic field treatment characteristics. The magnetic fields were obtained with superimposition of a static magnetic field with an alternating 50-Hz (0.02 s) magnetic field forming an intensity-modulated magnetic fields which total intensity ranges from 1 to 8 mT with a time total average of 5.5 mT. The total treatment time for daily session is 70 min.

tumor cells, when their intensity is higher than 1 mT and this does not depend upon magnetic field frequency in the studied frequency range (0–300 Hz). This suggested to the authors that, in agreement with the theory at the base of the entire project, the biophysical mechanism connected to the apoptosis like death induction may be more related to free radical recombination processes than to ion resonance like mechanisms. Free radical recombination processes are activated by a direct action of magnetic fields on electron spin energy state levels of atoms and molecules with unpaired electrons. It was in fact known that free radical recombination processes occur in a timescale of nanoseconds to microseconds, and in this timescale, the extremely low-frequency (0–300 Hz) magnetic fields are seen as static [32, 33]. In addition, the authors noted that the need for amplitude-modulated fields (the one that gave the best tumor growth inhibition) to increase the effect otherwise obtained using only static or extremely low-frequency magnetic fields observed in vitro and in vivo [31] is in agreement with the need for establishing optimal condition(s) for the singlet-triplet spin state conversion required for the free radical recombination processes [34]. Safety analysis, in agreement with the theoretical biophysical mechanism, shows no toxic morphological changes induced by the magnetic field exposure in renewing, slowly proliferating, or static normal cells.

Treatment time may exert also an important role: a 70 min per day treatment for 5 days a week for 4 weeks has shown an inhibition of tumor growth of about 50%. The same 70-min treatment used two times a day gave a tumor growth inhibition of almost 70%, suggesting that in analogy with a chemical treatment this type of physical treatment exerts a form of dose-response efficacy, considering the time treatment connected to dose response.

5.3. Survival, apoptosis and p53 studies

In another animal trial using the same tumor model, nude mice were exposed, once a day, 5 days a week for the entire life to study survival, tumor growth inhibition and immune-reactive p53 [35]. After almost 1 year of treatment, the treated mice improved significantly their life span and the correspondent Survival Index was 1.31, that is, 31% survival time increase (**Figure 7**).

Specimens from each experimental mouse (magnetic fields exposed and not magnetic fields exposed) after weighted underwent histopathology, immunohistochemistry and transmission electron microscopy analysis. The results show that exposure to magnetic fields inhibits tumor growth of mice bearing a subcutaneous WiDr human colon adenocarcinoma, in agreement with the previous study. In addition, significant variation (by about 50%) in mitotic index (decrease), apoptosis (increase) and mutant p53 protein (decrease) (**Figure 8**) in tumor tissue is analyzed at the end of exposure time.

The observed tumor growth inhibition appears to be associated with morphological changes only in transformed cells. No morphological changes in renewing (i.e., bone marrow cells), slowly proliferating (i.e., hepatocytes) and static (i.e., terminally differentiated neurons) normal cells were observed. In addition, no significant differences in the number and morphology of blood corpuscular elements, emunctory function of liver and kidney, and bone metabolism were detected, between the exposed and not-exposed animals. Authors' comments were

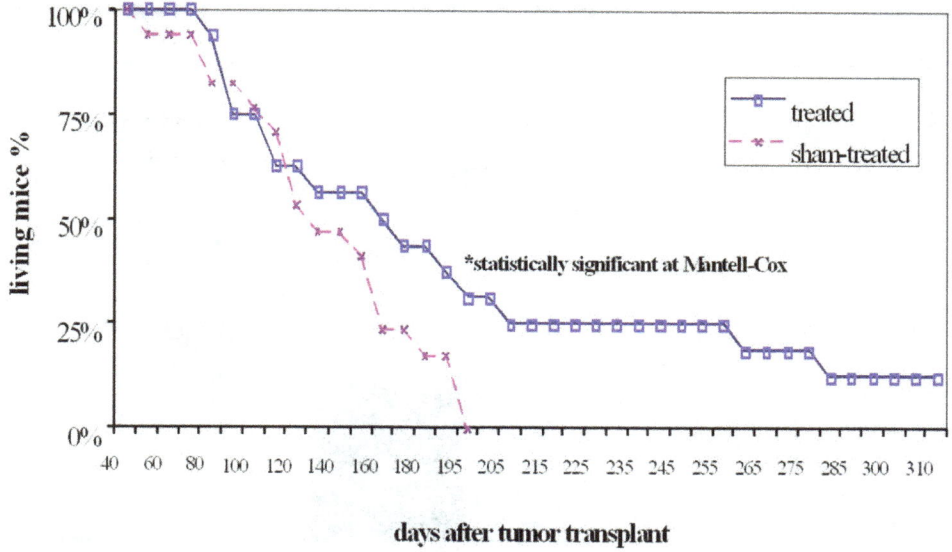

Figure 7. Survival time (days) of nude mice bearing human adenocarcinoma cancer and magnetic field treated (continue line) versus survival time (days) of nude mice bearing human tumor and not magnetic fields treated (dotted line). The magnetic field increases significantly the life span of nude mice bearing human cancer.

that the lack of adverse responses in normal cells and tissues suggests that the safety of this physical treatment may be related to its ability to interfere preferentially selectively with transformed cells. About p53 results they commented that from literature it is known that a loss of p53 functional status, due to either lack of gene expression or overexpression of its mutant form, leads to genomic instability and cancer [36]. The most frequently encountered mutations of p53 reduce its thermodynamic stability, determining the loss of the DNA binding conformation indispensable to the transcription regulation and tumor suppressor activity [37]. Pharmacological rescue of mutant p53 conformation and function has been also reported [38]. Others demonstrated that metal ions play a regulatory role in the control of p53 folding and DNA binding activity [39]. Specific DNA binding is influenced by redox regulation of p53, and binding of metal ions may directly affect p53 redox potential, either at the zinc binding cysteine residues or at other cysteine residue on the protein surface [40]. Thus, based on these data, authors suggest that the observed decrease of mutant p53 after magnetic field exposure, together with the increased apoptotic index and the slower growth of experimental tumors, could be explained by a rescue of wild-type p53. This phenomenon could be related to the effect of magnetic field exposure redox chemistry connected with metal ions.

5.4. Inhibition of metastatic spread and growth

Another important parameter to be evaluated in the assessment of potential antitumor efficacy of a treatment is its capability to inhibit the metastatic process. For this reason, a subsequent animal trial was conducted to evaluate the influence of the magnetic field treatment in the inhibition of metastatic spread and growth in a breast cancer model [41]. More specifically, a highly metastatic (in the lung) human cancer (MDA-MB-435) model, transplanted in nude mice, was used. Mice were exposed at the same magnetic field treatment regime (70 min a day for 5 days a

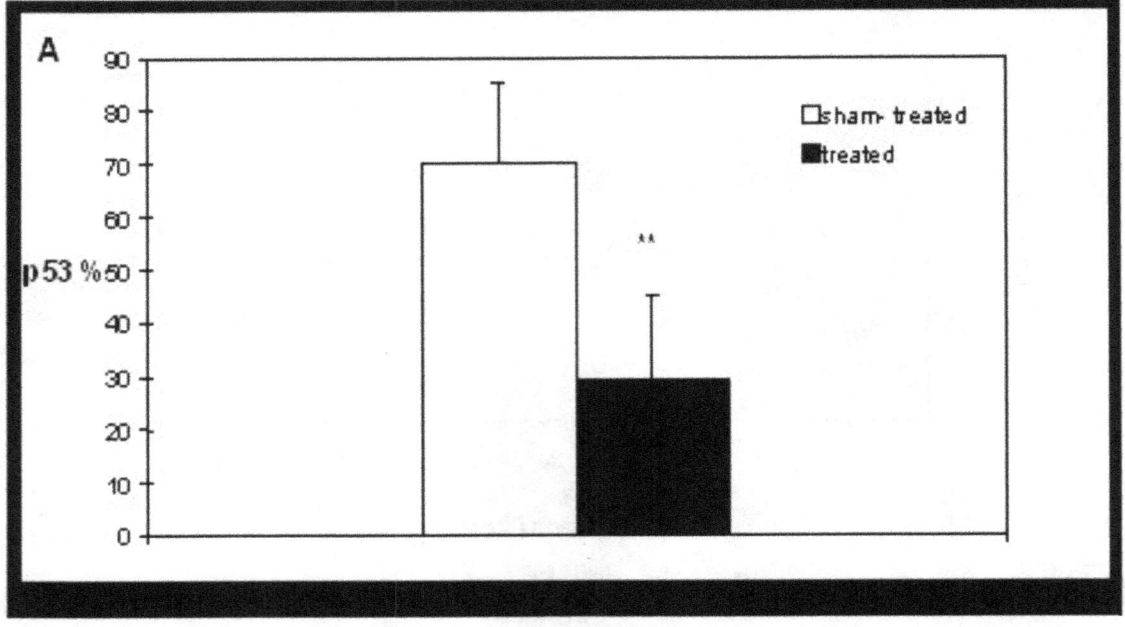

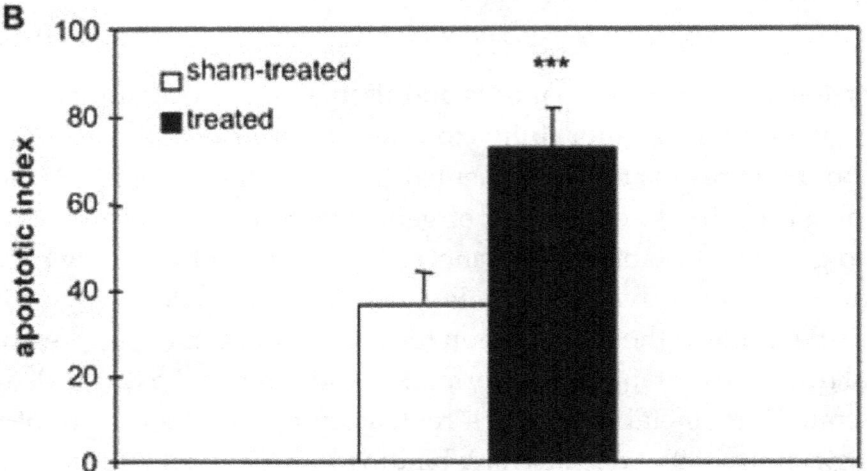

Figure 8. Influence of the magnetic field treatment on mutant p53 concentration (A) that markedly decreases, and on apoptosis (B) that markedly increases.

week) for 6 consecutive weeks. To allow a more complete evaluation of the potential antitumor efficacy of the magnetic field treatment, a positive control group treated with a chemotherapeutic agent (cyclophosphamide) was also used. At the end of the experiment, separate sections from each lung were examined at the microscope to determine the incidence of the different treatments (magnetic fields and cyclophosphamide) on number and sizes of metastases. Lung metastases were histologically counted, and each one was scored on the basis of the number of tumor cells. The size of each metastasis was evaluated by classifying the metastases in three categories (<10, 10–100, and >100) according to the total number of cells contained. As shown in **Figure 9**, both magnetic fields and cyclophosphamide treatments significantly decreased the number of lung metastases, classified according to the number of cell contained. In addition, the magnetic field treatment performed significantly better than cyclophosphamide.

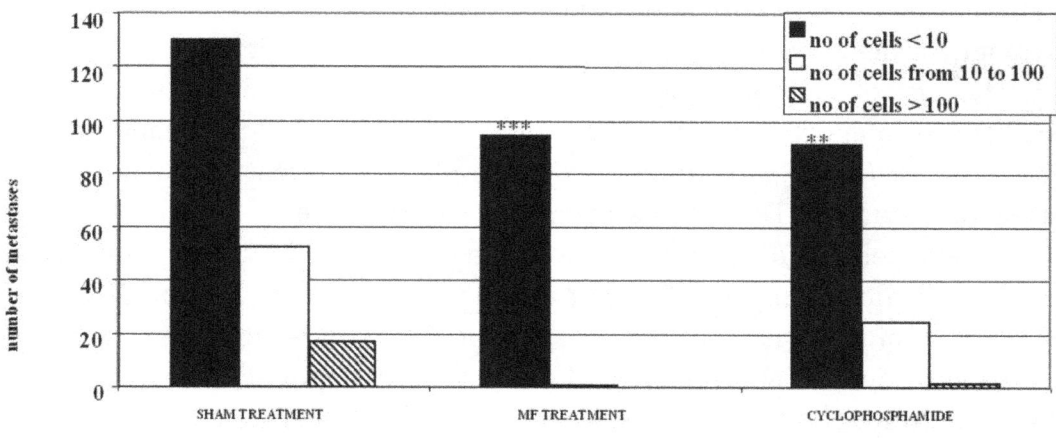

Test chi2:   **   p = 0.01   ***   p = 0.0001

Figure 9. Effect of magnetic field (MF) in spread and growth of lung metastasis in nude mice bearing human metastatic breast cancer. Results are compared with those coming from the same experiment where the other group, of the same nude mice bearing the same human cancer, was treated with cyclophosphamide, a known chemotherapeutic agent. Results, in terms of small-size metastasis (black bars), medium-size metastasis (white bars) and large-size metastasis (black and white bars), show that the magnetic field treatment is more efficient than cyclophosphamide in inhibiting spread and growth of metastasis.

In fact, while magnetic field treatment and cyclophosphamide-treated mice reported almost the same number of metastases in the lowest cell content category (<10 cells), magnetic field-treated and cyclophosphamide-treated mice in the medium cell-content category (10–100 cells) reported 98% and 50% reduction in the number of metastases, respectively, while in the high cell-content category (>100 cells) was 100% and 90% for the magnetic field treated and cyclophosphamide-treated mice, respectively, compared to the control mice. Safety analysis was performed in all experimental animals. Results were in agreement with those observed in the previous trials confirming the safety of the treatment. In fact, gross pathology at necroscopy, hematoclinical/hematological, and histological examination did not show any toxic or abnormal effects.

5.5. Synergism with chemotherapeutic agent atomic biology

The following trial was conducted to enquire about the possible synergism between magnetic field treatment and chemotherapeutic agents in terms of their influence on survival time [42]. Two animal models were tested, and immune-competent mice bearing murine Lewis Lung Carcinoma (LLCs) or B16 melanotic melanoma were exposed to magnetic fields treated with two commonly used anticancer drugs. The chemotherapeutic agents under investigation were cis-platin and cyclophosphamide, for the first and second models, respectively. The mice were exposed to the same magnetic fields used in the previous trials (static with the superimposition of extremely low-frequency magnetic field having a total time average intensity of 5.5 mT), provided daily (7 days a week) for the entire life. Synergistic activity was found only with cis-platin. In fact, the cis-platin antitumor efficacy was increased by magnetic field exposure, leading to significantly prolonged animal survival. The magnetic field treatment almost tripled the efficacy of cis-platin since the effect of cis-platin low dose (3 mg/Kg) used in combination with magnetic field exposure was similar to that of cis-platin high dose (10 mg/Kg) alone. Unfortunately, it is not possible to make a direct comparison between the presence/absence of synergism between magnetic fields and the anticancer activity of cis-platin and cyclophosphamide because the two drugs were tested on two completely different animal models (different mouse strains and tumors). The authors' comments were that the synergistic activity observed between magnetic field exposure and cis-platin can be explained by the hypothesized ability to influence free radical chemistry exerted by the magnetic field treatment [28]. Two mechanisms, alone or combined, may be at the base of the observed results. First the platinum ion stimulates superoxide radical production [43, 44], and the magnetic field exposure enhances active oxygen production. When this production occurs at the cell membranes, the respective permeability changes, influencing the cell drug intake [44]. Second, it has been shown that the rate of conversion of cis-platin to reactive species, able to bind to DNA, is increased by localized production (in our case possibly due to the magnetic field exposure) of free radicals [45].

5.6. Safety of the treatment and considerations on efficacy

This magnetic fields treatment was then used in a pilot study where, according with the authorization of the Ethical Committee instituted by law, patients with advanced neoplasm were exposed to magnetic fields to assess safety and acute toxicity [46]. Eleven patients were treated with the same magnetic field characteristics we used in animal trials (static with the superimposition of extremely low-frequency magnetic field having a total time average intensity of 5–5 mT). Treatment included neck, thoracic and abdomen areas. Two treatment protocols that differed in the length of daily exposure to magnetic fields were set. In the first, patients were treated for 20 min/day, 5 days a week, over 4 weeks; in the second, patients were treated for 70 min/day, 5 days/week, over 4 weeks. A minimum of two patients was introduced in each treatment plan; if intolerable toxicity was not observed, two to five additional were treated. The reported results show that human exposure to the used magnetic fields treatment is not associated with important toxic and adverse side effects. Different exposure regimes, exposing 20–70 min daily, respectively, appear to be associated only to small changes in some laboratory parameters. Authors of the study conclude that the overall data of this clinical study on safety in humans seem to be in agreement with safety and toxicity data from animal trials, showing no toxic or abnormal effects when gross pathology at necroscopy, blood and histological examination were performed [28, 31, 35, 41, 42]. In conclusion, the findings of this pilot study carried out in a small number of cancer patients support the possibility that the human exposure to magnetic fields with specific physical characteristics is associated with a favorable safety profile and good tolerability.

Based on all above-reported laboratory studies, it has been possible to confirm the antitumor efficacy of this new physical treatment that uses specific magnetic field characteristics. In fact, the reported data confirm the capability by magnetic fields to exert significant antitumor effects in different laboratory animal models as well as synergistic activity with chemotherapy without significant adverse effects. This may support the validity of this new approach to biological processes. More studies are necessary, mainly at the clinical level, to understand the real potential of this atomic approach in improving availability of cancer therapy. In addition, this approach may contribute to fulfill a knowledge gap facing biomedical science today, the one between the atomic level and the cellular level.

5.7. Result confirmation

The antitumor efficacy reported in the above illustrated papers was confirmed, years later, in a different laboratory, located within the Medical School of the Zhejiang University, China. This replica performed in a different laboratory located in a different continent, using the same exposure machine as well as the same magnetic field characteristics, gives to the old/previous project results the necessary scientific validity, scientific validity that is confirmed when the same results are reported in different laboratory using the same methodology. In this university, the antitumor efficacy of magnetic fields treatment has been studied in two pediatric tumors, nephroblastoma and neuroblastoma [47]. The antitumor efficacy exerted by this magnetic field treatment as well as its combined effect with cis-platin was studied in vitro and in vivo. In this Chinese study, the time-average intensity of the magnetic fields was slightly different from the previous studies, 5.1 mT instead of 5.5 mT. This is due to the modification of the time duration of each of the eight rounds constituting, as in the old project, one magnetic fields treatment session. In the old project, each round lasted different times [48]. Now, each round lasted 3.5 min, and consequently each exposure session of treatment lasted 28 min. One or more treatment sessions (up to 4) were administered daily. In addition to the use of the standard static with the superimposition of extremely low-frequency magnetic field having a total time average intensity of 5.1 mT, alternatively, only static magnetic fields were used, while the total time-average field intensity was kept to 5.1 mT to help understanding the biophysical mechanisms.

For the in vivo part of the study in China, mice magnetic field exposure was based on the same exposure system and with the same protocol except that each round lasted 10 min; thus, each session lasted 80 min instead of 70 min as in the old project. Mice received one session of treatment daily for 15 consecutive days. In vitro results show that after daily exposure of 2 h the cell number of nephroblastoma and neuroblastoma cell lines (G401, CHLA255, N2a) decreased significantly from day 2, and the inhibition rate reached to about 20% after 3 days of exposure. The inhibitory effect was positively associated with exposure time, and subtraction of the AC field decreased the inhibition rate. Furthermore, it was found that the field decreased cell proliferation and induced apoptosis. Combining of the field with chemotherapeutic cisplatin further increased the inhibition rate compared with single use of either cisplatin or MF. In G401 nephroblastoma tumor model in nude mice, daily exposure of 80 min per day combined with cisplatin resulted in significant decrease of the tumor mass. The side effect of combinational treatment was limited to mild liver injury (an increase in aminotransferase levels), while magnetic field exposure did not hamper liver and kidney functions by itself. In conclusion, this 50 Hz, static modulated magnetic field exhibited antitumor effect on neuroblastoma and nephroblastoma and had the potential to be used in combination with cis-platin for increased efficacy and reduced side effects in these two childhood malignancies.

These results from Zhejiang University are completely in agreement with the previous results of the multiannual, multi-disciplinary, multicenter research project, confirming the antitumor efficacy of the magnetic field treatment exerted in two new human cancers (nephroblastoma and neuroblastoma), its synergistic activity with the studied chemotherapeutic agent cis-platin, with no induction or trivial induction of adverse effects. This agreement confirms the scientific validity of the potential antitumor efficacy of this new physical treatment that uses magnetic fields (electromagnetic energy) and that comes from a new approach of biological processes based on quantum physics, and such approach considers the atomic structure as a key aspect in studying the biological activity possibly introducing to a new additional branch of medical science that might be called atomic biology in analogy with molecular biology.

5.8. Scientific consensus on the anticancer efficacy of magnetic fields

There has been a growing scientific consensus on the anticancer activity of static and extremely low-frequency magnetic fields. In the last decade, many authors have published different papers, reporting results that are in agreement with those analyzed above. We now will shortly analyze the content of these papers.

Specifically, tumor growth inhibition has been studied on nude mice bearing metastatic mouse breast tumor cells exposed to 100 mT, 1 Hz magnetic fields for different times a day (60, 180, and 360 min/day) for 4 weeks, observing a tumor growth inhibition as a function of the exposure time reaching the suppression of tumor growth when exposure was 360 min/day [49]. Tumor growth inhibition as well as metastasis inhibition was observed in mice bearing hepatocarcinoma cells exposed to 400 mT, 7.5 Hz magnetic fields, 120 min/day for 30 days, observing an inhibitory effect on tumor growth [50]. In another study, the application of 4.5 mT, 120 Hz magnetic fields, 50 min/day for 32 days inhibited preneoplastic lesions chemically induced in the liver of male rats by reducing cell proliferation [51]. The synergistic effect with anticancer drugs has been studied *in vivo* and *in vitro* by different authors. *In vivo*, El- Bialy *et al.* [52] studied female mice bearing an ascites carcinoma treated with 3 mg/Kg i.p. cis-platin and exposed to 10 mT, 50 Hz magnetic fields 60 min/day for 2 weeks, showing that extremely low-frequency magnetic fields enhanced the cytotoxic activity of cisplatin and potentiate the benefit of using a combination of low-dose cisplatin and extremely low-frequency magnetic fields in the treatment of ascites carcinoma. Chen W.F. *et al.* [53] studied human leukemic cells (K562) exposed *in vitro* to 8.8 mT static magnetic fields, treated with cis-platin at concentrations from 20 to 10 microg/ml, and the results suggest that the mechanism is correlated with the DNA damage model. Hao Q. *et al.* [54] reported results showing that an 8.8 mT static magnetic fields enhanced the cytotoxic potency of adriamycin (25 ng/ml) on K562 cells, and a decrease in P-gp expression may be one reason underlying this effect. Kakikawa M. *et al.* [55] reported results showing that 50 mT, 60 Hz magnetic fields enhanced the cytotoxicity both of mitomycin C and of cis-platin on *E. coli* bacterium; these results suggest that magnetic fields change the permeability of the cell membrane and affect drug intake. Results of a clinical trial devoted to studying the effects on palliation of general symptoms as well as survival were reported by C. Sun *et al.* [56] in 13 advanced nonsmall cell lung cancer (NSCLC) patients treated with 400 mT, 0–50 Hz magnetic fields 120 min/day for 6–10 weeks.

The authors observed prolonged survival and moderately improved general symptoms without any severe toxicity or side effects. More recently other three studies have been published enlarging the above scenario. Two hours of treatment with 50 Hz, 20 mT magnetic fields makes resistant cells of human ovarian carcinoma sensitive to cisplatin via p53 activation [57]. A metastatic melanoma mouse model exposed 400 mT, 7.5 Hz magnetic fields, 120 min/day for 27 days reported a significant growth inhibition of metastatic tumor burden of lung, showing that extremely low-frequency magnetic field exposure promoted the inhibitory effect of ROS on AKT pathway and decreased Foxp3 expression [58]. Three-hour exposure to 1 mT 50 Hz magnetic fields induces apoptosis on osteosarcoma cells via oxidative stress [59].

Part of the above-cited studies has been also considered in two reviews published in 2013, one devoted to analyze if radiotherapy could be enhanced by electromagnetic field treatment [60]. The first review concludes that the analyzed studies reflect encouraging results and corroborate the hypothesis that combined exposure to some chemical agents ionizing radiation should be used to increase DNA damage and help cancer treatment. The other review covers three areas of investigation connected to the use of magnetic fields, in particular free radical generation and oxidative stress, apoptosis, genotoxicity and cancer [61], concluding that magnetic field causes oxidative stress and, as a result, damages ion channels, leading to changes in cell morphology and expression of different genes and proteins and also changes in apoptosis and proliferation. In addition, about the use of magnetic fields in combination with other external factors, such as ionizing radiation and some chemicals, there is evidence strongly suggesting that magnetic fields modify their effects, improving cancer treatment. Finally, the authors stated that the analyzed studies provide valuable insight into the phenomenon of biomagnetism and open new avenues for the development of new medical applications. More recently, L. Montagnier, the 2008 Nobel Prize for Medicine assignee, has stressed, also on the base of the above scientific scenario, the importance of the use of magnetic fields in cancer treatment [62].

6. Comments and conclusions

All the reported reviews conclude that additional studies are necessary to better clarifying the biomolecular mechanism(s) and understand the real potential of this new possible medical treatment. The call for additional studies, included clinical ones, has been also suggested by the more recent review dealing with the capability of magnetic fields to influence genetic stability and the potentiality of their use in cancer treatment [25]. This last concludes that a number of papers reports on the correlation between static and extremely low-frequency magnetic fields and genetic instability. This correlation has been found in studies on gene expression and DNA damage due to oxidative stress, including double–strand breaks, chromosomal aberrations and micronucleus induction. This review also underlines that the analyzed literature makes it plausible to apply an atomic-level approach to biological processes (atomic biology approach) using electromagnetic energy as a bridge between the atomic level (spin energy levels) and the cellular level (oxidative stress, DNA damage, genetic instability, p53 status and apoptosis).

The content of present chapter, together with the consensus among the analyzed literature, supports the capability by magnetic fields to exert significant antitumor effects in different laboratory animal models as well as synergistic activity with chemotherapy. This, without significant adverse effects observed in the laboratory animal trials as well as in the limited human studies, highlights the potential validity of this new atomic based approach to biological processes.

We are only at the beginning of a scientific adventure of this new potential branch on biological/medical research that may be called atomic biology. The atomic (electron spin) based approach to cancer treatment has given promising results to foresee great potentiality of this approach to open new frontiers of biomolecular research and medical application, since magnetic fields, different from chemical products, have the capability of influencing in a very selective way only the desired spin state of a given biomolecule. The expected clinical results for this type of approach would hopefully be more selective, that is, with less adverse effects. More studies are necessary, mainly at the clinical level, to understand the real potential of this atomic approach in improving availability of cancer therapy.

Acknowledgements

The author wishes to express his gratitude to the many people who have helped in this long-lasting development of the project, among others: his wife Laura for her closeness and continuous encouragement during the entire project; his two sons Federico and Alessandro for having accepted some of their father's carelessness due to his activity in the project; Fausto Lanfranco for the continuous advice and helps and his wife Deanna whose farsightedness inspired the beginning of the project; Piero Ossola and Michele Berardelli for their important contributions for the physical aspects of the project; Flavio Ronchetto, Domenico Barone, Renzo Orlassino and Marcella Cintorino for their important contributions for the biological and medical aspects of the project; Xi Chen, for her commitment to continue the project at the Zhejiang University, China; Andrea Peruzzo for his encouragement and discussions; and Emanuela Noascone for her technical assistance during chapter preparation.

Author details

Santi Tofani

Address all correspondence to: santitofani@gmail.com

University of Turin and Ivrea Hospital, Piemonte, Italy

References

[1] Bucci M, Goodman C, Sheppard TL. A decade of chemical biology. Nature Chemical Biology. 2010;**6**:847-854. DOI: 10.1038/nchembio.489

[2] Braibant S, Giacomelli G, Spurio M. Particles and Fundamental Interactions: An Introduction to Particle Physics. 2nd ed. New York & Frankfurt: Springer; 2012. DOI: 10. 1007/978-94-007-2464-8

[3] Swart M. Costas M (Eds): Spin States in Biochemistry and Inorganic Chemistry: Influence on Structure and Reactivity. Ltd.: John Wiley & Sons; 2016. DOI: 10.1002/9781118898277

[4] Polyak K, Xia Y, Zweier JL, Kinzier KW, Volgestein BA. Model for p53-induced apoptosis. Nature. 1997;**389**:300-305. DOI: 10.1038/38525

[5] Liu B, Chen Y, St Clair DK. ROS and p53: A versatile partnership. Free Radical Biology and Medicine. 2008;**44**(8):1529-1535. DOI: 10.1016/j.freeradbiomed.2008.01.011

[6] Augustyn KE, Merino EJ, Barton JK. A role for DNA-mediated charge transport in regulating p53: Oxidation of the DNA-bound protein from a distance. PNAS. 2007;**104**(48): 18907-18912. DOI: 10.1073/pnas.0709326104

[7] Steiner UE, Ulrich T. Magnetic fields effects in chemical kinetics and related phenomena. Chemical Reviews. 1989;**89**:51-147. DOI: 10.1021/cr00091a003

[8] Bhat AV, Hora S, Pal A, Jha S, Taneja R. Stressing the (epi)genome: Dealing with ROS in cancer. Antioxidants & Redox Signaling. 2017 Aug 17. DOI: 10.1089/ars.2017.7158

[9] Ray PD, Huang B-W, Tsuji Y. Reactive oxygen species (ROS) homeostasis and redox regulation in cellular signaling. Cellular Signalling. 2012 May;**24**(5):981-990. DOI: 10.1016/j. cellsig.2012.01.008

[10] Che M, Wang R, Wang H-Y, Steven Zheng XF. Expanding roles of superoxide dismutases in cell regulation and cancer. Drug Discovery Today. 2016 January;**21**(1):143-149. DOI: 10.1016/j.drudis.2015.10.001

[11] Liu H, Liu X, Zhang C, Zhu H, Qian X, Youquan B, Lei Y. Redox imbalance in the development of colorectal cancer. Journal of Cancer. 2017;**8**(9):1586-1597. DOI: 10.7150/jca. 18735

[12] Cairns RA, Harris IS, Mak TW. Regulation of cancer cell metabolism. Nature Reviews Cancer. 2010;**11**:85-95. DOI: 10.1038/nrc2981

[13] Lio G-Y, Storz P. Reactive oxygen species in cancer. Free Radical Research. 2010;**44**(5). DOI: 10.3109/10715761003667554

[14] Bravard A, Sabatier L, Hoffschir F, Ricoul M, Luccioni C, Dutrillaux B. SOD2: A new type of tumor-suppressor gene? International Journal of Cancer. 1992;**51**:476-480. DOI: 10.1002/ijc.2910510323

[15] Hitchler MJ, Oberley LJ, Domann FJ. Epigenetic silencing of SOD2 by histone modifications in human breast cancer cells. Free Radical Biology and Medicine. 2008;**45**:1573-1580. DOI: 10.1016/j.freeradbiomed.2008.09.005

[16] Barnes FS, Greenebaum B. The effects of weak magnetic fields on radical pairs. Bioelectromagnetics. 2015;**36**:45-54. DOI: 10.1002/bem.21883

[17] Woodward JR, Foster TJ, Jones AR, Salauru AT, Scrutton NS. Time-resolved studies of radical pairs. Biochemical Society Transactions. 2009;**37**:358-362. DOI: 10.1042/BST0370358

[18] Canfield JM, Belford RL, Debrunner PG, Schulten K. A perturbation-theory treatment of oscillating magnetic-fields in the radical pair mechanism. Chemical Physics. 1994;**182**:1-18. DOI: 10.1016/0301-0104(93)E0442-X

[19] Schulten K, Staerk H, Weller A, Werner HJ, Nickel B. Magnetic-field dependence of geminate recombination of radical ion-pairs in polar-solvents. Zeitschrift für Physikalische Chemie. 1976;**101**:371-390. DOI: https://doi.org/10.1524/zpch.1976.101.1-6.371

[20] Usselman RJ, Chavarriaga C, Castello PR, Procopio M, Ritz T, Dratz EA, Singel DJ, Martino CF. The quantum biology of reactive oxygen species partitioning impacts cellular bioenergetics. Scientific Reports. 2016;**6**:38543. DOI: 10.1038/srep38543

[21] Schleicher E, Wenzel R, Ahmad M, Batschauer A, Essen LO, Hitomi K, Gettzoff ED, Bittl R, Weber S, Okafuji A. The electronic state of flavoproteins: Investigations with proton electron-nuclear double resonance. Applied Magnetic Resonance. 2010;**37**:339-352. DOI: https//doi.org/10.1007/s00723-009-0101-8

[22] Ritz T, Thalau P, Phillips JB, Wiltschko R, Wiltschko W. Resonance effects indicate a radical-pair mechanism for avian magnetic compass. Nature. 2004;**429**:177-180. DOI: 10.1038/nature02534

[23] Usselman RJ, Hill L, Singel DJ, Martino C. Spin biochemistry modulate reactive oxygen species (ROS) production by radio frequency magnetic fields. PLoS One. 2014;**9**(3). DOI: 10.1371/journal.pone.0093065

[24] Mattsson MO, Simkò M. Grouping of experimental conditions as an approach to evaluate effects of extremely low-frequency magnetic fields on oxidative response in in vitro studies. Frontiers in Public Health. 2014;**2**:132. DOI: 10.3389/fpubh.2014.00132

[25] Tofani S. Electromagnetic Energy as a Bridge Between Atomic and Cellular Levels in the Genetic Approach to Cancer Treatment. Current Topics in Medicinal Chemistry. 2015;**15**(6):572-578. DOI: 10.2174/1568026615666150225104217

[26] Lindahl T. Instability and decay of the primary structure of DNA. Nature. 1993;**362** (6422):709-715. DOI:10.1038/362709a0

[27] Fischer M. Census and evaluation of p53 target genes. Oncogene. 2017 Jul 13;**36**(28):3943-3956. DOI: 10.1038/onc.2016.502

[28] Tofani S. Physics may help chemistry to improve medicine: a possible mechanism for anticancer activity of static and ELF magnetic fields. Physica Medica. 1999;**15**(4):291-294 https://www.researchgate.net/publication/262487109

[29] Grissom CB. Magnetic field effects in biology: A survey of possible mechanisms with emphasis on radical-pair recombination. Chemical Reviews. 1995;**95**:3-24. DOI: 10.1021/cr00033a001

[30] Kattnig DR, Evans EW, Dejean V, Dodson CA, Wallace MI, Mackenzie SR, Timmel CR, Hore PJ. Chemical amplification of magnetic field effects relevant to avion magnetoreception. Nature Chemistry. 2016;**8**:384-390. DOI: 10.1038/nchem.2447

[31] Tofani S, Barone D, Cintorino M, de Santi M, Ferrara A, Orlassino R, Ossola P, Peroglio F, Rolfo K, Ronchetto F. Static and ELF magnetic fields induce tumor growth inhibition and apoptosis. Bioelectromagnetics. 2001;**22**(6):419-428. PMID: 11536283

[32] Scaiano JC, Cozens FL, McLean J. Model for the rationalization of magnetic field effects *in vivo*: application of the radical-pair mechanism to biological systems. Photochemistry and Photobiology. 1994;**59**:585-589. DOI: 10.1016/S0006-3495(96)79263-9

[33] Engström S. In: Barnes FS, Greenebaum B, editors. Handbook of Biological Effects of Electromagnetic Fields: Bioengineering and Biophysical Aspects of Electromagnetic Fields. Third ed. Boca Raton: CRC Press; 2007. pp. 157-168. ISBN: 9780849329524

[34] Polk C. Dosimetry of extremely-low-frequency magnetic fields. Bioelectromagnetics. 1992;**1**:209-235. DOI: 10.1002/bem.2250130720

[35] Tofani S, Cintorino M, Barone D, Berardelli M, De Santi MM, Ferrara A, Orlassino R, Ossola P, Rolfo K, Ronchetto F, Tripodi SA, Tosi P. Increased mouse survival, tumor growth inhibition and decreased immunoreactive p53 after exposure to magnetic fields. Bioelectromagnetics. 2002;**23**(3):230-238. PMID:11891753

[36] Sherr CJ. Cancer cell Cicle. Science. 1996;**274**:1672-1677. PMID: 8939849

[37] Bullock AN, Henckel J, DeDecker BS, Johnson CM, Nikolova PV, Proctor MR, Lane DP, Fersht AR. Thermodynamic stability of wild-type and mutant p53 core domain. Proceedings of the National Academy of Sciences of the United States of America. 1997;**94**:14338-14342. PMCID: PMC24967

[38] Foster BA, Coffey HA, Morin MJ, Rastinejad F. Pharmacological rescue of mutant p53 conformation and function. Science. 1999;**286**:2507-2510. PMID: 10617466

[39] Meplan C, Richard MJ, Hainaut P. Metalloregulation of the tumor suppressor protein p53: zinc mediates the renaturation of p53 after exposure to metal chelators in vitro and in intact cells. Oncogene. 2000;**19**:5227-5236. DOI: 10.1038/sj.onc.1203907

[40] Wu HH, Sherman M, Yuan YC, Momand J. Direct redox modulation of p53 protein: potential sources of redox control and potential outcomes. Gene Therapy and Molecular Biology. 1999;**4**:119-132. http://gtmb.org/volumes/Vol4/_11FC%20%20%20Momand%20p53%20119-132.pdf

[41] Tofani S, Barone D, Peano S, Ossola P, Ronchetto F, Cintorino M. Anticancer activity by magnetic fields: inhibition of metastatic spread and growth in a breast cancer model. IEEE Plasma Science. 2002;**30**(4):1552-1557. DOI: 10.1109/TPS.2002.804209

[42] Tofani S, Barone D, Berardelli M, Berno E, Cintorino M, Foglia L, Ossola P, Ronchetto F, Toso E, Eandi M. Static and ELF magnetic fields enhance the *in vivo* anti-tumor efficacy

of cis- platin against Lewis lung carcinoma, but not of cyclophosphamide against B 16 melanotic melanoma. Pharmacological Research. 2003;**48**(1):83-90. PMID: 12770519

[43] Masuda H, Tanaka T, Takahama U. Cisplatin generates superoxide anion by interaction with DNA in a cell-free system. Biochemical and Biophysical Research Communications. 1994;**203**:1175-1180. DOI: 10.1006/bbrc.1994.2306

[44] Maruyama M, Asano T, Nakagohri T, Uematsu T, Hasegawa M, Miyauchi H, et al. Application of high energy shock waves to cancer treatment in combination with cisplatin and ATX-70. Anticancer Research. 1999;**19**:1377-1383. PMID: 10470144

[45] Tonetti M, Giovine M, Gasparini A, Benatti U, De Flora A. Enhanced formation of reactive species from cis-diammine- (1,1-cyclobutanedicarboxylato)-platinum(II) (carbo-plati) in the presence of oxigen free radicals. Biochemical Pharmacology. 1993;**46**:1377-1383. PMID: 8240386

[46] Ronchetto F, Barone D, Cintorino M, Berardelli M, Lissolo S, Orlassino R, Ossola P, Tofani S. Extremely low frequency- modulated static magnetic fields to treat cancer: a pilot study on patients with advanced neoplasm to assess safety and acute toxicity. Bioelectromagnetics. 2004;**25**:563-571. DOI: 10.1002/bem.20029

[47] Yuan Lin-Qing, Wang Can, Zhu Kun, Li Hua-Mei, Gu Wei-Zhong, Zhou Dong-Ming, Lai Jia-Qi, Zhou Duo, Lv Yao. Tofani S, Chen Xi: The Antitumor Effect of 50 Hertz Modulated Static Magnetic Fields against Nephroblastoma and Neuroblastoma. Submitted to Bioelectromagnetics, June 2017

[48] Tofani S. Electromagnetic field exposure system for the study of possible anti-cancer activity. IEEE Transactions on Electromagnetic Compatibility. 2002;**44**(1):148-151. DOI: 10.1109/15.990721

[49] Tatarov I, Panda A, Petkov D, Kolappaswamy K, Thompson K, Kavirayani A, Lipsky MM, Elson E, Davis CC, Martin SS, DeTolla LJ. Effect of magnetic fields on tumour growth and viability. Comparative Medicine. 2011;**61**(4):339-345. PMCID: PMC3155400

[50] Nie Y, Du L, Mou Y, Xu Z, Weng L, Du Y, Zhu Y, Hou Y, Wang T. Effect of low frequency magnetic fields on melanoma: tumor inhibition and immune modulation. BMC Cancer. 2013;**13**:582. DOI: 10.1186/1471-2407-13-582

[51] Jiménez-García MN, Arellanes-Robledo J, Aparicio-Bautista DI, Rodríguez Segura MA, Villa-Treviño S, Godina-Nava JJ. Anti-proliferative effect of extremely low frequency electromagnetic field on preneoplastic lesions formation in the rat liver. BMC Cancer. 2010;**10**:159. DOI: https://doi.org/10.1186/1471-2407-10-159

[52] El-Bialy NS, Rageh MM. Extremely low-frequency magnetic fields enhances the therapeutic efficacy of low-dose cisplatin in the treatment of Ehrlich carcinoma. BioMed Research International. 2013;**2013**:189-352. http://dx.doi.org/10.1155/2013/189352

[53] Chen WF, Qi H, Sun RG, Liu Y, Zhang K, Liu JQ. Static magnetic fields enhanced the potency of cisplatin on k562 cells. Cancer Biotherapy & Radiopharmaceuticals. 2010;**25**(4): 401-408. DOI: 10.1089/cbr.2009.0743

[54] Hao Q, Wenfang C, Xia A, Qiang W, Ying L, Kun Z, Run-guang S. Effects of moderate-intensity static magnetic field and adriamycin on k562 cells. Bioelectromagnetics. 2011;**32**(3):191-199. DOI: 10.1002/bem.20625

[55] Kakikawa M, Yamada S. Effect of extremely low-frequency (ELF) magnetic field on anticancer drugs potency. IEEE Transactions on Magnetics. 2012;**48**:2869-2872. DOI: 10.1109/TMAG.2012.2200881

[56] Sun C, Yu H, Wang X, Han J. A pilot study of extremely low- frequency magnetic fields in advanced non-small cell lung cancer: Effects on survival and palliation of general symptoms. Oncology Letters. 2012;**4**:1130-1134. DOI: https://doi.org/10.3892/ol.2012.867

[57] Baharara J, Hosseini N, Farzin TR. Extremely low frequency electromagnetic field sensitizes cisplatin-resistant human ovarian adenocarcinoma cells via P53 activation. Cytotechnology. 2016 Aug;**68**(4):1403-1413. DOI: 10.1007/s10616-015-9900-y

[58] Tang R, Xu Y, Ma F, Ren J, Shen S, Du Y, Hou Y, Wang T. Extremely low frequency magnetic fields regulate differentiation of regulatory T cells: Potential role for ROS-mediated inhibition on AKT. Bioelectromagnetics. 2016 Feb;**37**(2):89-98. DOI: 10.1002/bem.21954

[59] Yang ML, Ye ZM. Extremely low frequency electromagnetic field induces apoptosis of osteosarcoma cells via oxidative stress. Zhejiang Da Xue Xue Bao. Yi Xue Ban. 2015;**44**:323-328. PMID: 26350014

[60] Artacho-Cordon F, Salinas-Asensio Mdel M, Calvente I, Rios-Arrabal S, Leon J, Roman-Marinetto E, Olea N, Nunez MI. Could radiotherapy effectiveness be enhanced by electromagnetic field treatment? International Journal of Molecular Sciences. 2013;**14**:14974-14995. DOI: 10.3390/ijms140714974

[61] Ghodbane S, Lahbib A, Sakly M, Abdelmelek H. Bioeffects of static magnetic fields: Oxidative stress, genotoxic effects, and cancer studies. BioMed Research International. 2013:602987. DOI: 10.1155/2013/602987

[62] Montagnier L. Method for Digital Transduction of DNA in Living Cells, US Patent Application 20160002620, January 7, 2016. https://www.google.com/patents/US20160002620

Treatment Decisions and Survival in Ovarian Cancer

Hugo de Seabra Martins Nunes, Alexandra Mayer,
Ana Francisca Jorge, Teresa Margarida Cunha,
Ana Opinião, António Guimarães and Fátima Vaz

Abstract

Objective: to review the most recent data on the impact of the primary treatment and individual factors on ovarian cancer patient survival and to study it in a real world population. **Methods/materials:** retrospective analysis of 147 consecutive ovarian cancer patients treated with platin-based chemotherapy, either after primary debulking surgery (PDS) (n = 94, 64%) or as neoadjuvant (NACT) treatment (53, 36%). **Results:** NACT patients were older (64.3 vs. 58.2 years), with radiologically unresectable disease (74%) and/or comorbidities (26%). Fifty-five percent of pts. submitted to PDS were staged III/IV. Serous carcinomas were equally distributed (PDS-57% vs. NACT-60%) but endometrioid (20 vs. 4%) and carcinomas not otherwise specified (6 vs. 30%) were more frequently diagnosed in the PDS and NACT group, respectively. Genetic diagnosis (24.4%): 11 BRCA1/2 and 1 RAD51C carriers identified. Residual disease after surgery was the only significant prognostic factor for both relapse (HR = 2267) and death (HR = 1847). Primary debulking surgery was associated with a significantly better PFS (HR = 0.541; p = 0.012) and with a trend to a better OS (HR = 0.714; p = 0.296). For pts. with III/IV disease OS was significantly superior in the PDS group. **Conclusion:** residual disease was the only significant prognostic factor. Primary surgery was associated with a significantly better PFS. The difference in OS was significant in stage III/IV patients. This reinforces the importance of maximal cytoreduction.

Keywords: epithelial ovarian cancer, neoadjuvant therapy, primary surgery

1. Introduction

Ovarian cancer (OC) is the most lethal gynaecological malignancy in developed countries, with over 225.000 new cases and more than 140.000 deaths every year worldwide [1].

Epithelial OC is currently divided into seven main subtypes: serous, endometrioid, clear cell, mucinous, transitional cell, mixed and undifferentiated and unclassified OC [2]. Due to inadequate screening and a lack of early clinical symptoms, 70% of women with OC present with advanced disease, associated with high morbidity and mortality [1, 3]. The standard of care for OC treatment comprises maximal cytoreductive resection aiming to remove all visible tumour tissue, followed by platinum-taxane chemotherapy [4]. However, most patients relapse within the first 5 years after diagnosis, with a median progression-free survival (PFS) of 11 to 18 months and a median overall survival (OS) of 24 to 38 months [5, 6]. Data from the EUROCARE show a 5-year age-standardised relative survival of 37.6% [7]. Data from the National Cancer Institute show a 5-year survival of 46.2% [8].

Many OC patient characteristics are associated with survival, like stage [9, 10], histology [10–14], residual disease and debulking status after cytoreductive surgery [10, 12, 14, 15], type of chemotherapy [6, 10, 13, 16] and BRCA status [17, 18]. Maximal surgery, even when total absence of residual disease cannot be obtained, seems to relate to survival advantage [19]. The expertise of the surgical team is important in providing optimal cytoreduction without compromising post-operative morbidity [20].

A subgroup of OC patients is found to have surgically unresectable cancer and prediction criteria for suboptimal cytoreduction are important in treatment decisions. Studies using computed tomography (CT) suggested that the presence of an omental cake extending to the spleen, a diaphragm coated by tumour or lesions >2 cm in the suprarenal, para-aortic lymph-nodes and porta hepatis, among others [21], were predictors of unresectable disease. Other features predicting the outcome of cytoreduction correspond to traditionally difficult anatomic locations, such as extensive upper abdominal disease [22]. Recently, the Society of Gynecologic Oncology and the American Society of Clinical Oncology published the latest guidelines on neoadjuvant chemotherapy (NACT), stating the predictors of suboptimal cytoreduction. These include radiological predictors, such as retroperitoneal lymph-nodes above the renal hilum >1 cm, diffuse small bowel adhesions or thickening, small bowel mesentery lesions >1 cm, root of the superior mesenteric artery lesions >1 cm, perisplenic lesions >1 cm, lesser sac lesions >1 cm, and ascites on at least two-thirds of CT scan slices; and clinical predictors such as age ≥ 60 years and CA-125 ≥ 500 U/mL [23].

Interval debulking surgery (IDS) after NACT for patients with unresectable disease criteria is still controversial. A meta-analysis [24] suggested that NACT was associated with a worse outcome, but in 2010 a study concluded that it was not inferior to primary debulking surgery (PDS) in bulky stage IIIC or IV OC [25]. Moreover, it was associated to significantly lower adverse effects, such as postoperative infections, venous complications, fistula and haemorrhage, as well as lower postoperative mortality rates [25–27]. Other studies, such as the SCORPION and the JCOG0602 trials, seem to confirm these findings [23]. Some phase III trials suggested that NACT would also lead to improved quality of life [28–30]. Preoperative predictors for complete cytoreduction and outcomes from NACT are needed and subject of research [31].

The decision of treating advanced OC patients with NACT became more frequent [32], but there are still unsolved issues. Staging is surgical and based on laparotomy findings. Residual disease after surgery is a major prognostic factor for survival [14, 25] and visual evaluation by the surgeon is critical to conclude about intra-abdominal tumour spread. Whether the surgeons' statement of complete tumour resection is equal in primary surgery and in IDS remains unclear. Microscopically carcinomatous areas may have a benign visual appearance after NACT [33] interfering with the visual evaluation of tumour extension and potentially leading to incomplete cytoreduction. Also, the possibility that NACT may induce platinum resistance [34, 35] remains unclear. A recent study revealed that although the proportion of platinum-resistant recurrence after NACT and IDS was superior, this difference was not significant. A significant difference was only observed when women who had a recurrence were retreated with platinum-based chemotherapy [36].

The highest risk associated with NACT may be that patients with significant side effects and refractory disease will lose the opportunity for debulking surgery [37], although it has been suggested that these patients have a poor prognosis and should be encouraged to participate in clinical trials or to discontinue active cancer therapy [23]. Another limitation of NACT is the insufficient data supporting the use of intraperitoneal (IP)/intravenous (IV) chemotherapy as adjuvant treatment after NACT [23]. Recent results from the OV21/ PETROC trial seem to support that a carboplatin-based IP regimen, after NACT and debulking surgery, is well tolerated and associated with a higher PFS compared to IV therapy (immature data) [38].

Besides patient characteristics, survival depends on treatment decisions and questions remain about the reproducibility of study data in routine clinical practice. We tried to review the most recent data on the primary treatment of OC and the factors that have impact on the survival of these patients. Therefore, our objective was to characterise a consecutive series of OC patients treated in our centre and to analyse the effect of patient variables and decision criteria on efficacy outcomes for patients treated with either PDS or primary NACT.

2. Material and methods

This study is a retrospective analysis. It includes all patients with epithelial OC observed in the Gynaecological Oncology multidisciplinary group of our centre and registered in the South Portuguese Cancer Registry (ROR-Sul), between January 2006 and December 2011. Medical records were reviewed, and demographic, clinical, surgical, pathologic, molecular and follow-up information obtained. Optimal cytoreduction was defined as no macroscopic residual disease at the end of surgery. Pathology data were collected from the pathology report after citoreductive surgery. The chemotherapy regimen used was the doublet of carboplatin (AUC = 6) and paclitaxel (175 mg/m² of body surface). Progression data were obtained from clinical notes: most were confirmed by CT scan and CA125 measurement criteria. In less than 5% of cases, progression was assumed by CA125 measurement and clinical examination. Information concerning molecular testing was obtained from patients previously counselled and given informed consent through procedures and forms approved by the Ethics Committee.

2.1. Statistics

Statistical analysis was performed with IBM SPSS Statistics software (version 23). Continuous data (presented as the means ± SD) that were normally distributed were analysed using Student's t-test, while data that were not normally distributed were analysed using the Mann–Whitney U test. The Pearson's exact chi-square or Fisher's exact test were used to compare the proportions between groups. Progression-free survival was defined as the time interval between the end of primary treatment and the date of progression. If there was no documented recurrence, PFS was calculated from the end of primary treatment to the date of last follow-up or death. Platinum-resistant relapse was defined as recurrence within 6 months of primary treatment. Overall survival was defined as the time interval between date of diagnosis and date of death or last follow-up. Progression free survival and OS were analysed by the log-rank test and the results were expressed as Kaplan–Meier plots. A Cox proportional hazards model was estimated to assess the impact of different prognostic variables on survival. A p value <0.05 was defined as statistically significant.

3. Results

3.1. Cases

Two hundred and fifty-seven patients were registered in the ROR-Sul database and 147 (58%) of those received systemic treatment and were included in this analysis. Excluded patients either were not submitted to surgery or chemotherapy in our centre, died without any specific treatment, had non-eligible neoplasia after surgery (3 mucinous adenocarcinomas of the appendix) or were diagnosed with early stage disease with low-risk features (**Figure 1**).

Demographic and clinical characteristics are summarised in **Table 1**. All 147 patients were treated with platin-based chemotherapy: either following primary surgery (n = 94, 64%) or in the neoadjuvant setting (n = 53, 36%). The mean age at diagnosis was 60.4 years (25–89; IC95% = [58.4–62.4]); patients in NACT group were older (64.3 vs. 58.2; p = 0.002) and we did not observe age differences between advanced versus non-advanced stages, different histologic subtypes or between platinum-resistant versus platinum-sensitive patients (p = 0.318; p = 0.108; p = 0.774, respectively). More cases of advanced disease were treated with NACT (6% stages IIIB, 83% IIIC-IV) as compared with primary surgery (27% stages IA-IC, 36% IIA-IIIB, 37% IIIC-IV). The median number of chemotherapy cycles was superior in the NACT group (8 vs. 6; p = 0.000). Macroscopic residual disease after debulking surgery (PDS or IDS) was present in 46% of all cases (IC95% = [37%; 54%]) and was not associated with the treatment modality (Pearson X2 = 0.001; p = 1.000). Most cases were serous, endometrioid or carcinomas not otherwise specified (NOS) (58.5, 14.3 and 15%, respectively); 9 patients (6%) had cancers with mucinous/clear cell histology. The proportion of serous carcinomas was similar between groups. In the PDS group, a significantly higher proportion of endometrioid tumours was observed (20 vs. 2%; p = 0.021) while carcinomas NOS were more frequent in the NACT group (16 vs. 6%; p = 0.021). Thirty-six patients (24.4%) had information of molecular testing: 23 in the PDS (7 BRCA carriers) and 13 in the NACT (4 BRCA carriers and 1 RAD51C carrier) groups.

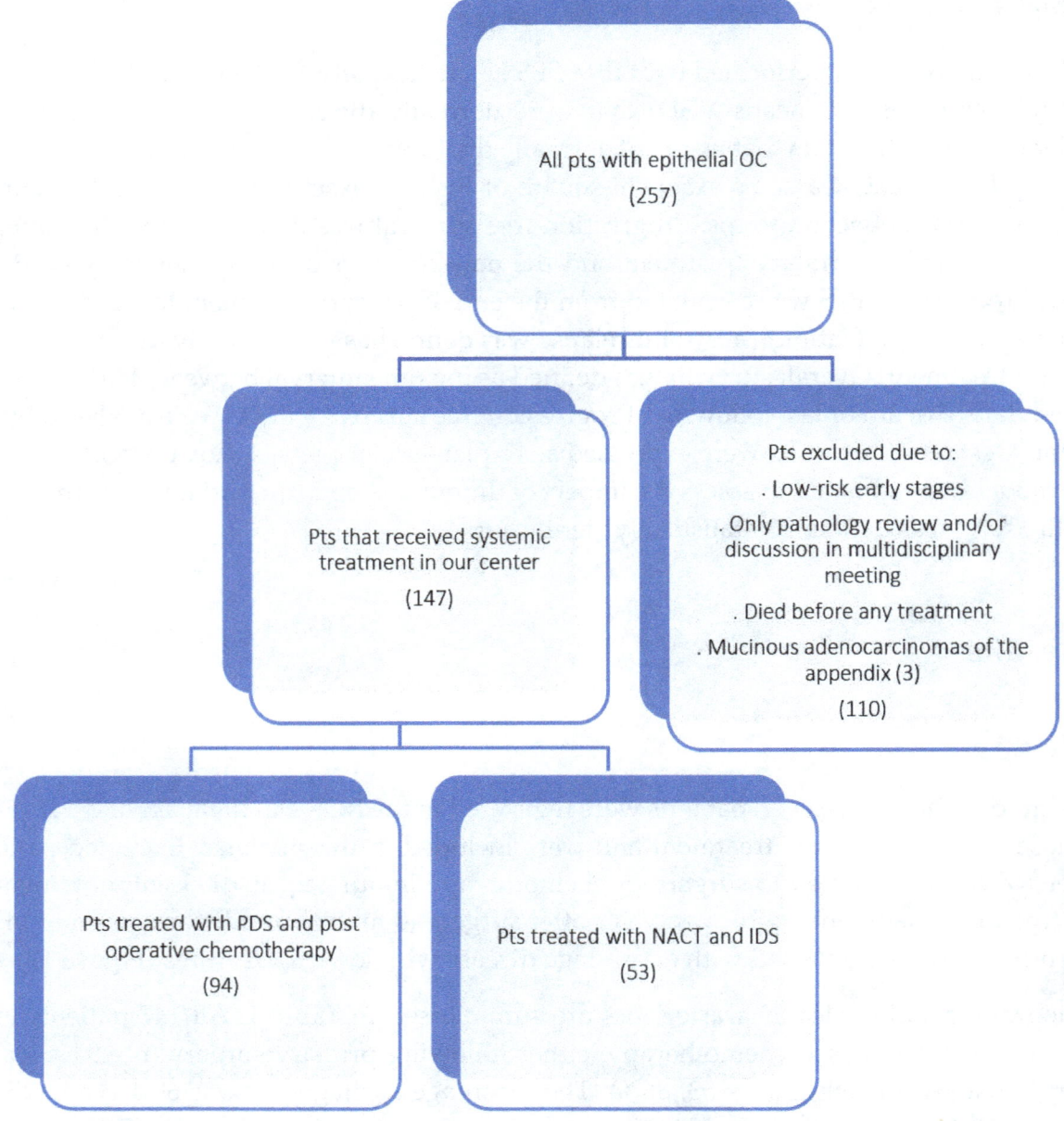

Figure 1. Study design. OC: Ovarian cancer; PDS: Primary debulking surgery; NACT: Neoadjuvant chemotherapy; IDS: Interval debulking surgery.

	PDS (N = 94)	NACT–IDS (N = 53)	P
Age (mean, years)	58 (±12)	64 (±10)	0.002
Histology [N(%)]			
Serous	54 (57.4)	32 (60.4)	0.021
Endometrioid	19 (20.4)	2 (3.8)	
Mucinous	3 (3.2)	1 (1.9)	
Clear cell	4 (4.3)	1 (1.9)	
Mixed	2 (2.1)	0 (0)	
Poorly differentiated	6 (6.4)	1 (1.9)	
Carcinoma NOS	6 (6.4)	16 (30.2)	

	PDS (N = 94)	NACT–IDS (N = 53)	P
FIGO Stage [N(%)]			
IA-IC	25 (26.6)	—	0.000
IIA-IIC	17 (18.1)	—	
IIIA	5 (5.3)	—	
IIIB	12 (12.8)	3 (5.7)	
IIIC	21 (22.3)	15 (28.3)	
IV	14 (14.9)	29 (54.7)	
Unknown	—	6 (11.3)	
Nr of cycles (median)	6 (±1.3)	8 (±2.7)	0.000
Residual disease after debulking surgery [N(%)]	60 (64)	29 (55)	1.000

Table 1. Demographic and clinical characteristics of the study population. PDS: Primary debulking surgery; NACT-IDS: Neoadjuvant chemotherapy and interval debulking surgery; NOS: Not otherwise specified; Values for continuous measurements are means, unless otherwise specified; FIGO: International Federation of Gynecology and Obstetrics.

3.2. Treatment decision

The decision for NACT was due mainly to radiological criteria: implants >2 cm outside the pelvis (18 pts; 34%), lymphadenopathies above renal hilum (12 pts; 23%), subcapsular or Parenchymal liver metastasis (8; 15%) or pre-sacred retroperitoneal disease (1 pt; 2%). In 14 pts (26%), comorbidities that contraindicated upfront surgery were also considered in the decision for NACT.

3.3. Efficacy analysis

For the total cohort, the median PFS and OS were 13.4 (IC95%= [9,3-17,5]) and 44.0 (IC95% = [29.7–58.3]) months, respectively. In the PDS group, PFS was significantly superior (23.4 vs. 13.8 months; p = 0.010), even when restricting analysis to advanced stages (21.4 vs. 12.5 months; p = 0.040). Patients with no macroscopic residual disease after debulking surgery had superior PFS (27.0 vs. 14.0 months; p = 0.000).

For patients treated with PDS, OS was significantly superior (48.4 vs. 30.9 months; p = 0.001), even when restricting the analysis to advanced stages (44.4 vs. 28.2 months; p = 0.014) (Figure 2).

Patients with no macroscopic residual disease after debulking surgery had superior OS (52.7 vs. 36.0 months; p = 0.002) (Figure 3), as well as those with non-advanced stage disease (52.5 vs. 37.1 months; p = 0.009). Moreover, patients with platinum-sensitive relapse (>6 months) had significantly superior OS (56.0 vs. 12.3 months; p = 0.000) (Figure 4), as compared to platinum resistant patients.

The Cox proportional hazards model (Table 2) allowed estimating the impact in survival of factors such as age at diagnosis, histology, stage, platinum free interval, residual disease after debulking surgery and therapeutic modality. Adjusting for these variables, the

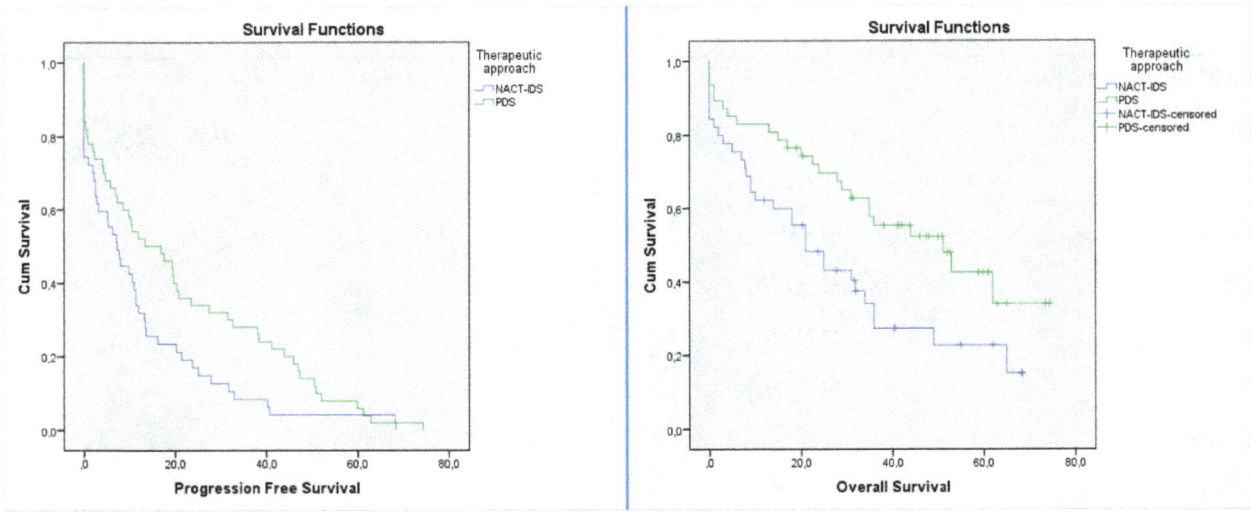

Figure 2. Kaplan–Meier survival curves showing the PFS and OS rates of patients in the NACT/IDS *vs.* PDS groups (only advanced stages) (7.3 *vs.* 13.4 months; p = 0.010 and 21.0 *vs.* 55.1 months; p = 0.001, respectively).

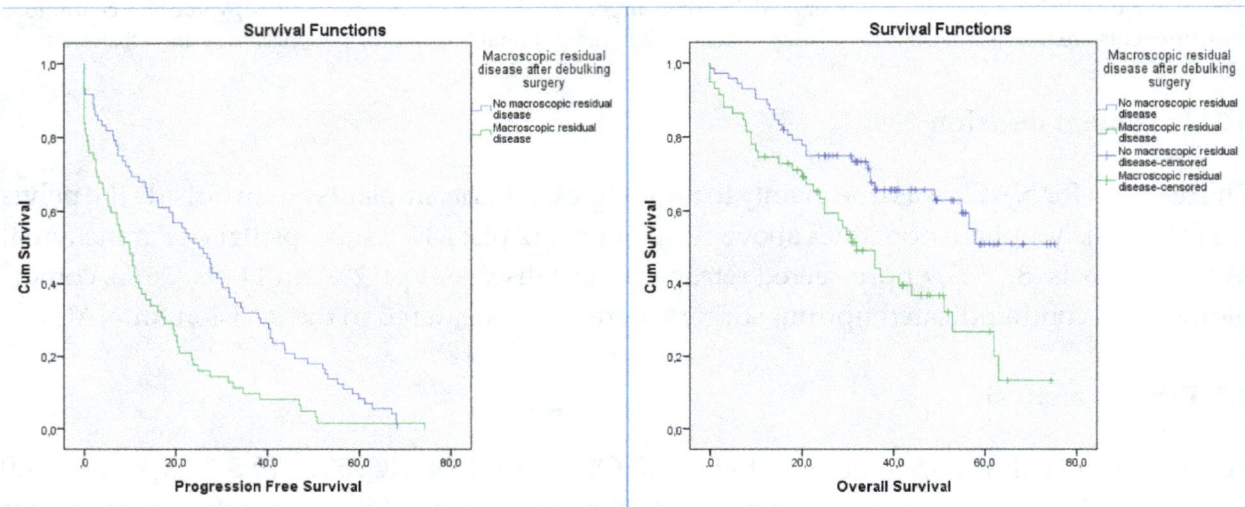

Figure 3. Kaplan–Meier survival curves showing the PFS and OS rates of patients with *vs.* without macroscopic residual disease after debulking surgery (PFS: 9.9 *vs.* 25.1 months, p = 0.000; as it did not fall below 50% at the time of the analysis, it is not possible to estimate median OS, p = 0.002).

only statistically significant prognostic factor for both relapse and death was the presence of macroscopic residual disease after surgery, with more than 2-fold higher risk of relapse (HR = 2267; p = 0.000) and 80% higher risk of death (HR = 1847; p = 0.036). Primary debulking surgery was associated to a significantly better outcome, but only in terms of PFS (HR = 0.541; p = 0.012), with no significant gain in OS compared to NACT, although there is a trend to a better outcome (HR = 0.714; p = 0.296). Other factors, such as age, histology or advanced stage did not have a significant effect on relapse. Platinum-resistant disease was associated with a 9-fold higher risk of death (HR = 8964; p = 0.000). There is a trend towards a worse prognosis of advanced stage disease (HR = 1293; p = 0.468) and towards a better outcome of serous histology (HR = 0.847; p = 0.560).

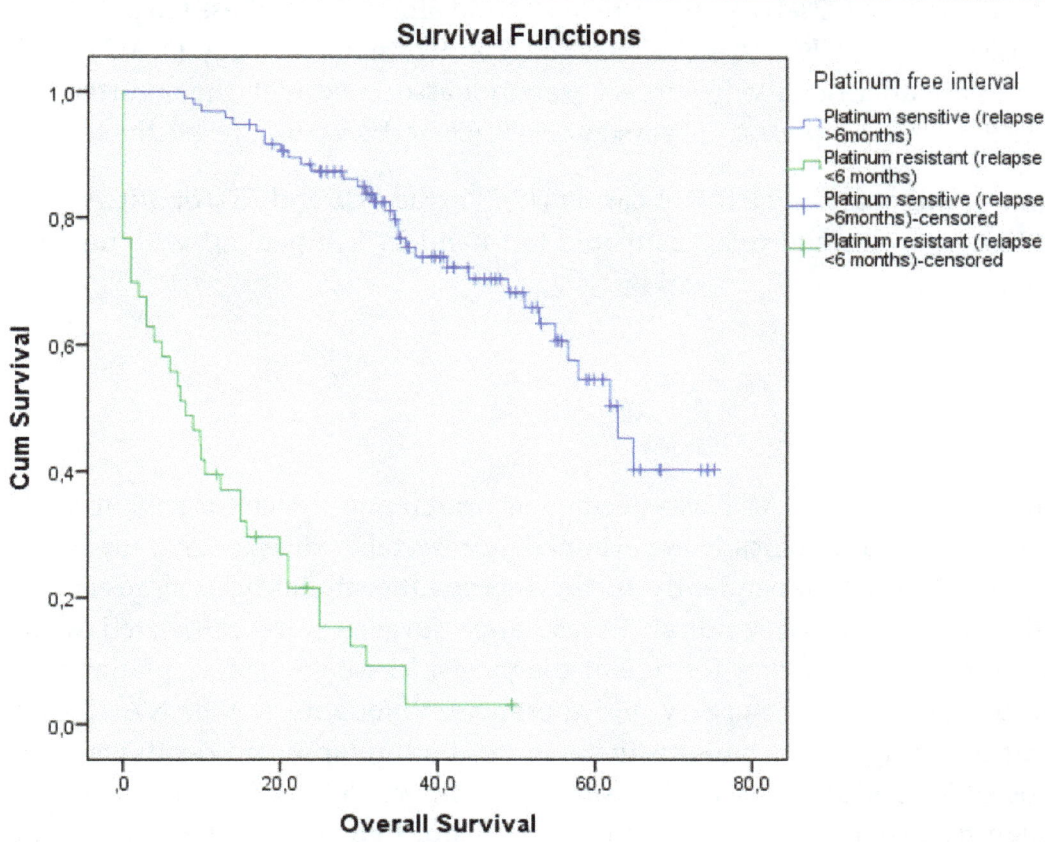

Figure 4. Kaplan–Meier survival curves showing OS rates of patients with platinum-sensitive *vs.* platinum-resistant relapse after primary treatment (63.0 *vs.* 8.0 months, p = 0.000).

	OS				PFS			
	Coefficient	SE	P	HR (95% CI)	Coefficient	SE	P	HR (95% CI)
Age	0.021	0.012	0.097	1021 (0.996–1046)	0.004	0.008	0.559	1004 (0.990–1020)
Serous histology (*vs* nonserous)	−0.166	0.285	0.560	0.847 (0.484–1481)	0.323	0.194	0.096	1381 (0.944–2020)
Advanced stage (stage III-IV *vs.* I-II)	0.257	0.354	0.468	1293 (0.646–2590)	−0.315	0.243	0.195	0.730 (0.453–1176)
Residual disease	0.603	0.293	0.036	1847 (1040–3278)	0.818	0.219	0.000	2267 (1504–3416)
PDS (*vs* NACT)	−0.337	0.322	0.296	0.714 (0.380–1344)	−0.615	0.244	0.012	0.541 (0.335–0.873)
Platinum resistant disease	2193	0.300	0.000	8964 (4976–16.147)	—	—	—	—

Table 2. Multivariate Cox regression model. OS: overall survival; PFS: progression-free survival; SE: standard error; HR: hazard ratio; CI: confidence interval; PDS (vs NACT): primary debulking surgery (vs neoadjuvant chemotherapy).

Ninety seven percent (97%) of patients relapsed and almost 1/3 of these (46 pts) had platinum-resistant disease (31%; IC95% = [23%; 39%]). The treatment strategy (NACT vs. PDS) and residual disease after debulking surgery were not associated with the occurrence of relapse (Pearson X2 = 2318 and p = 0.297; Pearson X2 = 0.708 and p = 0.625, respectively).

At the time of this analysis, all BRCA carriers (7/7) in the PDS and 75% of BRCA carriers in the NACT (3/4) group were alive as compared to 54 and 36% of patients with unknown BRCA status, respectively.

4. Discussion

Between 2006 and 2011, NACT was decided as primary approach for advanced OC, mostly for patients with radiologically determined unresectable disease and for older patients with comorbidities. Independently of the therapeutic modality, non-advanced stage at diagnosis and absence of residual disease after surgery were associated with progression free survival. Adjusting for age at diagnosis, histology, stage, platinum free interval, residual disease after surgery and therapeutic modality (either NACT or PDS), the only statistically significant prognostic factor for both relapse and death was the presence of macroscopic residual disease after surgery. Primary debulking surgery was associated with a significantly better outcome only in terms of PFS, although a trend to a better OS was also observed. When analysis was restricted to stages III and IV OS was significantly superior in the PDS group, as compared with the NACT group. BRCA status was known for a small proportion of patients in both groups, which limits statistical analysis and conclusions. However, it's interesting to note that all known BRCA carriers in the PDS group were alive at the time of this analysis, compared to only 75% after NACT-IDS. That happens for unknown BRCA status patients as well, but with a smaller difference between groups (54 vs. 36%). Recent observations suggest a selection of tumour cell clones without somatic loss of heterozygosity (LOH) for the wild-type allele of BRCA genes, during neoadjuvant therapy [39].

Patients treated with PDS had better outcome in terms of PFS. This is not unexpected since this group included patients with less advanced disease, but suggests that the cytotoxic treatment before primary surgery in the NACT group could not counteract the bad prognosis associated with advanced stage. This was observed even if patients in the NACT group received a higher number of chemotherapy cycles (8 vs. 6; p = 0.000). Some authors have expressed concern about the selection of resistant clones in patients submitted to NACT [34–36] but we did not observe an association between the platinum free interval and the chosen treatment approach (Pearson X2 = 3955 and p = 0.058). Patients with platinum-sensitive relapse (>6 months) had significantly superior OS (56.0 vs. 12.3 months; p = 0.000), as compared to platinum resistant patients. This was confirmed in the multivariate survival analysis, with Cox model showing that platinum-resistant disease was associated with a 9-fold higher risk of death (HR = 8964; p = 0.000). These findings should be carefully interpreted, since further lines of treatment widely vary between platinum-sensitive and platinum-resistant populations.

There is evidence that longer platinum-chemotherapy-free interval is associated with better survival (especially PFS after further lines of treatment) [40], but although the platinum-free interval is defined as the period of time from the last date of platinum dose until progressive disease is documented, it does not take into account how progression is defined (CA125 alone, radiological and symptomatic recurrence) [41].

The PDS group had a significantly higher number of patients with endometrioid histology. This factor and more advanced cases in the NACT group, may have contributed to the better outcomes in patients submitted to upfront surgery. The higher proportion of carcinoma NOS in NACT group (16 vs. 6%; p = 0.021) is a limitation of our study, since consecutive pathology review was not done. However, this finding is not unexpected in pathology reports of surgical specimens after NACT.

We did not observe an improvement of optimal debulking rates with NACT, as macroscopic residual disease after debulking surgery (PDS or IDS) was not associated with the treatment strategy (Pearson X2 = 0.001; p = 1.000). In the 2010 EORTC-NCIC trial, no gross residual tumour after PDS was achieved in 19% of patients and after IDS in 51% of patients [25]. Progression-free survival and OS for both arms were 12 and 30 months, respectively. In our cohort, cytoreduction was higher (36%) in the PDS group, as well as PFS and OS (13.4 and 55.1 months, respectively). Cytoreduction rate for our NACT group (45%) was closer to the rate described in the EORTC trial but our observations for PFS and OS were lower (7.3 and 21.0 months, respectively). Besides the expected differences between a randomised trial and an observational study, stage IV patients were well-balanced between arms in the EORTC trial but predominated in the NACT group (55 vs. 15%) of our study. In the CHORUS trial the complete cytoreduction rate was inferior to the one in our cohort, both in PDS and NACT groups (15 vs. 35%) but PFS and OS outcomes with NACT were better (10 and 23 months, respectively) than with PDS (12 and 25 months, respectively) [42]. However, a recent observational trial [32] showed NACT to be inferior to PDS in stage IIIC but superior in stage IV. It is important to remember that, for this analysis, we considered complete cytoreduction as the absence of macroscopic residual disease, even if, this was not the case for other studies [25, 32, 42].

Although retrospective, our study reflects how decisional criteria for both modalities were applied in a group of consecutive, non-selected OC patients. Statistical methodologies were selected according to the retrospective nature of the study: univariate analysis first identified factors influencing the outcomes of these patients (other than primary treatment); these factors were then integrated in the multivariate analysis (Cox regression model), to ascertain the efficacy of each strategy, adjusting to variables previously identified as an influence to prognosis. Limitations to this study are possible selection and recall bias, as well as unknown confounding variables that may have a negative impact on the accuracy of the results. One example is the limited accuracy in determining performance status and comorbidities as criteria for the decision of upfront treatment, although notes from multidisciplinary meetings were carefully reviewed. As for the assessment of residual disease after debulking surgery, heterogeneity was observed due to changing criteria for the classification of ideal resection during the period covered by our study.

In conclusion, the only significant prognostic factor for both relapse and death was the presence of macroscopic residual disease after surgery, which enhances the importance of maximal cytoreduction in the primary treatment. As for the influence of treatment modality on outcomes, PDS was associated to a significantly better PFS and a non-significant trend to a better OS. Other factors, such as age, histology or advanced stage did not have a significant effect on relapse. Our findings are in agreement with other studies [19, 20, 25, 32, 42, 43] about the impact of optimal debulking surgery in survival of OC patients. This is observed whether complete debulking is attained with easily resectable disease or extensive surgery. It has also been shown that the impact of potentially negative biologic factors such as grade and histology can be overcome by surgical debulking [43]. This is why surgical expertise plus supportive management (antibiotics, blood banking, and intensive care) should parallel the development of better systemic therapies.

Author details

Hugo de Seabra Martins Nunes[1]*, Alexandra Mayer[2], Ana Francisca Jorge[3], Teresa Margarida Cunha[4], Ana Opinião[1], António Guimarães[1] and Fátima Vaz[1]

*Address all correspondence to: hugosmnunes@gmail.com

1 Department of Medical Oncology, Portuguese Institute of Oncology Lisbon Francisco Gentil, Lisbon, Portugal

2 Southern Portugal Cancer Registry (ROR-Sul), Portuguese Institute of Oncology Lisbon Francisco Gentil, Lisbon, Portugal

3 Department of Gynaecology, Portuguese Institute of Oncology Lisbon Francisco Gentil, Lisbon, Portugal

4 Department of Radiology, Portuguese Institute of Oncology Lisbon Francisco Gentil, Lisbon, Portugal

References

[1] Jemal A, Bray F, Ferlay J. Global cancer statistics: 2011. CA: a Cancer Journal for Clinicians. 2011;**61**(2):69-90

[2] Kurman R, Carcangiu M, Herrington C, Young R, Curto G, Longo G, et al. WHO Classification of Tumours of Female Reproductive Organs. 4th ed. Lyon, France: IARC WHO Classif Tumours; 2014

[3] Cannistra SA. Cancer of the ovary. The New England Journal of Medicine. 2004;**351**: 2519-2529

[4] Ledermann J, Raja F, Fotopoulou C, Gonzalez-Martin A, Colombo N, Sessa C, et al. Newly diagnosed and relapsed epithelial ovarian carcinoma: ESMO clinical practice guidelines for diagnosis, treatment and follow-up. Annals of Oncology. 2013;**24**(Suppl. 6):vi24-vi32

[5]   Piccart M, Bertelsen K, James K, Cassidy J, Mangioni C, Simonsen E, et al. Randomized intergroup trial of Cisplatin-paclitaxel versus Cisplatin-cyclophosphamide in women with advanced epithelial ovarian cancer: Three-year results. Journal of the National Cancer Institute. 2000;**92**(9):699-708

[6]   Mcguire W, Hoskins W, Brady M, Kucera P, Partridge E, Look K, et al. Cyclophosphamide and cisplatin compared with paclitaxel and cisplatin in patients with stage III and stage IV ovarian cancer. The New England Journal of Medicine. 1996;**334**(1):1-6

[7]   De Angelis R, Sant M, Coleman MP, Francisci S, Baili P, Pierannunzio D, et al. Cancer survival in Europe 1999-2007 by country and age: Results of EUROCARE-5 - a population-based study. The Lancet Oncology. 2016;**15**(1):23-34

[8]   Howlader N, Noone A, Krapcho M, Miller D, Bishop K, Altekruse S, et al. SEER Cancer Statistics Review. Bethesda, MD: Natl Cancer Institute; 1975-2013

[9]   Rubin SC, Randall TC, Armstrong KA, Chi DS, Hoskins WJ, Curto F, et al. Ten-year follow-up of ovarian cancer patients after second-look laparotomy with negative findings. Obstetrics and Gynecology. 1999;**93**(1):21-24

[10] Omura GA, Brady MF, Homesley HD, Yordan E, Major FJ, Buchsbaum HJ, et al. Long-term follow-up and prognostic factor analysis in advanced ovarian carcinoma: The gynecologic oncology group experience. Journal of Clinical Oncology. 1991;**9**(7): 1138-1150

[11] Halperin R, Zehavi S, Langer R, Hadas E, Bukovsky I, Schneider D, et al. Primary peritoneal serous papillary carcinoma: A new epidemiologic trend? A matched-case comparison with ovarian serous papillary cancer. International Journal of Gynecological Cancer. 2001;**11**(5):403-408

[12] Hoskins W, Bundy B, Thigpen J, Omura G, Curto G, Longo H, et al. The influence of cytoreductive surgery on recurrence-free interval and survival in small-volume stage III epithelial ovarian cancer: A gynecologic oncology group study. Gynecologic Oncology. 1992;**47**(2):159-166

[13] Marszalek A, Alran S, Scholl S, Fourchotte V, Plancher C, Rosty C, et al. Outcome in advanced ovarian cancer following an appropriate and comprehensive effort at upfront cytoreduction: A twenty-year experience in a single cancer institute. International Journal of Surgical Oncology. 2010;**2010**:214919

[14] Winter WE, Maxwell GL, Tian C, Carlson JW, Ozols RF, Rose PG, et al. Prognostic factors for stage III epithelial ovarian cancer: A gynecologic oncology group study. Journal of Clinical Oncology. 2007;**25**(24):3621-3627

[15] Gerestein CG, Eijkemans MJC, De Jong D, Van Der Burg MEL, Dykgraaf RHM, Kooi GS, et al. The prediction of progression-free and overall survival in women with an advanced stage of epithelial ovarian carcinoma. BJOG: An International Journal of Obstetrics & Gynaecology. 2009;**116**(3):372-380

[16] Burger RA, Brady MF, Bookman MA, Fleming GF, Monk BJ, Huang H, et al. Incorporation of bevacizumab in the primary treatment of ovarian cancer. Obstetrical & Gynecological Survey. 2012;**67**(5):289-290

[17] Bolton KL. Association between BRCA1 and BRCA2 mutations and survival in women with invasive epithelial ovarian cancer. Journal of the American Medical Association. 2012;**307**(4):382-390

[18] Alsop K, Fereday S, Meldrum C, DeFazio A, Emmanuel C, George J, et al. BRCA mutation frequency and patterns of treatment response in BRCA mutation-positive women with ovarian cancer: A report from the Australian ovarian cancer study group. Journal of Clinical Oncology. 2012;**30**(21):2654-2663

[19] Wallace S, Kumar A, Mc Gree M, Weaver A, Mariani A, Langstraat C, et al. Efforts at maximal cytoreduction improve survival in ovarian cancer patients, even when complete gross resection is not feasible. Gynecologic Oncology. 2017;**145**(1):21-26

[20] Giede KC, Kieser K, Dodge J, Rosen B, Curto G, Longo F, et al. Who should operate on patients with ovarian cancer? An evidence-based review. Gynecologic Oncology. 2005;**99**(2): 447-461

[21] Nelson BE, Rosenfield AT, Schwartz PE. Preoperative abdominopelvic computed tomographic prediction of optimal cytoreduction in epithelial ovarian carcinoma. Journal of Clinical Oncology. 1993;**11**(1):166-172

[22] Bristow R, Duska L, Lambrou N, Fishman E, O'Neill M, Trimble E, et al. A model for predicting surgical outcome in patients with advanced ovarian carcinoma using computed tomography. Cancer. 2000;**89**:1532-1540

[23] Wright AA, Bohlke K, Armstrong DK, Bookman MA, Cliby WA, Coleman RL, et al. Neoadjuvant chemotherapy for newly diagnosed, advanced ovarian cancer: Society of Gynecologic Oncology and American Society of clinical oncology clinical practice guideline. Journal of Clinical Oncology. 2016;**34**(28):3460-3473

[24] Bristow RE, Chi DS. Platinum-based neoadjuvant chemotherapy and interval surgical cytoreduction for advanced ovarian cancer : A meta-analysis. Gynecologic Oncology. 2006;**103**:1070-1076

[25] Vergote I, Tropé C, Amant F, Kristensen G, Ehlen T, Johnson N, et al. Neoadjuvant chemotherapy or primary surgery in stage IIIC or IV ovarian cancer. The New England Journal of Medicine. 2010;**363**:943-953

[26] Van der Burg M, Van Lent M, Buyse M, Kobierska A, Colombo N, Favalli G, et al. The effect of debulking surgery after induction chemotherapy on the prognosis in advanced apithelial ovarian cancer. The New England Journal of Medicine. 1995;**332**(10)

[27] Rose P, Nerenstone S, Brady M, Clarke-pearson D, Olt G, Rubin S, et al. Secondary surgical Cytoreduction for advanced ovarian carcinoma. The New England Journal of Medicine. 2004;**351**:2489-2497

[28] Rustin GJS, Van Der Burg MEL, Griffin CL, Guthrie D, Lamont A, Jayson GC, et al. Early versus delayed treatment of relapsed ovarian cancer (MRC OV05/EORTC 55955): A randomised trial. Lancet. 2010;**376**(9747):1155-1163

[29] Wenzel L, Huang HQ, Monk BJ, Rose PG, Cella D, Mackey D, et al. Quality-of-life comparisons in a randomized trial of interval secondary cytoreduction in advanced ovarian carcinoma: A gynecologic oncology group study. Journal of Clinical Oncology. 2005;**23**(24):5605-5612

[30] Bezjak A, Tu D, Bacon M, Osoba D, Zee B, Stuart G, et al. Quality of life in ovarian cancer patients: Comparison of paclitaxel plus cisplatin, with cyclophosphamide plus cisplatin in a randomized study. Journal of Clinical Oncology. 2004;**22**(22):4595-4603

[31] Baek M-H, Lee S-W, Park J-Y, Rhim CC, Kim D-Y, Suh D-S, et al. Preoperative predictive factors for complete cytoreduction and survival outcome in epithelial ovarian, tubal, and peritoneal cancer after neoadjuvant chemotherapy. International Journal of Gynecological Cancer. 2017;**27**(3):420-429

[32] Meyer LA, Cronin AM, Sun CC, Bixel K, Bookman MA, Cristea MC, et al. Use and effectiveness of neoadjuvant chemotherapy for treatment of ovarian cancer. Journal of Clinical Oncology. 2016 Nov 10;**34**(32):3854-3863

[33] Hynninen J, Lavonius M, Oksa S, Grénman S, Carpén O, Auranen A, et al. Is perioperative visual estimation of intra-abdominal tumor spread reliable in ovarian cancer surgery after neoadjuvant chemotherapy? Gynecologic Oncology. 2013;**128**(2):229-232

[34] Matsuo K, Eno ML, Im DD, Rosenshein NB, Curto H, Longo H, et al. Chemotherapy time interval and development of platinum and taxane resistance in ovarian, fallopian, and peritoneal carcinomas. Archives of Gynecology and Obstetrics. 2010;**281**(2):325-328

[35] Chi DS, Musa F, Dao F, Zivanovic O, Sonoda Y, Leitao MM, et al. An analysis of patients with bulky advanced stage ovarian, tubal, and peritoneal carcinoma treated with primary debulking surgery (PDS) during an identical time period as the randomized EORTC-NCIC trial of PDS vs neoadjuvant chemotherapy (NACT). Gynecologic Oncology. 2012;**124**(1):10-14

[36] Rauh-Hain JA, Nitschmann CC, Worley MJ, Bradford LS, Berkowitz RS, Schorge JO, et al. Platinum resistance after neoadjuvant chemotherapy compared to primary surgery in patients with advanced epithelial ovarian carcinoma. Gynecologic Oncology. 2013;**129**(1):63-68

[37] Sato S, Itamochi H. Neoadjuvant chemotherapy in advanced ovarian cancer: Latest results and place in therapy. Therapeutic Advances in Medical Oncology. 2014;**6**(6):293-304

[38] Mackay H, Gallagher C, Parulekar W, Ledermann J, Armstrong D, Gourley C, et al. OV21/PETROC: A randomized gynecologic cancer intergroup (GCIG) phase II study of intraperitoneal (IP) versus intravenous (IV) chemotherapy following neoadjuvant chemotherapy and optimal debulking surgery in epithelial ovarian cancer (EOC). Journal of Clinical Oncology. 2016;**34** (suppl; abstr LBA5503)

[39] Gorodnova TV, Sokolenko AP, Ivantsov AO, Iyevleva AG, Suspitsin EN, Aleksakhina SN, et al. High response rates to neoadjuvant platinum-based therapy in ovarian cancer patients carrying germ-line BRCA mutation. Cancer Letters. 2015;**369**(2):363-367

[40] Lee CK, Simes RJ, Brown C, Gebski V, Pfisterer J, Swart AM, et al. A prognostic nomogram to predict overall survival in patients with platinum-sensitive recurrent ovarian cancer. Annals of Oncology. 2013;**24**(4):937-943

[41] Pujade-Lauraine E. How to approach patients in relapse. Annals of Oncology. 2012; **23**(Suppl. 10):23-26

[42] Kehoe S, Hook J, Nankivell M, Jayson GC, Kitchener H, Lopes T, et al. Primary chemotherapy versus primary surgery for newly diagnosed advanced ovarian cancer (CHORUS): An open-label, randomised, controlled, non-inferiority trial. Lancet. 2015;**6736**(14):1-9

[43] du Bois A, Reuss A, Pujade-Lauraine E, Harter P, Ray-Coquard I, Pfisterer J, et al. Role of surgical outcome as prognostic factor in advanced epithelial ovarian cancer: A combined exploratory analysis of 3 prospectively randomized phase 3 multicenter trials: By the Arbeitsgemeinschaft Gynaekologische Onkologie Studiengruppe Ovarialkarzin. Cancer. 2009;**115**(6):1234-1244

Targeted Therapies in Platinum-Resistant Ovarian Cancer: Advances in Immunotherapy Combination Strategies

Arkene Levy and Patricia C. Rose

Abstract

Platinum-resistant ovarian cancer (OC) is one of the most lethal gynecological malignancies that has shown minimal improvement in 5 year overall survival rates for the past 15 years. This chapter discusses the current targeted therapies that are being used or evaluated as monotherapy and/or adjuvants to chemotherapeutic regimens in platinum-resistant ovarian cancer. These therapeutics include focal adhesion kinase inhibitors (FAK) such as defactinib, anti-angiogenic agents such as bevacizumab, poly(adenosine diphosphate [ADP] ribose) polymerase (PARP) inhibitors such as olaparib, epidermal growth factor receptor family targeting agents such as erlotinib, folate receptor antagonists such as farletuzumab, and insulin growth factor receptor inhibitors such as linsitinib. The rationale for using immunotherapeutic agents will also be discussed. The importance of combination strategies utilizing immunotherapies will be highlighted with specific focus on immune checkpoint inhibitors that are currently in multiple clinical trials assessing synergistic effects with targeted agents such as PARP inhibitors in platinum-resistant OC. These therapeutic combinations have the potential to produce substantial improvements in platinum-resistant OC treatment outcomes in the future. Finally, the major challenges and limitation associated with these combination therapies and strategies to overcome them will be explored.

Keywords: ovarian cancer, platinum resistance, targeted therapy, immunotherapy, combination strategies

1. Introduction

Ovarian cancer (OC) is the leading cause of death from gynecologic malignancies in the United States [1]. It is estimated that 22,240 women will be diagnosed with OC, and 14,080 women will die of the disease in 2017 [1]. Ovarian malignancies can be primary (arising from normal structures within the ovary) or secondary (arising from non-ovarian tissue). Approximately 90% of all primary OC are epithelial carcinomas [2]. Epithelial ovarian cancer (EOC) is sensitive to many chemotherapeutic agents, and the current standard treatment consists of cytoreductive surgery followed by chemotherapy with platinum compounds such as cisplatin or carboplatin and a taxane agent such as paclitaxel [3]. A high percentage of patients with advanced EOC however, eventually develop recurrent disease within 3 years and only 10–30% of patients presenting with stage III or IV disease survive 5 years following initial diagnosis [3, 4]. This poor survival rate is mainly due to the development of chemotherapy resistance following several rounds of treatment. In many cases, initial recurrences are platinum-sensitive but the disease eventually becomes platinum-resistant; which is defined as disease progressing within 6 months of platinum-based therapy [4, 5]. Platinum-resistant patients are subsequently limited to non-platinum and non-taxane chemotherapy treatment options such as topotecan, gemcitabine, and pegylated liposomal doxorubicin which have shown moderate therapeutic success [6]. Alternative treatment options for platinum-resistant disease are, therefore, constantly being explored and immunotherapy and targeted agents are increasingly undergoing clinical trials which are showing positive results.

2. Platinum compounds and mechanisms of resistance

The serendipitous discovery that platinum coordination complexes blocked bacterial replication led to the hypothesis that these complexes could be of great clinical value as anti-tumor agents [7]. Cis-diamminedichloroplatinum II (cisplatin) was the first drug in its class successfully marketed followed by carboplatin and oxaliplatin. All three drugs have similar mechanisms of action. Cisplatin and carboplatin are approved for the treatment of OC; while tumor cell resistance mechanisms to both drugs are similar they differ in their pharmacokinetic and toxicity profiles [8]. Oxaliplatin is highly effective in colorectal cancers because it's mechanism of action (MOA) is not limited to that of the other platinum compounds [8].

Cisplatin, the prototype platinum compound, is taken up into cells by passive diffusion or via the active copper transporter 1 (CTR1) [9]. The subsequent activation of cisplatin is mediated by the displacement of chloride atoms by water to form a highly reactive electrophile that targets nucleophilic sites on DNA and DNA-associated proteins. The N-7 guanine base is most susceptible, although the O-6 guanine, N1, N3 adenine, and N3 cytosine are also targeted. Cisplatin DNA interactions result in the formation of both mono- and bifunctional adducts with the latter forming cis-Pt (NH3)2-d(GpG) at twice the rate of cis-Pt (NH3)2-d(ApG). Interstrand crosslinks are not as common. The bulky adducts between DNA and cisplatin can bend the helix and unwind DNA. The critical importance is the recognition of DNA-cisplatin adducts by proteins that either initiate DNA repair by nucleotide excision repair (NER) or inhibit repair through high mobility group (HMG) proteins. Platinum compounds are cell cycle non-specific (CCNS) causing arrest in S/G2 [9].

Multiple mechanisms are thought to play a role in tumor cell resistance to cisplatin due to the heterogeneity of the disease. Resistance to cisplatin typically confers resistance to carboplatin, but not to oxaliplatin. Some common mechanisms of tumor cell resistance to cisplatin in OC includes increased repair to damaged DNA [10], drug efflux by copper efflux transporters ATP7A [11] and ATP7B [12], reduced uptake by CTR1 [13], and increased expression of glutathione and GSH-S-transferase, which are electron donors forming conjugates with cisplatin and rendering it inactive [10]. Both increased efflux and reduced uptake result in reduced drug accumulation. Overexpression of epidermal growth factor (EGF) and its receptor (EGFR) in cancer cells are critical for growth and survival and EGFR overactivity using autocrine and/or paracrine signals is associated with platinum resistance [14]. The overexpression of the tyrosine kinase; focal adhesion kinase, has also been linked to platinum resistance in OC through several mechanisms including increased expression of the transcription factor OCT4 and the cell surface protein N-cadherin, as well as increased aldehyde dehydrogenase (ALDH) activity [15, 16].

3. Targeted therapies in platinum-resistant ovarian cancer

Although there are many chemotherapeutic agents available, the level of response of platinum-resistant ovarian cancer (OC-Pt) to these drugs is increasingly diminished as the disease progresses [17]. In the past decade, this has fueled a consistent increase in the development of targeted therapies aimed at either supplementing chemotherapeutic regimens or providing novel monotherapy in OC-Pt [17]. Categories of targeted drugs that are undergoing clinical trials or have received FDA approval for OC-Pt include focal adhesion kinase (FAK) inhibitors, poly(adenosine diphosphate [ADP] ribose) polymerase (PARP) inhibitors, anti-angiogenic agents, epidermal growth factor receptor targeting agents, folate receptor antagonists, and insulin growth factor receptor inhibitors.

3.1. PARP inhibitors

PARP inhibitors are a group of targeted drugs that have been at the forefront of emerging OC-Pt therapeutics over the past decade [18, 19]. Human PARPs comprise a total of 17 enzymes [20]. The PARP-1 isoform was the first member of the family to be described and it is the major active PARP enzyme in human cells with the remainder of activity mainly attributed to the PARP-2 isoform [21]. Both PARP-1 and PARP-2 are DNA damage repair enzymes [21]. Human PARP-1 (113 kDa) is a nuclear protein/enzyme which binds with DNA and promotes DNA repair by releasing PARP-1 from DNA and allows recruitment of proteins involved in both base excisional repair (BER) and homologous recombination [22]. Human PARP-2 (62 kDa) is a nuclear protein that binds less efficiently to DNA single-strand breaks but instead recognizes gaps and flap structures [23]. These DNA repair properties of PARPs have made them important anticancer targets in a variety of cancers including OC.

The inhibition of PARP enzymes, especially PARP-1, results in an excess of single-strand breaks, which subsequently causes double-strand breaks to occur as DNA replicates [24]. Under normal circumstances, defects such as double-strand breaks are usually repaired by the homologous recombination process that involves breast cancer type susceptibility (BRCA) proteins. Tumors with defective homologous recombination, including BRCA1/2-mutated OCs, are therefore very sensitive to PARP inhibition [25].

PARP inhibitor drugs are able to cause cancer cell death by inhibiting repair of single-strand breaks and subsequently trapping PARP on DNA, forming cytotoxic PARP-DNA complexes [25]. Several small molecular PARP inhibitor drugs are now undergoing clinical trials and two of them (olaparib and rucaparib) have already been approved by the FDA for use in OC-Pt.

Olaparib (Lynparza), a product of AstraZeneca, received approval from the U.S. Food and Drug Administration (FDA) in December 2014. Olaparib is an inhibitor of several PARP enzymes, including PARP1, PARP2, and PARP3 [26]. The orally administered drug is used for monotherapy in patients with germline BRCA-mutated advanced recurrent OC-Pt [26]. Phase II clinical trials have shown that olaparib significantly improves progression-free survival (PFS) in OC-Pt with similar rates of response reported in patients with BRCA1- and BRCA2-mutated disease [26]. The most common side effects observed with olaparib were mild gastrointestinal irritation, anemia, and severe fatigue.

Rucaparib (Rubraca), a product of Clovis Oncology, was granted accelerated approval from the FDA on December 19, 2016 for the treatment of patients with deleterious BRCA mutation (germline and/or somatic) associated with advanced OC, which had been treated with two or more chemotherapies that included those with OC-Pt. Rucaparib is also a non-specific inhibitor of several PARP enzymes, including PARP1, PARP2, and PARP3 [27]. The ARIEL2 and Study 10 clinical trials produced critical integrated efficacy and safety data in OC-Pt patients which showed that the average response rate was approximately 25% with minimal differences between patients who harbored a BRCA1 mutation, and those who harbored a BRCA2 mutation [27]. Adverse reactions to the drug included fatigue, anemia, dysgeusia, and decreased appetite [27].

A third PARP inhibitor niraparib (Zejula), a product of Tesaro, was approved on March 27, 2017 to maintain treatment of adult patients with recurrent epithelial ovarian and fallopian tube cancer that is completely or partially responsive to platinum-based chemotherapy. Niraparib inhibits both PARP1 and PARP2 and currently has no specific indications in OC-Pt [28].

It is generally accepted that the major categories of cancers that are sensitive to PARP inhibitors are BRCA-mutated cancers. Interestingly, drug resistance to PARP inhibitors have been linked to the development of secondary mutations in the BRCA gene themselves [29]. These secondary mutations can restore functional BRCA1 or BRCA2 genes leading to deleterious consequences in patients with cancer [29]. Other mechanisms of resistance to PARP inhibitors include increased multi drug resistance protein-1 (MDR-1) activity, which leads to increased drug efflux from cancer cells as well as reduced expression of tumor suppressor p53-binding protein 1 (TP53BP1), which is required for non-homologous end-joining DNA repair [30]. Many of these resistance mechanisms are active in OC-Pt [10–16] and therefore can potentially circumvent the therapeutic effects of PARP inhibitors. Nonetheless, PARP inhibitors show much promise in OC-Pt therapeutics.

3.2. Anti-angiogenic therapies

Solid tumors rely on neovascularization for growth and survival in hypoxic environments. The process of angiogenesis is critical for normal ovarian function and for growth, development, and metastasis of OC cells [31]. The hypoxic environment drives angiogenesis in solid tumors which requires continual and persistent growth of new blood vessels [32]. Data strongly suggest a close correlation between increased levels of hypoxia-inducible factor 1-α (HIF 1-α); a transcription factor stabilized during hypoxia and vascular endothelial growth factor (VEGF) in EOC [33]. VEGF is a potent pro-angiogenic growth factor that is upregulated during hypoxia and is elevated in epithelial ovarian neoplasms [33]. VEGF-A is a major pro-angiogenic growth factor that binds to VEGF receptor-1 (VEGFR-1) and VEGF receptor-2 (VEGFR-2), although VEGFR2 is considered the major target. The VEGF-A/VEGFR-2 interaction activates the RAF/MAPK and PI3K/AKT signaling pathways favoring both proliferation and survival of endothelial cells. Intratumoral protein levels of VEGFR-2 were found to be significantly higher in platinum-resistant OC compared to platinum-sensitive OC patient tumors [34]. Many agents targeting angiogenesis have been developed and several have shown some degree of clinical efficacy in OC-Pt. The anti-angiogenic group of drugs include bevacizumab, aflibercept, nintedanib, trebananib, pazopanib, sunitinib, sorafenib, and cediranib.

Bevacizumab (Avastin), a monoclonal antibody that binds to the vascular endothelial growth factor (VEGF)-receptor ligand VEGF-A, is the most extensively investigated anti-angiogenic agent in clinical OC research. Currently, it is the only anti-angiogenic drug that is FDA approved for the treatment of OC as monotherapy or in combination regimens with paclitaxel, topotecan, doxorubicin (pegylated), carboplatin, or gemcitabine for recurrent OC-Pt [35]. Bevacizumab potentiates the cytotoxic effect of chemotherapeutic agents by reducing interstitial fluid pressure and vascular permeability to increase delivery of cytotoxic drugs to cancer cells [35].

A phase II trial of bevacizumab as a single agent in OC-Pt reported that 40.3% of these patients survived progression free for at least 6 months while median PFS and overall survival were 4.7 and 17 months, respectively [36]. Common adverse effects related to bevacizumab were hematologic and gastrointestinal [36].

Subsequent randomized phase III clinical trials focused on the use of bevacizumab with standard chemotherapeutic regimens as first-line treatment in both platinum-sensitive and platinum-resistant OC. AURELIA was the first randomized phase III trial (Study ID#: NCT00976911) to evaluate combined bevacizumab with chemotherapy in OC-Pt [37]. All patients received standard chemotherapy with either paclitaxel or topotecan or liposomal doxorubicin. Patients randomized to arm 2 of the study received bevacizumab (10 mg/kg IV every 2 weeks or 15 mg/kg IV every 3 weeks) concomitantly. The study showed improved PFS and overall response rate with no new safety concerns. The percentage of adverse events associated with chemotherapy + bevacizumab was 57.0% versus 40.3% (chemotherapy alone). Proteinuria and hypertension had the highest incidence rate, whereas gastrointestinal perforations were comparable 2% (bevacizumab) versus 0% (bevacizumab + chemotherapy). Treatment arms that consisted of a higher exposure to chemotherapy in the bevacizumab + chemotherapy combined study group, had a higher incidence rate of hand-foot syndrome and peripheral sensory neuropathy.

The topoisomerase I inhibitor Irinotecan (Camptosar), in combination with bevacizumab was evaluated in recurrent OC in an open-label randomized phase III trial (Study ID#: NCT01091259) [38]. This cohort included 19 patients with OC-Pt. The objective response rate for all patients entered was 27.6% and the clinical benefit rate was 72.4%. Adverse events with the addition of bevacizumab relative to GI toxicity was limited to <3% and considered acceptable [38]. These studies show that it is clinically proven that bevacizumab + chemotherapy demonstrate efficacy in OC-Pt and that safety can be achieved with the right dose and combination of drugs.

Pazopanib (Votrient) is an oral anti-angiogenic multi-targeted tyrosine kinase inhibitor with activity against VEGFR-1, 2, and 3. Pazopanib is currently FDA approved for advanced renal cell carcinoma and soft tissue carcinoma. The PACOVAR study (Study ID#: NCT01238770) evaluated pazopanib in combination with metronomic cyclophosphamide in 16 patients with platinum-resistant EOC [39]. Metronomic chemotherapy is the close, regular administration of chemotherapy drugs at low, minimally toxic doses, with no prolonged break periods. In the PACOVAR study, median PFS and overall survival were 8.35 and 24.95 months, respectively. The most common adverse events were elevation of liver enzymes, leukopenia, diarrhea, and fatigue. Altogether, five serious adverse events developed in four patients. The study concluded that pazopanib + metronomic cyclophosphamide was a feasible regimen for patients with recurrent OC-Pt.

Pazopanib has also shown promising results in mice injected with a highly aggressive cisplatin-resistant SKOV-3 clone of OC cells in combination with metronomic oral topotecan (toperisomerase I inhibitor) [40].

Aflibercept (Ziv-aflibercept/VEGF-trap) mimics the VEGF receptor and has similar ligand binding components to VEGFR-1 and VEGFR-2 [41]. Aflibercept binds to circulating VEGFs and acts like a "VEGF trap" [42]. This primarily results in suppression of VEGF-A and VEGF-B activity and subsequently inhibits the growth of new blood vessels in tumors [42]. Aflibercept was administered at two doses in a randomized, double-blind, phase II trial that assessed response evaluation criteria in solid tumor response rates, as a single agent treatment in recurrent OC-Pt (Study ID#: NCT00327171). The study concluded that the treatment was well tolerated by the patients but the required objective response rate endpoint was not achieved [43]. The participants in this study had received 3–4 prior chemotherapy lines and were resistant to liposomal doxorubicin or topotecan. Hypertension was the most common toxicity observed.

3.3. Focal adhesion kinase (FAK) inhibitors

Focal adhesion kinase (FAK) is a non-receptor cytoplasmic tyrosine kinase that is encoded by the protein tyrosine kinase 2 (PTK2) gene, and is found in most tissues in the human body [44]. PTK2 gene amplification with subsequent increased activation through phosphorylation occurs in many OCs, where it is involved in promoting cancer cell migration, invasion, adhesion, proliferation, and survival [45–47]. High FAK activity is generally associated with worse overall cancer patient survival [48, 49]. Several studies have shown that FAK expression is significantly increased in OC-Pt, and that this platinum resistance is associated with increased tumor-associated aldehyde dehydrogenase (ALDH) activity, as well as overexpression of X-linked inhibitor of apoptosis (XIAP) [16, 50]. We have also demonstrated in our studies that platinum-resistant OC cells are resensitized to cisplatin when co-treated with a FAK inhibitor [15].

Several FAK inhibitors have been developed to prevent FAK activation by blocking its phosphorylation sites; which halts its downstream signaling pathways with subsequent reduction in ovarian tumorigenesis and cancer progression. A few of these drugs are now in clinical trials. The FAK inhibitor defactinib from Verastem was evaluated in a phase I study (Study ID#: NCT00787033) which found that OC-Pt patients achieved a prolonged PFS [51]. Defactinib produced grade 1–2 adverse events that were easily managed and reversible, even with continued dosing [51]. A phase I/Ib, open-label (Study ID#: NCT01778803) multi-center, dose-escalation trial of paclitaxel in combination with defactinib was subsequently initiated in OC-Pt patients with advanced cancers [52]. The combination was found to be efficacious with no apparent increase in the severity and incidence of paclitaxel-related toxicities.

A phase I/Ib, open-label, multi-center, dose-escalation, and dose expansion trial (Study ID#: NCT02943317) to evaluate the safety, efficacy, pharmacokinetics, and pharmacodynamics of defactinib in combination with the human monoclonal PD-L1 antibody avelumab in recurrent or refractory stage III–IV OC is currently ongoing, and is expected to enroll approximately 100 patients at up to 15 sites across the United States. The FAK inhibitor GSK2256098 was also evaluated in a phase I clinical trial (Study ID#: NCT01138033) in patients with advanced solid tumors including OC-Pt [53]. GSK2256098 significantly reduced FAK activity in tumors of patients that received the drug at a dose of 750 mg twice daily.

FAK inhibition is still an emerging area in OC-Pt therapeutics and many clinical trials are underway that will provide more insight into their efficacy in different histological types of OC.

3.4. Folate receptor antagonists

Folate receptors (FRs) are proteins that bind folate with high affinity. The FR-α and FR-β isoforms are well characterized as membrane-bound receptors that facilitate the binding and subsequent internalization of folate compounds and their chemical derivatives [54]. The FR-α receptor is significantly overexpressed in EOC where it promotes tumor growth by either an aberrant folate uptake mechanism or dysregulated signaling pathways [55]. The FR-α receptor can also induce platinum resistance by regulating the expression of apoptosis-related molecules; Bcl-2 and Bax and a higher expression of FR-α level has been linked to poor prognosis in OC patients [56]. These properties of the FR-α receptor makes it a prime therapeutic target for OC. In recent years, two drugs (vintafolide and farletuzumab) have gained relevance as FR-α receptor antagonist applicable in OC-Pt. Farletuzumab (MORAb-003), a monoclonal antibody to FR-α was evaluated in a phase III trial (Study ID#: NCT00738699) in combination with paclitaxel for advanced OC-Pt patients [57]. The drug was developed by Morphotek and the study was unfortunately discontinued because of minimal changes in PFS and the occurrence of serious adverse events including neutropenia and atrial fibrillation [57].

Vintafolide (originally known as EC145), is a water-soluble derivative of folic acid that is conjugated to the vinca alkaloid 'desacetylvinblastine hydrazide' [58]. The combination of vintafolide with pegylated liposomal doxorubicin (PLD) produced a statistically significant increase in PFS for OC-Pt patients [59]. This result was the outcome of the PRECEDENT trial; a randomized phase II study, that compared the combination of vintafolide + PLD with PLD alone [59]. Patients with FR positive cancer showed improved PFS compared to no PFS benefits in FR negative patients. After this successful phase II trial, a phase III trial called the PROCEED study was initiated (Study ID#: NCT01170650) to further evaluate the efficacy and safety of the vintafolide + PLD (Doxil) combination in OC-Pt patients. The main goal of the study is to determine PFS using version 1.1 of the response evaluation criteria in solid tumor (RECIST), and etarfolatide imaging to determine patients FR status [55]. Etarfolatide is a non-invasive, folate receptor-targeting companion imaging agent, which consists of a small molecule targeting the folate receptor and an imaging agent, which is based on technetium-99 m [55].

The targeting of the FR receptor appears to be promising strategy for OC-Pt cancer subsets that significantly overexpress these receptors. New folate conjugates are in development and this area of therapeutics is expected to consistently improve.

3.5. Insulin-like growth factor receptor inhibitors

The insulin-like growth factor (IGF) system consists of IGF-I, IGF-II, their target receptors (IGF-IR, IGF-IIR, insulin receptor (IR), and the insulin-related receptor (IRR)) as well as a family of six different IGF-binding proteins (IGFBPs) [60]. Upon binding of IGFs to IGF-1R and IR (but not IRR and IGF-2R), many signaling pathways can be activated. These downstream signaling mechanisms include the Ras-Raf-MAPK and PI3K-Akt transduction pathways. These transduction mechanisms result in stimulation of cell proliferation, motility, and inhibition of apoptosis [60]. All IGF-signaling system components are expressed in OC and likewise stimulate cell proliferation, invasive, and angiogenic activity of OC cells [61]. More importantly, IGF-1R/IR inhibition in platinum-resistant ovarian cancer cells resensitizes them to the cytotoxic effects of cisplatin; indicating a role of the IGF system in OC-Pt [62]. This highlights a therapeutic opportunity for insulin and insulin-like growth factor receptor inhibition.

In the past few years, a number of inhibitors targeting the IGFR/IR have been developed, including antibodies against the receptors and small molecule receptor kinase inhibitors [63]. A trial (Study ID#: NCT01708161) with ganitumab (developed by Amgen), a human mono-clonal antibody against IGF-IR, has been completed in patients with solid tumors including OC-Pts. This was a multi-center, open-label, phase Ib/II study. The aim of the phase Ib arm, was to estimate the median toxic doses and/or identify the recommended phase II dose(s) for the combination of BYL719 (a PI3K inhibitor) and ganitumab [64]. The phase II arm assessed the clinical efficacy and safety of the combination in OC patient populations including PIK3CA-mutated or -amplified OCs [64]. Data from this study are yet to be released, but will provide insight on the effect of ganitumab in OC-Pt.

A phase I/II trial (Study ID#: NCT00889382) with the small molecule, dual IGF-1R/IR tyro-sine kinase inhibitor linsitinib (OSI-906) has also been completed [65]. The study evaluated intermittent and continuous linsitinib dosing and weekly paclitaxel in patients with recurrent EOCs including OC-Pts as well as other solid cancer types (endometrial and primary perito-neal) [65]. Of the 58 patients treated in the study, 3 OC patients showed a partial response, and stable disease was achieved in 10 OC patients. Pharmacokinetic studies showed no significant interactions when linsitinib was administered 2 h prior to paclitaxel. The most common drug-related toxicities were fatigue, nausea, hyperglycemia and drug eruption. Other details of the study outcomes related to PFS have not yet been published.

Many compounds are constantly being screened for IGF-IR inhibitory activity, but the simi-larity between the IGF-IR and the IR receptor presents a challenge for developing selective inhibitors for the IGF-IR. The main concern with this lack of selectivity is that dual inhibitors of IR and IGF-IR, has resulted in hyperglycemia in many clinical trials. This is a major hurdle to overcome in this area of OC therapeutics.

3.6. Epidermal growth factor receptor/human epidermal growth factor receptor family

The epidermal growth factor receptor (EGFR) is a member of the tyrosine kinase family of growth factor receptors. These receptors play a direct role in regulating cell proliferation, apoptosis, survival, cell differentiation, and migration [14]. The ERbB family of receptor tyrosine kinases includes EGFR (also known as HER1/ErbB1), EGFR2 (HER2/neu/ERbB2), HER3/ErbB3, and HER4/ErbB4 [66]. Dysregulation of the EGFR function has been linked to the pathology of OC [14] but evidence is conflicting; as other studies have not found strong evidence of a direct link between EGFR expression and function and OC progres-sion. Many factors have been suggested for the mixed results; these include variability in experimental methods, detection procedures, and scoring metrics. Despite the variable study outcomes in OC, evidence supports dysregulated EGFR ligand and receptor expression, heterologous regulation by GPCR ligands, and other non-ligand stimuli initiating chronic activation of EGFRs [14]. This chronic stimulation favors tumor development and progression [14].

The current therapeutic strategy is to inhibit EGFR activity using small molecule tyrosine kinase inhibitors or monoclonal antibodies [67]. Clinical trials have been conducted using the following agents alone and in combination: cetuximab, gefitinib, erlotinib, trastuzumab, and pertuzumab. These treatment regimens were evaluated in patients with recurrent or progressive disease, platinum-sensitive disease, and platinum-resistant/refractory disease among others [67].

Of note, the PENELOPE phase III trial investigated the efficacy of pertuzumab in combination with chemotherapy (single-agent topotecan, weekly paclitaxel, or gemcitabine) for treatment of platinum-resistant patients with downregulated human epidermal growth factor 3 (HER3) mRNA expression [68]. The results showed no significant improvement in PFS for the primary analysis (stratified hazard ratio, 0.74; 95% CI, 0.50–1.11; $P = 0.14$; median PFS, 4.3 months for pertuzumab plus chemotherapy versus 2.6 months for placebo plus chemotherapy). The study concluded that pertuzumab has the potential to be investigated further despite the lack of significance. To date, clinical trials evaluating anti-EGFR and HER therapies have shown minimal improvement in OC-Pt treatment outcome. Further studies evaluating inhibitors of downstream signaling and simultaneous antagonism of the EGFR and HER have been recommended [66].

4. Immunotherapy and advances in immunotherapeutic combination strategies in ovarian cancer

Current chemotherapeutic regimens for OC-Pt patients whether monotherapy or combinatorial are inadequate. Immunotherapeutic approaches are now being increasingly explored for these patients where a therapeutic ceiling has been reached with standard chemotherapy. Immunotherapy in OC-Pt patients is just emerging and is currently restricted to clinical trials that have shown promising results. The American Cancer Society defines cancer immunotherapy as 'treatment that uses your body's own immune system to help fight cancer'. Within the tumor microenvironment, the pathological interactions between cancer cells and immune cells is complex and most events spiral into an immunosuppression that causes tumor cells to proliferate and evade immune system attack [69]. There are several categories of immunotherapeutic agents that either stimulate the body's immune system's ability to eradicate cancer cells (e.g. cancer vaccines and adoptive T cell transfer), target proteins on the surface of T cells that prevent them from attacking cancer cells (e.g. immune checkpoint inhibitors), or identify specific abnormalities on the surface of cancer cells that render them susceptible to targeted agents (e.g. monoclonal antibodies) [69]. Many of these drugs are being evaluated in OC-Pt patients and are discussed below.

4.1. Immune checkpoint inhibitors

Checkpoint proteins are molecules found on the surface of T cells that prevent them from attacking cancer cells [70]. Two such proteins are cytotoxic T lymphocyte antigen-4 (CTLA-4) and programmed death-1 (PD-1) [71]. PD-1 is expressed on the surface of activated T cells and its ligands, PD-L1 and PD-L2 are found on the surface of dendritic cells or macrophages [70]. Interaction of PD-1 with either PD-L1 or PD-L2 results in inhibition of T cell signaling, reduction in T cell numbers, and increased susceptibility of T cells to apoptosis [71]. CTLA-4 regulates T cell priming and activation in the initiation phase of the immune response [71]. The high expression of PD-L1 and PD-L2 on OC cells is associated with shorter PFS [72]. Similarly, evidence suggests that OC patients with low CTLA-4-mediated signals have a better prognosis than patients with high CTLA-4 activity [73].

4.1.1. Anti-PD-1/PD-L1 antibodies

Several antibodies directed against PD-1 (pembrolizumab, nivolumab, and avelumab), PD-L1 (atezolizumab and durvalumab), and CTLA-4 (ipilimumab) have been evaluated in OC. Nivolumab (Opdivo) is a fully humanized IgG4 antibody that blocks the engagement of PD-1-by-PD-1 ligands [74]. Nivolumab was administered every 2 weeks to patients with advanced or relapsed OC-Pt and response rate was assessed by RECIST [74]. The study included 15 OC-Pt patients and the drug showed encouraging clinical efficacy. Some adverse drug reactions including fever, disorientation, and gait disturbance were observed. A dose escalation study (Study ID#: UMIN000005714) is now under way as a second arm of this trial.

Avelumab (Bavencio) is a fully human monoclonal antibody of isotype IgG1 that targets PD-L1. It was evaluated in a phase Ib (Study ID#: NCT01772004) expansion study in 75 patients with recurrent/refractory OC which included OC-Pt [75]. Of this cohort, 8 patients showed a partial response and 33 patients displayed stable disease, which was reported as a disease control rate of 54.7%.

One other phase Ib study (KEYNOTE-028/Study ID#: NCT02054806) evaluated the anti-tumor activity and safety of pembrolizumab (Keytruda) in patients with PD-L1 positive advanced OC which included patients refractory to platinum therapy [76]. Pembrolizumab is a humanized antibody that binds to and blocks PD-1. PD-1 blockade with pembrolizumab was well tolerated and displayed anti-tumor activity. Of the 26 patients enrolled in the study, 1 achieved complete response, 2 partial response, and 6 had stable disease. The most common adverse events were fatigue (42.3%), anemia (30.8%), and decreased appetite (30.8%).

The role of the PD-1/PD-L1 axis is continuously been studied and characterized in OC and with new information on OC-Pt immunogenicity emerging consistently, this disease is expected to remain a focused target of PD-1/PD-L1 based therapeutics.

4.1.2. Anti-CTLA4 antibodies

Inhibition of CTLA-4 during the T cell priming/activation step leads to dysregulated expansion of auto-reactive T cells, including tumor-specific T cells [73]. The anti-CTLA 4 monoclonal antibody ipilimumab (Yervoy) has shown anti-tumor effect in stage IV OC. Ipilimumab is a recombinant human monoclonal antibody (IgG1 kappa immunoglobin) that antagonizes the CTLA-4 immune checkpoint. The administration of ipilimumab to 11 stage IV OC patients previously vaccinated with granulocyte-macrophage colony-stimulating factor (GM-CSF)-modified irradiated autologous tumor cells showed promising results [77]. Ipilimumab caused a reduction or stabilization of CA-125 levels in these patients and no serious toxicities directly attributable to the antibody were observed.

Tremelimumab is a fully human IgG2 monoclonal antibody to CTLA-4. The combination of tremelimumab with the immunotherapeutic agent durvalumab is currently undergoing a phase I trial (Study ID#: NCT01975831) which includes OC-Pt patients [78]. The primary endpoints of this study are to evaluate safety and identify the maximum tolerated dose of the combination. The secondary objectives are to determine effects on tumor response and PFS. Preliminary data show that the combination has a manageable safety profile, with evidence of clinical activity. Trials with anti-CTLA-4 inhibitors in other cancer types have been associated with significant immune-related toxicities [79], and this might be the major limitation in terms of advancing their application in OC-Pt. More clinical trials are needed in this area of OC-Pt therapeutics.

4.2. Cancer vaccines

The aim of vaccinations in cancer patients is to sensitize the immune system to recognize, target, and eradicate tumor cells in an approach that employs both adaptive and innate immunity [80]. Vaccines aim to provoke a tumor-specific immune response by increasing tumor-associated antigen (TAA) presentation by antigen-presenting cells (APCs) which subsequently generates tumor-antigen specific cytotoxic T lymphocytes [80].

Dendritic cell, peptide, and recombinant viral vaccines are the main types currently undergoing clinical trials for OC. One promising TAA for dendritic cell vaccines is mucin 1 (MUC-1). MUC-1 is a heavily glycosylated, type 1 transmembrane protein that is overexpressed in a large number of cancers including OCs [81]. While multiple MUC-1 vaccines are now in development, CVac (developed by Prima BioMed) is the leading candidate for OC. In the CAN-003 phase II study, 63 confirmed Stage III or IV OC patients received CVac [82]. While the study cohort did not disclose if the patient cohort included OC-Pts, CVac demonstrated positive trends in progression free survival and immune responses and further studies in OC-Pt patients are warranted.

A dendritic cell vaccine pulsed with autologous hypochlorous acid-oxidized OC lysate was also evaluated in a pilot study (Study ID#: NCT01132014) of five subjects with recurrent OC [83]. Of the five patients who received the DC vaccine, two had PFS of 24 months or more.

Peptide vaccines rely primarily on the immunogenicity of the injected peptides to stimulate an immune response. In the cancer setting, the peptides chosen for the vaccine are TAAs.

A phase I trial of the NY-ESO-1 OLP vaccine showed promising results in advanced OC patients that initially received chemotherapy with at least one platinum-based chemotherapy regimen [84]. NY-ESO-1 OLP contains synthetic overlapping long peptides (OLP) from the cancer-testis antigen NY-ESO-1 [84]. The vaccine was found to be safe and rapidly induced consistent integrated immune responses in nearly all vaccinated patients. A phase I/IIb multi-center study was also conducted to evaluate the safety and immunogenicity of the anti-idio-typic antibody vaccine ACA125 in 119 patients with advanced ovarian carcinoma (including OC-Pt patients) [85]. ACA125 functionally imitates the tumor antigen CA125. Preliminary evidence demonstrated safety and immunogenicity of the vaccine. The study data has not reveal conclusions regarding OC-Pt subgroups and this requires further evaluation.

Recombinant viral vaccines utilize genetically modified viruses as vectors for introducing TAA-encoding DNA into cells within the body. PANVAC is a vaccine with payload delivered through two viral vectors: recombinant vaccinia and recombinant fowlpox [86]. The vectors contain transgenes for the tumor-associated antigens epithelial mucin 1 (MUC-1) and carci-noembryonic antigen (CEA). Overexpression of MUC-1 and CEA is seen in OC [87, 88]. In a pilot study of PANVAC in 14 OC patients (including OC-Pt), median time to progression was 2 months and median OS was 15.0 months [86].

4.3. Adoptive cell therapy

Adoptive cell therapy (ACT) involves the infusion of tumor antigen cells to stimulate innate anti-tumor immunity and induce cancer regression [89]. A pilot study in which seven patients with recurrent local OC were given multiple cycles of intraperitoneal infusions of autologous MUC1 peptide-stimulated cytotoxic T lymphocytes has been completed [90]. Clinical benefit was seen in only one patient who was disease free >12 years. While it is difficult to interpret this information in the context of OC-Pt, the study is worth mentioning as at least one patient had received prior platinum therapy.

A phase I clinical trial of adoptive transfer of folate receptor-alpha-redirected autologous T cells for recurrent OC cancer was initiated to establish the safety and proof of concept of autologous FRα-redirected T cells administered intravenously, in subjects with recurrent stage II to IV FRα-positive epithelial ovarian carcinoma (including OC-Pt subgroups) [91]. It is also possible that ACT can be used in combination strategies but the challenge with solid tumors such as OCs; is that tumor microenvironment immunity can cause immunosuppres-sion and render ACT ineffective.

4.4. Toll-like receptors agonists (TLRs)

Toll-like receptors (TLRs) comprise a family of 13 receptors found on hematopoietic and non-hematopoietic cells [92]. The TLR8 subtype is mainly found in monocytes and dendritic cells and it plays an important role in the immune response by recognizing single-stranded RNAs as its natural ligand. Motolimod (Motolid/formerly known as VTX2337) is a synthetic, small molecule, selective agonist of TLR8 that stimulates natural killer cell activity and enhances antibody-dependent cellular cytotoxicity [92]. A phase II randomized, double-blind, placebo-controlled study (Study ID#: NCT01294293), evaluated chemo-immunotherapy combination using motolimod with PLD in recurrent or persistent OC [92]. While the addition of moto-limod to PLD did not significantly improve overall survival or PFS, the combination was well tolerated, with no synergistic or unexpected serious toxicity. Another phase II study is also now underway (Study ID#: NCT01666444) in patients with recurrent or persistent epi-thelial ovarian, fallopian tube, or primary peritoneal cancer. The purpose of this study is to compare the overall survival of patients treated with motolimod + PLD versus those treated with PLD alone in women with recurrent or persistent, epithelial ovarian, fallopian tube, or primary peritoneal cancer. This study will provide further insight on the future of motolimod in OC-Pt.

5. Combination strategies with immunotherapy

Over the past decade we have learned that OC in general responds poorly (11–25% over-all) to single-agent immunotherapy; especially checkpoint blocking strategies [93]. There is very limited data regarding response rates of OC-Pt subgroups specifically, but in most cases these cohorts of patients are integrated in general OC study data, suggesting similar patterns of response. When reviewed collectively, the data suggest that efficient anti-tumor immune response is likely to require combinatorial therapeutic strategies that simultaneously target different stages of tumor escape. Combinations involving immune checkpoint inhibi-tors, anti-angiogenic agents, and PARP inhibitors are gaining momentum in clinical OC-Pt research and are highlighted below.

5.1. Checkpoint inhibitor + PARP inhibitor

Currently, several trials combining PARP and immune checkpoint inhibitors are ongoing [94]. An open-label dose escalation study (Study ID#: NCT02485990) of tremelimumab alone or combined with olaparib for recurrent or persistent OC is currently recruiting participants. This study is aimed at determining what dose of tremelimumab and olaparib is safe and effec-tive in patients with persistent OC including those with OC-Pt.

A phase I/II Study (Study ID#: NCT02484404) of durvalumab in combination with olaparib and/or cediranib for advanced solid tumors including OC-Pt is currently recruiting. The aim of the phase I arm is to determine the safety of the combination of durvalumab with olaparib or cediranib. Phase II studies will determine the efficacy of these combination in treating OC.

The TOPACIO trial (Study ID#: NCT02657889) will evaluate niraparib in combination with pembrolizumab in patients with triple-negative breast cancer or OC-Pt. The primary outcome measures are to determine dose-limiting toxicities of combination treatment with niraparib and pembrolizumab and to determine the objective response rate using RECISTv1.1.

5.2. PARP inhibitor + anti-angiogenic agent

The OCTOVA study (Study ID#: NCT03117933), is currently recruiting participants for a randomized phase II trial investigating the efficacy of chemotherapy plus olaparib and cediranib combination therapy in patients with BRCA-mutated OC-Pt. Patients will be randomized to one of three treatment groups: olaparib only, olaparib and cediranib, and the control group paclitaxel. The aim is to compare efficacy and tolerability of the three treatments.

5.3. Checkpoint inhibitor + anti-angiogenic agent

A phase II study (Study ID#: NCT02659384) to evaluate the combination of atezolizumab plus bevacizumab and acetylsalicylic acid in recurrent OC-Pt is currently recruiting. The primary aim is to determine PFS at 6 months by RECIST.

5.4. Checkpoint inhibitors + cancer vaccine

The administration of ipilimumab in 11 patients with metastatic ovarian carcinoma after vaccination with irradiated autologous tumor cells engineered to secrete GM-CSF (GVAX), showed promising results [95]. Three patients achieved stable disease as measured by CA-125 levels, and one patient achieved an objective response by radiographic criteria and maintained disease control over 4 years with regular infusions of anti-CTLA-4 antibody.

6. Challenges and future perspectives

There are still many hurdles to overcome in the treatment of OC-Pt but some progress has been made in recent years, especially with the development of new immunotherapeutic agents. The good news is that OC cancer is a targetable tumor and although the OC-Pt subgroup of patients have biologically distinct tumors, both targeted therapies and immunotherapy offer an opportunity to uniquely address these differences. As new agents are developed in these categories, the main challenge with existing and future clinical trials will be the risk of adverse events and toxicities, especially with combination immunotherapeutic regimens, where there is an elevated risk for adverse immune events. A second challenge is the optimization of the dose and schedule of immunotherapeutic combinations in order to maximize the overall risk-benefit profile of a given combination. This requires multiple clinical trials with dose escalation studies that can be expensive. This approach is necessary however, especially in the setting of platinum-resistant OC cancer where much research is still needed.

Author details

Arkene Levy* and Patricia C. Rose

*Address all correspondence to: alevy1@nova.edu

Nova Southeastern University, Florida, USA

References

[1] Siegel RL, Miller KD, Jemal A. Cancer statistics, 2017. CA: A Cancer Journal for Clinicians. 2017;**67**(1):7-30. DOI: 10.3322/caac.21387

[2] Prat J. New insights into ovarian cancer pathology. Annals of Oncology. 2012;**23**(suppl 10): x111-x117. DOI: 10.1093/annonc/mds300

[3] Cannistra SA. Cancer of the ovary. The New England Journal of Medicine. 2004;**351**:2519-2529. DOI: 10.1056/NEJMra041842

[4] Pfisterer J, Ledermann JA. Management of platinum-sensitive recurrent ovarian cancer. Seminars in Oncology. 2006;**33**(suppl 6):12-16. DOI: https://doi.org/10.1053/j.seminoncol.2006.03.012

[5] Cannistra SA. Is there a "best" choice of second-line agent in the treatment of recurrent, potentially platinum-sensitive ovarian cancer? Journal of Clinical Oncology. 2002;**20**:1158-1160. DOI: 10.1200/JCO.2002.20.5.1158

[6] Karabulut B, Sezgin C, Terek M, et al. Topotecan in platinum-resistant epithelial ovarian cancer. Chemotherapy. 2005;**51**:347-351. DOI: 10.1159/000088959

[7] Rosenberg B. Noble metal complexes in cancer chemotherapy. Advances in Experimental Medicine and Biology. 1977;**91**:129-150

[8] Johnstone TC, Suntharalingam K, Lippard SJ. The next generation of platinum drugs: Targeted Pt(II) agents, nanoparticle delivery, and Pt(IV) prodrugs. Chemical Review. 2016;**116**(5):3436-3486. DOI: 10.1021/acs.chemrev.5b00597

[9] Johnstone TC, Park GY, Lippard SJ. Understanding and improving platinum anticancer drugs—Phenanthriplatin. Anticancer Research. 2014;**34**(1):471-476

[10] Kartalou M, Essigmann J. Mechanisms of resistance to cisplatin. Mutation Research. 2001;**478**(1-2):23-43. DOI: https://doi.org/10.1016/S0027-5107(01)00141-5

[11] Samimi G, Varki NM, Wilczynski S, Safaei R, Alberts DS, Howell SB. Increase in expression of the copper transporter ATP7A during platinum drug-based treatment is associated with poor survival in ovarian cancer patients. Clinical Cancer Research. 2003; **9**(16 Pt 1):5853-5859

[12] Komatsu M, Sumizawa T, Mutoh M, Chen ZS, Terada K, Furukawa T, Yang XL, Gao H, Miura N, Sugiyama T, Akiyama S. Copper-transporting P-type adenosine triphosphatase (ATP7B) is associated with cisplatin resistance. Cancer Research. 2000;**60**(5):1312-1316

[13] Song I, Savaraj N, Siddik Z, Liu P, Wei Y, Wu C, Kuo M. Role of human copper transporter Ctr1 in the transport of platinum-based antitumor agents in cisplatin-sensitive and cisplatin-resistant cells. Molecular Cancer Therapeutics. 2004;**3**(12):1543-1549

[14] Hudson LG, Zeineldin R, Silberberg M, Stack MS. Activated epidermal growth factor receptor in ovarian cancer. Cancer Treatment and Research. 2009;**149**:203-226. DOI: 10.1007/978-0-387-98094-2_10

[15] Reboe M, Levy A, Dhandyuthapani S, Rathinavelu A. Y15 enhances the cytotoxic profile of cisplatin, paclitaxel and vitamin E in platinum resistant ovarian cancer cells. The Faseb Journal. 2015;**29**:785.1

[16] Bean LM, Sulzmaier FJ, Tancioni I, Uryu S, Jean C, Chen XL, Kleinschmidt EG, Anderson KM, Cordasco EA, Axelrod J, et al. FAK inhibition re-sensitizes platinum-resistant serous ovarian cancer. American Journal of Cancer Research. 2016;**76**(14):3812. DOI: 10.1158/1538-7445.AM2016-3812

[17] Vaughan S, Coward JI, Bast RC Jr, et al. Rethinking ovarian cancer: Recommendations for improving outcomes. Nature Reviews. Cancer. 2011;**11**(10):719-725. DOI: 10.1038/nrc3144

[18] Farmer H, McCabe N, Lord CJ, et al. Targeting the DNA repair defect in BRCA mutant cells as a therapeutic strategy. Nature. 2005;**434**(7035):917-921. DOI: 10.1038/nature03445

[19] Bryant HE, Schultz N, Thomas HD, et al. Specific killing of BRCA2-deficient tumours with inhibitors of poly(ADP-ribose) polymerase. Nature. 2005;**434**(7035):913-917. DOI: 10.1038/nature03443

[20] Krishnakumar R, Kraus WL. The PARP side of the nucleus: Molecular actions, physiological outcomes, and clinical targets. Molecular Cell. 2010;**39**:8-24. DOI: 10.1016/j.molcel.2010.06.017

[21] Virág L, Szabó C. The therapeutic potential of poly(ADP-ribose) polymerase inhibitors. Pharmacological Reviews. 2002;**54**(3):375-429

[22] Houtgraaf JH, Versmissen J, van der Giessen WJ. A concise review of DNA damage checkpoints and repair in mammalian cells. Cardiovascular Revascularization Medicine. 2006;**7**(3):165-172. DOI: 10.1016/j.carrev.2006.02.002

[23] Berghammer H, Ebner M, Marksteiner R, Auer B. pADPRT-2: A novel mammalian polymerizing (ADP-ribosyl) transferase gene related to truncated pADPRT homologues in plants and *Caenorhabditis elegans*. FEBS Letters. 1999;**449**:259-263

[24] Coward JI, Middleton K, Murphy F. New perspectives on targeted therapy in ovarian cancer. International Journal of Women's Health. 2015;7:189-203. DOI: http://doi.org/10.2147/IJWH.S52379

[25] Murai J, Huang SY, Das BB, et al. Trapping of PARP1 and PARP2 by clinical PARP inhibitors. Cancer Research. 2012;72(21):5588-5599. DOI: 10.1158/0008-5472.CAN-12-2753

[26] Munroe M, Kolesar J. Olaparib for the treatment of BRCA-mutated advanced ovarian cancer. American Journal of Health-System Pharmacy. 2016;73(14):1037-1041. DOI: 10.2146/ajhp150550

[27] Oza AM, Tinker AV, Oaknin A, Shapira-Frommer R, McNeish IA, Swisher EM, Ray-Coquard I, Bell-McGuinn K, et al. Antitumor activity and safety of the PARP inhibitor rucaparib in patients with high-grade ovarian carcinoma and a germline or somatic BRCA1 or BRCA2 mutation: Integrated analysis of data from Study 10 and ARIEL2. Gynecologic Oncology. 2017; pii: S0090-8258(17)31260-X. DOI: 10.1016/j.ygyno.2017.08.022

[28] Sandhu SK, Schelman WR, Wilding G, et al. The poly(ADP-ribose) polymerase inhibitor niraparib (MK4827) in BRCA mutation carriers and patients with sporadic cancer: A phase 1 dose-escalation trial. The Lancet Oncology. 2013;14(9):882-892. DOI: 10.1016/S1470-2045(13)70240-7

[29] Issaeva N et al. 6-thioguanine selectively kills BRCA2-defective tumors and overcomes PARP inhibitor resistance. Cancer Research. 2010;70:6268-6276. DOI: 10.1158/0008-5472.CAN-09-3416

[30] Lord CJ, Ashworth A. Mechanisms of resistance to therapies targeting BRCA-mutant cancers. Nature Medicine. 2013;19(11):1381-1388. DOI: 10.1038/nm.3369

[31] Spannuth WA, Nick AM, Jennings NB, Armaiz-Pena GN, Mangala LS, Danes CG, Lin YG, Merritt WM, Thaker PH, Kamat AA, Han LY, Tonra JR, Coleman RL, Ellis LM, Sood AK. Functional significance of VEGFR-2 on ovarian cancer cells. International Journal of Cancer. 2009;124(5):1045-1053. DOI: 10.1002/ijc.24028

[32] Shweiki D, Itin A, Soffer D, Keshet E. Vascular endothelial growth factor induced by hypoxia may mediate hypoxia initiated angiogenesis. Nature. 1992;359:843-845. DOI: 10.1038/359843a0

[33] Wong C, Wellman TL, Lounsbury KM. VEGF and HIF-1 alpha expression are increased in advanced stages of epithelial ovarian cancer. Gynecologic Oncology. 2003;91:513-517

[34] Avril S et al. Increased PDGFR-beta and VEGFR-2 protein levels are associated with resistance to platinum-based chemotherapy and adverse outcome of ovarian cancer patients. Oncotarget. 2017. Available from: https://doi.org/10.18632/oncotarget.18415 [Accessed: September 12, 2017]

[35] Chase DM, Chaplin DJ, Monk BJ. The development and use of vascular targeted therapy in ovarian cancer. Gynecologic Oncology 2017;145:393-406. DOI: http://dx.doi.org/10.1016/j.ygyno.2017.01.031

[36] Burger RA, Sill MW, Monk BJ, Greer BE, Sorosky JI. Phase II trial of bevacizumab in persistent or recurrent epithelial ovarian cancer or primary peritoneal cancer: A gynecologic oncology group study. Journal of Clinical Oncology. 2007;**25**(33):5165-5171. DOI: 10.1200/JCO.2007.11.5345

[37] Pujade-Lauraine E et al. Bevacizumab combined with chemotherapy for platinum-resistant recurrent ovarian cancer: The AURELIA open-label randomized phase III trial. Journal of Clinical Oncology. 2014;**32**:1302-1308. DOI: 10.1200/JCO.2013.51.4489

[38] Musa F, et al. Phase II study of irinotecan in combination with bevacizumab in recurrent ovarian cancer. Gynecologic Oncology 2017;**144**(2):279-284. DOI: http://dx.doi.org/10.1016/j.ygyno.2016.11.043

[39] Dinkic C et al. Pazopanib (GW786034) and cyclophosphamide in patients with platinum-resistant, recurrent, pre-treated ovarian cancer—Results of the PACOVAR-trial. Gynecologic Oncology. 2017;**146**(2):279-284. DOI: 10.1016/j.ygyno.2017.05.013

[40] Hashimoto K, Man S, Xu P, Cruz-Munoz W, Tang T, Kumar R, Kerbel RS. Potent preclinical impact of metronomic low-dose oral topotecan combined with the antiangiogenic drug pazopanib for the treatment of ovarian cancer. Molecular Cancer Therapeutics. 2010;**9**(4):996-1006. DOI: 10.1158/1535-7163.MCT-09-0960

[41] Kumaran GC, Jayson GC, Clamp AR. Antiangiogenic drugs in ovarian cancer. British Journal of Cancer. 2009;**100**(1):1-7. DOI: 10.1038/sj.bjc.6604767

[42] Fraser HM, Wilson H, Rudge JS, Wiegand SJ. Single injections of vascular endothelial growth factor trap block ovulation in the macaque and produce a prolonged, dose-related suppression of ovarian function. The Journal of Clinical Endocrinology and Metabolism. 2005;**90**:1114-1122. DOI: 10.1210/jc.2004-1572

[43] Tew WP, Colombo N, Ray-Coquard I, del Campo JM, Oza A, Pereira D, Mammoliti S, et al. Intravenous aflibercept in patients with platinum-resistant, advanced ovarian cancer: Results of a randomized, double-blind, phase II, parallel-arm study. Cancer. 2014;**120**:335-343. DOI: 10.1002/cncr.28406

[44] Schaller MD, Borgman CA, Cobb BS, Vines RR, Reynolds AB, Parsons JT. pp125FAK a structurally distinctive protein-tyrosine kinase associated with focal adhesions. Proceedings of the National Academy of Sciences of the United States of America. 1992;**89**:5192-5196

[45] Hungerford JE, Compton MT, Matter ML, Hoffstrom BG, Otey CA. Inhibition of pp125FAK in cultured fibroblasts results in apoptosis. The Journal of Cell Biology. 1996;**135**:1383-1390

[46] Frisch SM, Vuori K, Ruoslahti E, Chan-Hui PY. Control of adhesion-dependent cell survival by focal adhesion kinase. The Journal of Cell Biology. 1996;**134**:793-799

[47] Sood AK, Coffin JE, Schneider GB, Fletcher MS, DeYoung BR, Gruman LM, Gershenson DM, Schaller MD, Hendrix MJC. Biological significance of focal adhesion kinase in ovarian

cancer: Role in migration and invasion. American Journal of Pathology. 2004;**165**:1087-1095. DOI: 10.1016/S0002-9440(10)63370-6

[48] Bonome T, Lee JY, Park DC, et al. Expression profiling of serous low malignant potential, low-grade, and high-grade tumors of the ovary. Cancer Research. 2005;**65**:10602-10612. DOI: 10.1158/0008-5472.CAN-05-2240

[49] Ward KK, Tancioni I, Lawson C, Miller NLG, Jean C, Chen XL, et al. Inhibition of focal adhesion kinase (FAK) activity prevents anchorage-independent ovarian carcinoma cell growth and tumor progression. Clinical & Experimental Metastasis. 2013;**30**(5):579-594. DOI: http://doi.org/10.1007/s10585-012-9562-5

[50] Fraser M, Leung B, Jahani-Asl A, Yan X, Thompson WE, Tsang BK. Chemoresistance in human ovarian cancer: The role of apoptotic regulators. Reproductive Biology and Endocrinology. 2003;**1**:66. DOI: 10.1186/1477-7827-1-66

[51] Jones SF, Siu LL, Bendell JC, et al. Investigational New Drugs. 2015;**33**:1100. DOI: 10.1007/s10637-015-0282-y

[52] Patel MR, Infante JR, Moore KN, Keegan M, Poli A, Padval M, Fields Jones S, Horobin J, Burris HA. Phase I/Ib study of the FAK inhibitor defactinib (VS-6063) in combination with weekly paclitaxel for advanced ovarian cancer. In: Proceedings of the AACR-NCI-EORTC International Conference: Molecular Targets and Cancer Therapeutics (AACR 2013); 19-23 October 2013; Boston, MA. Philadelphia (PA). Molecular Cancer Therapeutics. 2013;**12**(11 Suppl):Abstract nr A69

[53] Soria JC, Gan HK, Blagden SP, Plummer R, Arkenau HT, Ranson M, Evans TRJ, Zalcman G, Bahleda R, et al. A phase I, pharmacokinetic and pharmacodynamic study of GSK2256098, a focal adhesion kinase inhibitor, in patients with advanced solid tumors. Annals of Oncology. 2016;**27**(12):2268-2274. DOI: 10.1093/annonc/mdw427

[54] Wu M, Fan J, Gunning W, Ratnam M. Clustering of GPI-anchored folate receptor independent of both cross-linking and association with caveolin. The Journal of Membrane Biology. 1997;**159**(2):137-147

[55] Serpe L, Gallicchio M, Canaparo R, Dosio F. Targeted treatment of folate receptor-positive platinum-resistant ovarian cancer and companion diagnostics, with specific focus on vintafolide and etarfolatide. Pharmacogenomics and Personalized Medicine. 2014;**7**:31-42. DOI: 10.2147/PGPM.S58374

[56] Chen Y-L, Chang M-C, Huang C-Y, et al. Serous ovarian carcinoma patients with high alpha-folate receptor had reducing survival and cytotoxic chemo-response. Molecular Oncology. 2012;**6**(3):360-369. DOI: 10.1016/j.molonc.2011.11.010

[57] Morphotek—An efficacy and safety study of MORAb-003 in platinum-resistant or refractory relapsed ovarian cancer (FAR-122). Available from: http://clinicaltrials.gov/show/NCT00738699. NLM identifier: NCT00738699. [Accessed: September 1, 2017]

[58] Dosio F, Milla P, Cattel L. EC-145, a folate-targeted vinca alkaloid conjugate for the potential treatment of folate receptor-expressing cancers. Current Opinion in Investigational Drugs. 2010;**11**(12):1424-1433

[59] Naumann W, Coleman R, Robert A, Burger R, Sausville E, Kutarska E, Ghamande S, Gabrail N, DePasquale S, et al. PRECEDENT: A randomized phase II trial comparing vintafolide (EC145) and pegylated liposomal doxorubicin (PLD) in combination versus PLD alone in patients with platinum-resistant ovarian cancer. Journal of Clinical Oncology. 2013;**31**(35):4400-4406. DOI: 10.1200/JCO.2013.49.7685

[60] Yunusova NV, Villert AB, Spirina LV, Frolova AE, Kolomiets LA, Kondakova IV. Insulin-like growth factors and their binding proteins in tumors and ascites of ovarian cancer patients: Association with response to Neoadjuvant chemotherapy. Asian Pacific Journal of Cancer Prevention. 2016;**17**(12):5315-5320. DOI: http://doi.org/10.22034/APJCP.2016.17.12.5315

[61] Shao M, Hollar S, Chambliss D, Schmitt J, Emerson R, Chelladurai B, et al. Targeting the insulin growth factor and the vascular endothelial growth factor pathways in ovarian cancer. Molecular Cancer Therapeutics. 2012;**11**:1576-1586. DOI: 10.1158/1535-7163.MCT-11-0961

[62] Gotlieb WH, Bruchim I, Gu J, Shi Y, Camirand A, Blouin MJ, et al. Insulin-like growth factor receptor I targeting in epithelial ovarian cancer. Gynecologic Oncology. 2006;**100**:389-396. DOI: 10.1016/j.ygyno.2005.09.048

[63] Beauchamp MC, Yasmeen A, Knafo A, Gotlieb WH. Targeting insulin and insulin-like growth factor pathways in epithelial ovarian cancer. Journal of Oncology. 2010;**2010**:257058. DOI: 10.1155/2010/257058

[64] A Phase Ib/II Study of the Combination of BYL719 Plus AMG 479 in Adult Patients With Selected Solid Tumors. Available from: http://clinicaltrials.gov/show/ NCT01708161. NLM identifier: NCT01708161 [Accessed: September 1, 2017]

[65] Harb WA, Sessa C, Hirte HW, Kaye SB, Banerjee SN, Christinat A, et al. Final results of a phase I study evaluating the combination of linsitinib, a dual inhibitor of insulin-like growth factor-1 receptor (IGF-1R), and insulin receptor (IR) with weekly paclitaxel (PAC) in patients (Pts) with advanced solid tumors. Journal of Clinical Oncology. 2013;**31**(15_suppl):e13502-e13502. DOI: 10.1200/jco.2013.31.15_suppl.e13502

[66] Teplinsky E, Muggia F. EGFR and HER2: Is there a role in ovarian cancer? Translational Cancer Research. 2015;**4**(1):107-117. DOI: 10.3978/j.issn.2218-676X.2015.01.01

[67] Siwak DR, Carey M, Hennessy BT, et al. Targeting the epidermal growth factor receptor in epithelial ovarian cancer: Current knowledge and future challenges. Journal of Oncology. 2010;**2010**. DOI: 10.1155/2010/568938

[68] Kurzeder C, Bover I, Marme F, et al. Double-blind, placebo-controlled, randomized phase III trial evaluating pertuzumab combined with chemotherapy for low tumor

human epidermal growth factor receptor 3 mRNA-expressing platinum-resistant ovarian cancer (PENELOPE). Journal of Clinical Oncology. 2016;**34**:2516-2525. DOI: 10.1200/JCO.2015.66.0787

[69] Khalil DN, Smith EL, Brentjens RJ, Wolchok JD. The future of cancer treatment: Immunomodulation, CARs and combination immunotherapy. Nature Reviews. Clinical Oncology. 2016;**13**:273-290. DOI: 10.1038/nrclinonc.2016.25

[70] Pardoll DM. The blockade of immune checkpoints in cancer immunotherapy. Nature Reviews. Cancer. 2012;**12**:252-264. DOI: 10.1038/nrc3239

[71] Gaillard SL, Secord AA, Monk B. The role of immune checkpoint inhibition in the treatment of ovarian cancer. Gynecologic Oncology Research and Practice. 2016;**3**:11. DOI: https://doi.org/10.1186/s40661-016-0033-6

[72] Eng KH, Weir I, Tsuji T, Odunsi K. Immuno-stimultory/regulatory gene expression patterns in advanced ovarian cancer. Genes & Cancer. 2015;**6**(9-10):399-407. DOI: 10.18632/genesandcancer

[73] Heong V, Ngoi N, Tan DSP. Update on immune checkpoint inhibitors in gynecological cancers. Journal of Gynecologic Oncology. 2017;**28**(2):e20. DOI: 10.3802/jgo.2017.28.e20

[74] Hamanishi J et al. Efficacy and safety of anti-PD-1 antibody (Nivolumab: BMS-936558, ONO-4538) in patients with platinum resistant ovarian cancer. Journal of Clinical Oncology. 2014;**32**(suppl):5511. DOI: 10.1200/jco.2014.32.15_suppl.5511

[75] Disis ML, Patel MR, Pant S, Infante JR, Lockhart AC, Kelly K, et al. Avelumab (MSB0010718 C), an anti-PD-L1 antibody, in patients with previously treated, recurrent or refractory ovarian cancer: A phase Ib, open-label expansion trial. Asco Meet Abstr. 2015;**33**(suppl 15):5509

[76] Varga A, Piha-Paul SA, Ott PA, Mehnert JM, Berton-Rigaud D, Johnson EA, et al. Antitumor activity and safety of pembrolizumab in patients (pts) with PD-L1 positive advanced ovarian cancer: Interim results from a phase Ib study. Asco Meet Abstr. 2015;**33**(suppl 15):5510

[77] Hodi FS, Mihm MC, Soiffer RJ, Haluska FG, Butler M, Seiden MV, Davis T, Henry-Spires R, MacRae S, Willman A, Padera R, Jaklitsch MT, Shankar S, Chen TC, Korman A, Allison JP, Dranoff G. Biologic activity of cytotoxic T lymphocyte-associated antigen 4 antibody blockade in previously vaccinated metastatic melanoma and ovarian carcinoma patients. Proceedings of the National Academy of Sciences of the United States of America. 2003 Apr 15;**100**(8):4712-4717

[78] Callahan MK. A phase I study to evaluate the safety and tolerability of MEDI4736, an anti-PD-L1 antibody, in combination with tremelimumab in patients with advanced solid tumors. In: Proceedings of the ASCO Annual Meeting, 2014, http://meetinglibrary.asco.org/content/130062-144

[79] Di Giacomoa AM, Biagiolib M, Maioa M. The emerging toxicity profiles of anti-CTLA-4 antibodies. Seminars in Oncology. 2010;**37**(5):499-507. DOI: 10.1053/j.seminoncol.2010. 09.007

[80] Chester C, Dorigo O, Berek J, Kohrt H. Immunotherapeutic approaches to ovarian cancer treatment. Journal for Immunotherapy of Cancer. 2015;**3**:7. DOI: https://doi.org/10.1186/ s40425-015-0051-7

[81] Gray H, Gargosky S. Progression-free survival in ovarian cancer patients in second remission with mucin-1 autologous dendritic cell therapy. Abstract #5504. Oral Presentation, ASCO Annual Meeting. 2014

[82] Mitchell P, Quinn M, Grant P, Allen D, Jobling T, White S, Zhao A, Karanikas V, Vaughan H, Pietersz G, McKenzie I, Gargosky S, Loveland BE. A phase II, single-arm study of an autologous dendritic cell treatment against mucin 1 in patients with advanced epithelial ovarian cancer. Journal for Immunotherapy of Cancer. 2015;**2**:16. DOI: 10.1186/2051-1426-2-16

[83] hiang CL, Kandalaft LE, Tanyi J, Hagemann AR, Motz GT, Svoronos N, et al. A dendritic cell vaccine pulsed with autologous hypochlorous acid-oxidized ovarian cancer lysate primes effective broad antitumor immunity: From bench to bedside. Clinical Cancer Research. 2013;**9**:4801-4815. DOI: 10.1158/1078-0432.CCR-13-1185

[84] Sabbatini P, Tsuji T, Ferran L, Ritter E, Sedrak C, Tuballes K, et al. Phase I trial of overlapping long peptides from a tumor self-antigen and poly-ICLC shows rapid induction of integrated immune response in ovarian cancer patients. Clinical Cancer Research. 2012;**18**:6497-6508. DOI: 10.1158/1078-0432.CCR-12-2189

[85] Reinartz S, Köhler S, Schlebusch H, Krista K, Giffels P, Renke K, et al. Vaccination of patients with advanced ovarian carcinoma with the anti-idiotype ACA125: Immunological response and survival (phase Ib/II). Clinical Cancer Research. 2004;**10**:1580-1587. DOI: 10.1158/1078-0432.CCR-03-0056

[86] Mohebtash M, Tsang KY, Madan RA, Huen NY, Poole DJ, Jochems C, et al. A pilot study of MUC-1/CEA/TRICOM poxviral-based vaccine in patients with metastatic breast and ovarian cancer. Clinical Cancer Research. 2011;**17**:7164-7173. DOI: 10.1158/1078-0432. CCR-11-0649

[87] Engelstaedter V, Heublein S, Schumacher AL, Lenhard M, Engelstaedter H, Andergassen U, et al. Mucin-1 and its relation to grade, stage and survival in ovarian carcinoma patients. BMC Cancer. 2012;**12**:600. DOI: https://doi.org/10.1186/1471-2407-12-600

[88] Yurkovetsky Z, Skates S, Lomakin A, Nolen B, Pulsipher T, Modugno F, Marks J, Godwin A, Gorelik E, Jacobs I, Menon U, Lu K, Badgwell D, Bast RC Jr, Lokshin AE. Development of a multimarker assay for early detection of ovarian cancer. Journal of Clinical Oncology 2010;**28**(13):2159-2166. DOI: 10.1200/JCO.2008.19.2484

[89] Drerup JM, Liu Y, Padron AS, Murthy K, Hurez V, Zhang B, Curiel TJ. Immunotherapy for ovarian cancer. Current Treatment Options in Oncology. 2015;**16**(1):317. DOI: http://doi.org/10.1007/s11864-014-0317-1

[90] Wright SE, Rewers-Felkins KA, Quinlin IS, Phillips CA, Townsend M, Philip R, Dobrzanski MJ, Lockwood-Cooke PR, Robinson W. Cytotoxic T-lymphocyte immunotherapy for ovarian cancer: A pilot study. Journal of Immunotherapy. 2012; Feb-Mar;**35**(2):196-204. DOI: 10.1097/CJI.0b013e318243f213

[91] Kandalaft LE, Powell DJ, Coukos G. A phase I clinical trial of adoptive transfer of folate receptor-alpha redirected autologous T cells for recurrent ovarian cancer. Journal of Translational Medicine. 2012;**10**:157. DOI: 10.1186/1479-5876-10-157

[92] Monk BJ, Brady MF, Aghajanian C, Lankes HA, Rizack T, Leach J, Fowler JM, Higgins R, et al. A phase II, randomized, double-blind, placebo-controlled study of chemo-immunotherapy combination using motolimod with pegylated liposomal doxorubicin in recurrent or persistent ovarian cancer: A gynecologic oncology group partners study. Annals of Oncology. 01-05-2017;**28**(5):996-1004. DOI: 10.1093/annonc/mdx049

[93] De Felice F, Marchetti C, Palaia I, Musio D, Muzii L, Tombolini V, Panici PB. Immunotherapy of ovarian cancer: The role of checkpoint inhibitors. Journal of Immunology Research 2015; 2015. DOI: http://dx.doi.org/10.1155/2015/191832

[94] Konstantinopoulos P, Moore K, Sachdev J, Mita M, Vinayak S, Seward S, et al. Phase I/II study of niraparib plus pembrolizumab in patients with triple-negative breast cancer or recurrent ovarian cancer (KEYNOTE-162). Journal of Clinical Oncology. 2016;**34** abstract TPS5599

[95] Hodi FS, Butler M, Oble DA, Seiden MV, Haluska FG, Kruse A, et al. Immunologic and clinical effects of antibody blockade of cytotoxic T lymphocyte-associated antigen 4 in previously vaccinated cancer patients. Proceedings of the National Academy of Sciences. 2008;**105**:3005-3010. DOI: 10.1073/pnas.0712237105

4

Radiation Therapy for Non-Small Cell Lung Cancer in the Twenty-First Century

Alejandro Santini Blasco, Cristian Valdez Cortes,
Veronica Sepúlveda Arcuch,
Ricardo Baeza Letelier and Sergio Bustos Caprio

Abstract

Lung cancer is the biggest oncologic problem for global health, as it is the most deadly and prevalent pathology after skin cancer. Two million patients are diagnosed every year, and around 80% of them die due to the disease. Radiotherapy has been practiced for decades to treat these patients, but recently, there has been important advances on this treatment on early stages (I and II), as stereotactic radiation therapy is becoming crucial. There has also been an increase on the importance of this treatment on more advanced stages (III), since intensity-modulated radiation therapy has achieved the reduction of undesirable side effects. The performance of stereotactic radiation at metastasis stages on patients with oligometastasis has accomplished great results. Likewise, hypofractionated treatments on polymetastatic patients have increased their quality of life.

Keywords: lung cancer, radiotherapy, IMRT, SBRT

1. Introduction

Lung cancer (LC) is the main cause of oncologic death in the world. It is a very important public health problem, having over two million new cases diagnosed every year in the world and almost 60% of them on undeveloped countries [1].

Rates vary around the world, Europe has the highest (53.5/100 thousand inhabitants) and Africa the lowest (2/100 thousand inhabitants). In Uruguay, sadly, the incidence on men is similar to that on Eastern Europe (50.11/100 thousand inhabitants). However, incidence on

Advances on diagnosis	• Timely diagnosis: screening with low-intensity scanner
	• Precise staging: PET-CT on lung cancer. Fiber optic bronchoscopy on EBUS
Advances on staging	• New TNM classification
	• Molecular classification of lung cancer (study of mutation EGFR, ALK, PD-L1, etc.)
Advances on surgical procedures	• Less invasive surgery. Video-assisted thoracoscopic surgery (VATS), video-assisted mediastinoscopic lymphadenectomy (VAMLA), transcervical extended mediastinal lymphadenectomy (TEMNLA)
Advances on systematic treatments	• New chemotherapy drugs
	• Targeted treatments:
	• Tumors with EGFR gene mutations—ITKS drugs (gefitinib, afatinib, erlotinib)
	• Tumors with ALK gene changes (crizotinib)
	• Antiangiogenesis agent (bevacizumab)
	• Immunotherapy: PD-L1 tumors (nivolumab)
Advances on radiotherapy treatment	• Stereotactic body radiation therapy on patients with early tumors, stage I–IIA
	• Radiosurgery on patients with oligometastasis
	• Intensity-modulated radiation therapy for stage II and III patients
	• Breathing control techniques. Four-dimensional computed tomography

Table 1. Advances on diagnosis and treatment of lung cancer.

women is significantly lower (9.95/100 thousand inhabitants), although with a tendency to grow [2]. Even though the incidence and death rate for lung cancer on women is lower than men, it has been acknowledged to be higher than breast cancer in some countries [3].

Usually, lung cancer patients are diagnosed at advanced stages, due to the fact that most of the disease's natural history develops asymptomatically. In these cases, the treatments have not been sufficiently effective, and the death rate remains very high. However, in the last decades, multiple advances have been made, which include diagnosis, assignation of subgroups, surgical treatments, systematic treatments (chemotherapy and targeted therapies), and radiotherapy. All of these facts have helped lung cancer to become the main subject of discussion in recent scientific meetings and oncologic congresses.

In **Table 1**, we will describe the main recent advances on the diagnosis and treatment of lung cancer.

Radiotherapy is the most used treatment for lung cancer patients, because of its role on both early (used exclusively or combined with chemotherapy, process of curative aim) and advanced stages (palliative treatment). It is estimated that 80% of patients with lung cancer diagnosis will receive radiotherapy at some point on their treatment [4, 5].

In this study, we will explain the new advances of radiotherapy on non-small cell lung cancer.

2. Radiotherapy on the treatment of lung cancer

Nowadays, radiotherapy plays an essential role in every stage of lung cancer treatment. On each of these stages, advances have been made that enhance the results. These advances thanks to better protection of the normal tissues, better definition of the tumors' therapeutic target, that moves normally with breathing, as well as an effective association with different drugs (chemotherapy, targeted drugs, and immunotherapy). In **Table 2**, we will explain the standard treatments and the new advances of radiotherapy according to the different stages of AJCC [6, 7].

Stage	Standard treatment	Advances (advantages)
Stage I–IIA (tumors < 5 cm)	1. Surgical resection 2. Traditional radiotherapy (60–66 Gy/30–33 Fr)	SBRT (1–5 fractions, less death rate, higher local control)
Stage IIB–III (big-sized tumors or with enlarged lymph nodes)	1. Surgical resection 2. 3D-CRT + QT	IMRT VMAT 4DCRT (better tolerance, higher local control, unpleasant side effects reduced)
Stage IV (brain metastasis)	1. Surgical resection 2. Whole brain and spinal cord radiation therapy	Stereotactic radiotherapy (SRT). Stereotactic radiosurgery (SRS) Hippocampus protection in radiotherapy treatment (noninvasive treatment, higher local control, unpleasant side effects reduced)
Stage IV (oligometastasis)	1. Chemotherapy 2. Targeted cancer therapies 3. Palliative radiotherapy	SBRT on oligometastasis SBRT + immunotherapy (better control on the disease, higher survival rate)

Table 2. Standard radiotherapy treatments and advances on each stage of lung cancer.

3. Advances on the treatment of early LC (stereotactic body radiation therapy, SBRT)

In most countries, the standard treatment for patients with early LC (I–IIA, less than 5 cm size tumors, with absence of nodal involvement) remains to be surgery (lobectomy plus hilar and ipsilateral mediastinal lymph node dissection) [6–12] (**Figure 1**). With this treatment, the 5-year survival rate is between 60–80% for patients at stage I and 30–50% for patients at stage II. For those not apt for surgery, the standard treatment, until a couple years ago, was fractionated radiotherapy for 6–7 weeks, with control rates of 30–70% [13].

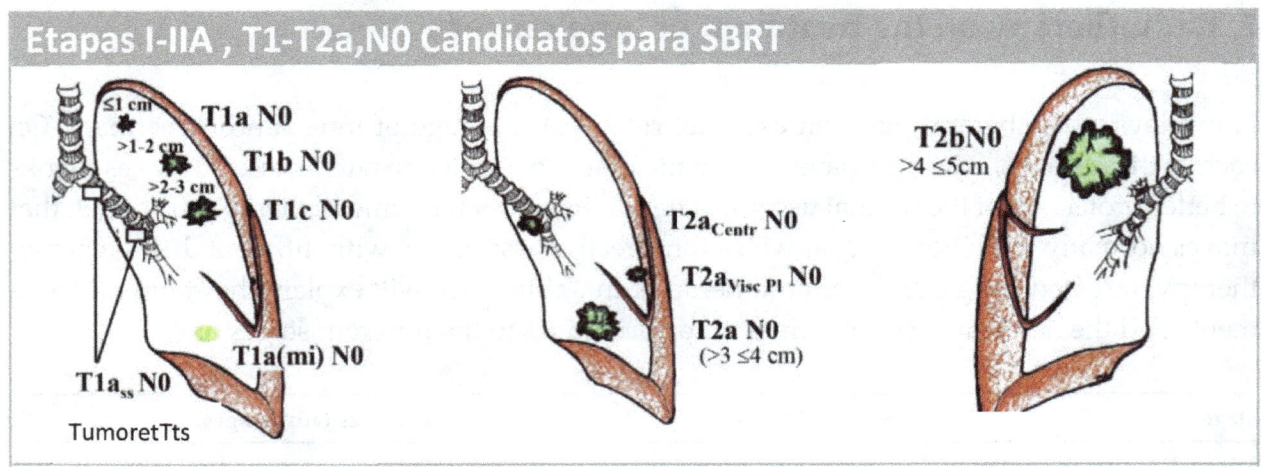

Figure 1. SBRT indications according to the stages of TNM UICC 8th edition (I–IIA).

In the last decade, a new technique has been developed, called stereotactic body radiation therapy (SBRT). After being used in malignant and benign intracranial injuries, it was extended to other physical wounds. SBRT consists of the delivery of extremely high doses of radiation, in little fractions, but with a precise delimitation of the treatment's targets. This technique has the potential of accomplishing similar results to those obtained with surgery but with very low morbidity and mortality rates. It is performed on an outpatient basis and in 1–5 fractions of 1 h each, during approximately a week. In **Figure 2**, it is clearly illustrated the difference between three-dimensional radiation therapy (3D-CRT) and SBRT in the distribution of doses.

This technique was first used for treating lung cancer in 1995, and the results obtained so far have been very encouraging [14]. In the past years, an increasing number of papers showing similar results to those obtained with surgery have been published. This has coined the concept of "conservatory lung cancer treatment," similar to what happened with breast cancer in the 1980s [15]. Nowadays, not only is this technique the most adequate to LC patients that are not candidates to surgery, but it is also considered by some authors as a second "Gold Standard" [16]. Recently, on a revision of the participant centers in the elaboration of the NCCN (National Comprehensive Cancer Network) Guidelines, the existence of a wide variation in the local treatment of these patients was proved, which confirms a clear lack of level I evidence to decide which treatment, surgery or SBRT, is the most adequate [17].

Around the same time, various studies that prove how important of a role does the low-intensity scanner plays in the early diagnose of lung cancer have been published [18]. In most clinical guidelines, there is a clear indication and a precise group of patients who are benefited from this screening study; therefore, we hope that in our country, as well as in the rest of Latin America, this procedure will become usual so that we can treat more patients at an early stage of the disease. The upcoming situation will determine a challenge for the health authorities, so an outpatient treatment of one to five applications with almost no death rate is perceived as utterly interesting [19, 20].

The SBRT has permitted an increase in the number of patients who are treated with a curative aim, and the undesired effect rates are very low (especially pneumonitis, 3–6%), even for those patients whose lung function is compromised, compared to radiotherapy in its three dimensions [21–24].

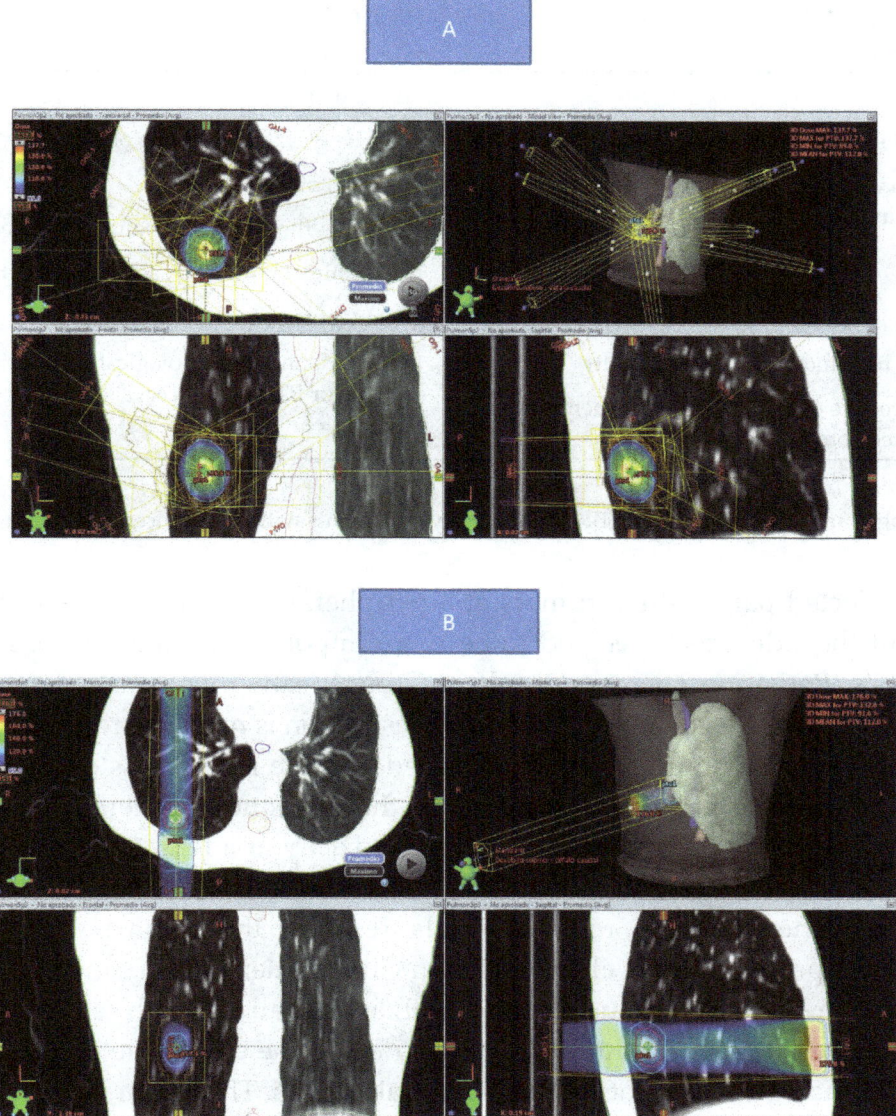

Figure 2. (A) Dose distribution and treatment beam on lung cancer T1bc (2.1 mm) N0 M0 treated with SBRT. (B) Same case, with radiotherapy planning conformed of 3D. Note the difference and volume of the treated lung.

Recently, Stenan et al. have analyzed the advantages and disadvantages of both surgery and SBRT that are explained in **Table 3** [20].

To date, there are various retrospective studies that demonstrate tumor control rates higher than 80%, with morbidity and mortality rates at a minimum (**Table 4**). A recent revision at SEER (Surveillance, Epidemiology, and End Results Program) by Yale University's group was published by Yu et al. It includes a group of patients over age 67, treated between 2007 and 2009 with LC at an early stage [30]. More than 1000 patients were checked, 367 treated with SBRT and 711 treated with surgery. The acute toxicity (0–1 month) was 7.9% for SBRT and 54.9% for surgery (p < 0.001). At 24 months, the difference in toxicity was not that significative (69% against 73.9% p = 0.31). The IRR of toxicity for SBRT against surgery was 0.74 (95% CI of 0.64–0.87). The mortality rate was lower for SBRT (23.3% vs. 40.1% p < 0.001). The main complications carried by surgery in this study were, besides the pain caused to the patient, IAM, cardiac arrhythmias, TVP, PTE, and pneumonia that are not registered at surgical operations. Every patient that was subjected to surgery needed a hospitalization of at least 3 days in case no complications occurred.

Surgery (lobectomy + hilum and mediastinal lymphadenectomy)	SRBT
Advantages:	Advantages:
• Definite pathological diagnosis	• Five-year survival rate of 90%
• Allows the diagnosis of lymph node involvement, which is redundant for selecting patients for adjuvant treatment	• Outpatient treatment
	• Lung function and quality of life are preserved
	• Minimal morbidity, almost no mortality
Disadvantages:	Disadvantages:
• Procedure of high morbidity and mortality	• No definitive pathological verification. Local fibrosis for RT may conceal a local recurrence
• Invasive procedure on patients who frequently suffer from associated comorbidities	

Table 3. Advantages and disadvantages of SBRT and surgery on patients with lung cancer at early stages (I and IIA).

Initially, the selected patients had tumors at a peripheral level, due to the fact that, at first, the analysis of the side effects seemed to be more important on the central injury [31–33]. Even at RTOG's (Radiation Therapy Oncology Group) team, there was a denominated zone of exclusion called "no fly zone." However, this restriction is not that strong anymore, owing to the fact that the fractionation must be adjusted and the restrictions of the organs at risk maintained within the established limits [34]. In the first studies where some patients with central tumors were included, some cases of high toxicity at a long run were described [35, 36]. Nevertheless, in most recent publications, where the number of fractions is higher and the doses for each one are slightly reduced, similar results to those from peripheral tumors are obtained. **Table 5** presents in detail works that include patients with central tumors [37–42]. Baba et al. made a revision of 20 studies on more than 500 patients with central injuries treated with SBRT. The toxicity levels III and IV were 8.6% and the death rate of the treatment was 2%, a bit higher than those patients with peripheral tumors. The 3-year local control rate was 60–100% and the survival rate was 50–75% [43].

Study	No. of patients	Treatment	Result	Drawbacks
Brown et al. [25]	59	15–67 Gy on 1–5 Fr	Five-year survival rate, free from disease, of 90%	Pneumonitis G3, 7%
Negata et al. [26]	104	12 Gy on 1–14 Fr	Three-year survival rate, free of progression, of 70%	Dyspnea G3, 9%
				Pneumonitis, 7%
				Pain, 2%
Onishi et al. [27]	257	30–84 Gy on 1–14 Fr	Five-year survival rate of 84%	Lung complications G3, 5.4%
				Esophageal complications, 1%
Senthi et al. [28]	676	3–8 Fr (54–60 Gy)	Five-year survival rate of 89%	No significant drawbacks
Ven der Voort et al. [29]	70	12–15 Gy × 3 Fr	Two-year survival rate of 92%	Late toxicity G3, 10%

Table 4. Initial retrospective studies. Fragmentation and results. SRBT on patients with lung cancer on stages I and IIA.

Author	No. of patients	Tumor characteristics	Dosage	Local control	Survival rate
Chang et al. [27]	27	48% T1–T2 52% recurrence	40–50 Gy/5 Fr	3 patients (40 Gy)	
Milano et al. [38]	53	66% T1–T2 36% NSCLC with metastasis	20–55 Gy/1–18 Fr	73% to 3 years	72% to 2 years (T1–T2)
Haasbeek et al. [39]	63	No T1–T3	60 Gy/8 Fr	92.5% to 5 years	DFS 71% SR 49.7%
Rowe et al. [40]	47	59% T1–T2 41% NSCLC	50 Gy/4 Fr	Two local failures	PFS 24% to 2 years
Oshiro et al. [41]	21	95% recurrence of NSCLC	25–39 Gy/1–10 Fr	60% to 2 years	SR 62.2% to 2 years
Unger et al. [42]	20	85% NSCLC with metastasis	30–40 Gy/5 Fr	63% to 1 year	SR 54% to 2 years

Table 5. SBRT results on patients with non-small cell lung cancer (NSCLC) with focal injuries.

Table 6 describes the recommended treatment schemes for SBRT according to NCCN's Clinical Guidelines. It also details the differences between the doses for each fraction on central and peripheral tumors [9].

To date, it has not been published any randomized study that compares surgery to SBRT on patients eligible for surgery, so the recommendations are based on retrospective works or on a series of cases which mainly include noncandidate patients due to their comorbidity. Mahmood et al. revised 19 works where high-risk surgery patients were submitted to suboptimal resection (sublobar or wedge resection) or SBRT [44]. In this revision, it was proved a local control of 90% with SBRT, similar results to those obtained with lobectomy on patients with low risk but very much superior to the results obtained with suboptimal surgery. The rate of local recurrence was 4% for SBRT and 20% for surgery (p = 0.07).

Most of the results obtained with SBRT on patients with low surgical risk come from information given by patients who rejected surgery. To date at least three different studies have been published that add a total of 260 cases. In these, the local control rate was 93% for T1 and 73%

Doses	No. of fractions	Indication
25–34 Gy	1	Small (<2 cm) peripheral tumors. More than 2 cm between chest wall
45–60 Gy	3	Small peripheral tumors. Less than 2 cm between the chest wall
48–50 Gy	4	Central or peripheral tumors, smaller than 4–5 cm, and less than 1 cm between the chest wall
50–55 Gy	5	Central or peripheral tumors less than 1 cm between the chest wall
60–70 Gy	8–10	Central tumors

Table 6. Fractioning on SBRT. Modified from NCCN [7].

for T2. The 5-year survival rate was 72 and 62%, respectively, and the local and distant recurrence rate was 20% [45–47].

Zheng et al. published a meta-analysis in 2014 that includes every study published on non-small cell lung cancer's treatment between 2000 and 2012 [48]. Forty publications regarding SBRT are included, from which 30 were retrospective (4800 patients) and 23 on surgery. The average age was 74 years old for SBRT and 66 years old for surgery. The 1-year survival rate was 83.4% against 92.5%, 2-year survival rate was 56.6% against 77%, and 5-year survival rate was 41.2% against 66.1%. These results seemed to show a slight advantage for surgery patients. Nevertheless, when the operable patients are studied and the data are organized by age, the chance of survival and nonrecurrence is similar. These prove that the selection of treatments depends on the patients' age; the youngers are usually treated with surgery and the older with SBRT.

To compare these two procedures directly, some randomized works have been developed, among them, the "STAR" protocol, directed by MD Anderson's team; the "ROSEL" protocol, directed by a Dutch and German team; and, lastly, one by RTOG [46, 49, 50]. All of them include patients with non-small cell lung cancer at stage I and tried to compare standard surgery, lobectomy, and lymphoganglionar hilar-mediastinal dissection with SBRT. The three studies were finished before time due to the difficulty in the inclusion of the patients, most of them rejected the randomization to evaluate both treatments, of which none was better than the other, but one implied a surgical intervention that the other did not. Chang et al. analyzed patients who were included in two of these frustrated protocols, they were randomized, and the results were published as a whole [51, 52]. Only 58 patients were included (31 for SBRT and 27 for surgery), the average follow-up was 40.2 months, and the 3-year survival rate was 95% for SBRT and 79% for surgery (p = 0.54). In the group conformed by patients on SBRT, 10% (three individuals) presented some type of minimal adverse effect (chest pain 10%, dyspnea or cough 6%, and only one patient presented rib fracture). On the other hand, in the group conformed by those who were treated with surgery, one patient passed owing to complications during surgery (4%), and 44% (12 patients) presented some complications regarding G3-4 (RTOG's Toxicity Scale). This author concludes that even though the quantity of patients is low and requires more complex work, the SBRT is a clear valid option for treating non-small cell lung cancer patients at an early stage. Other authors who reanalyzed the results obtained by these three studies wonder whether the failure of inclusion of patients maintains the question or if it is an answer by itself.

Rusthoven et al. proposed that these results prove that similar changes to those occurred to breast cancer's conservatory treatments during the 1980s will happen to non-small cell lung cancer's treatments. It could be compared as well to localized and low-risk prostate cancer, where radiotherapy and surgery are valid alternatives with very little difference between them, even though there are no randomized works that compare them directly [53, 54]. This situation in concern with the implementation of the low-intensity scanner on risk groups will absolutely change the epidemiology, so a higher number of patients with lung cancer will be treated with a curative aim at the radiotherapy units.

Nowadays, there are various works in course: the RTOG 013 that analyzes a dose escalation on focal tumors, smaller than 5 cm; the RTOG 0915 that compares different treatment schemes, 34Gy/1 fraction against 48 Gy in 4 fractions; the VALOR (Veterans Affair Lung Cancer Surgery Or Stereotactic Radiotherapy) protocol from the USA; and the SABRTooth in the UK that tries to answer various current questions [55, 56].

Finally, studies have begun to question the necessity of a histological confirmation previous to SBRT on patients with a suspicious lump on their lung and at high risk. In this sense, for those who are submitted to lung cancer screening with a low-intensity scanner (older than 50–55 years old, younger than 74, and tobacco use exceeding 30 pack-years) and are as well discovered a suspicious lung lump and submitted to surgery, many authors do not perform a histological confirmation before the thoracotomy, due to the fact that the probability of malignancy is higher than 65% and also the complication rate from the needle biopsy is high [57]. The importance of this situation increases for those patients who are SBRT candidates, as they usually have higher comorbidity rates [58, 59]. Therefore, in recent publications, the necessity of previous biopsy to SBRT is analyzed. The performance of algorithms that employ at least two serial scans to evaluate the evolution of the patient, added to the use of PET-CT, benefits the achievement of a high positive predictive factor. Recent studies show that the long-term survival results from patients treated with SBRT with or without the previous biopsy are similar, contrary to the popular belief that one may hope a higher survival rate for those not confirmed for inclusion in this group without an oncologic pathology [60].

To sum up, we could say that patients with localized lung cancer, T1 and T2, without lymph node involvement, conform a growing group due to the implementation of screening studies. Radiotherapy with SBRT technique is one of the electable treatments, with encouraging results and a low morbidity and mortality rate.

4. Advances on the treatment of advanced local nonmetastatic non-small cell lung cancer: stages II and III

4.1. Intensity-modulated radiotherapy (IMRT)

4.1.1. Volumetric arc therapy (VMAT)

The standard treatment for patients with locally advanced NSCLC, on stages II and III, is surgery. For those who are not eligible for it, the preferred treatment is combined chemotherapy and radiotherapy [9, 61]. The most used drugs are explained in **Table 7**, but the analysis of the different schemes is beyond the scope of this paper.

Chemotherapy schemes combined with radiotherapy, recommended by NCCN

Cisplatin 50 mg/m^2 days 1, 8, 29, and 36 + etoposide 50 mg/m^2 days 1–5, 29–33

Cisplatin 100 mg/m^2 days 1 and 29 + vinblastine 5 mg/m^2/weekly × 5

Carboplatin AUC 5 day 1 + pemetrexed 500 mg/m^2 day 1 every 21 days × 4 cycles (nonsquamous cancer)

Cisplatin 75 mg/m^2 day 1 + pemetrexed 500 mg/m^2 day 1 every 21 days × 3 cycles (nonsquamous cancer) ± 4 cycles of pemetrexed 500 mg/m^2

Paclitaxel 45–50 mg/m^2 weekly + carboplatin AUC 2 ± 2 additional cycles of paclitaxel 200 mg/m^2 and carboplatin AUC 6

Table 7. Schemes and drugs used on combined radiotherapy and chemotherapy on patients with non-small cell lung cancer.

Radiotherapy is typically delivered in 30–35 fractions, five times a week until reaching a total dose of 60–66 Gy [62–64]. Distant metastases are the main cause of failure on the treatment, but 45% of the patients also present a persistence or local failure [64]. SBRT is not feasible for this group of patients due to its volume.

For these patients, intensity-modulated radiotherapy (IMRT) and, more recently, volumetric arc therapy (VMAT) have been established as electable techniques, due to its possibility to improve tolerance, fundamentally by limiting the doses delivered to the esophagus (acute toxicity) and to the lung parenchyma (late toxicity) [65] (**Figure 3**).

The combination of these treatment planning techniques added to the improvements on the delimitation of volumes like scanner simulation on 4D, or the guided RT with images with cone beam CT (a scanner in the same machine of treatment), allows to decrease the toxicity and ensure a better distribution of doses on the treatment's volumes [66].

Various studies that compare the different treatments, more precisely 3D-CRT (radiotherapy conformed in three dimensions) vs. IMRT or VMAT*(VMAT, sophisticated RT IMRT technique characterized for the use of at least one dynamic arc that allows the quick delivery of doses on irregular volumes), clearly show the advantages of the modern techniques in terms of the medium dose on a healthy lung, lung V20, dose on the spinal cord, and dose on the esophagus and heart [67, 68]. These modern techniques have spread very quickly to most of the centers of reference. Most of the clinical comparisons between IMRT and 3DCRT are retrospective studies from separate institutions, with the limitations entailed to that notion [66]. An analysis from the National Cancer Database from the USA shows that, with the use of 3DCRT or IMRT, an improvement on the survival rate is obtained, compared to 2D techniques [69]. However, when we compare the 3D with IMRT in a separate way, the differences are not so clear. On an analysis of the subgroups on patients at T3 and T4, the differences on favor to IMRT are more evident [70].

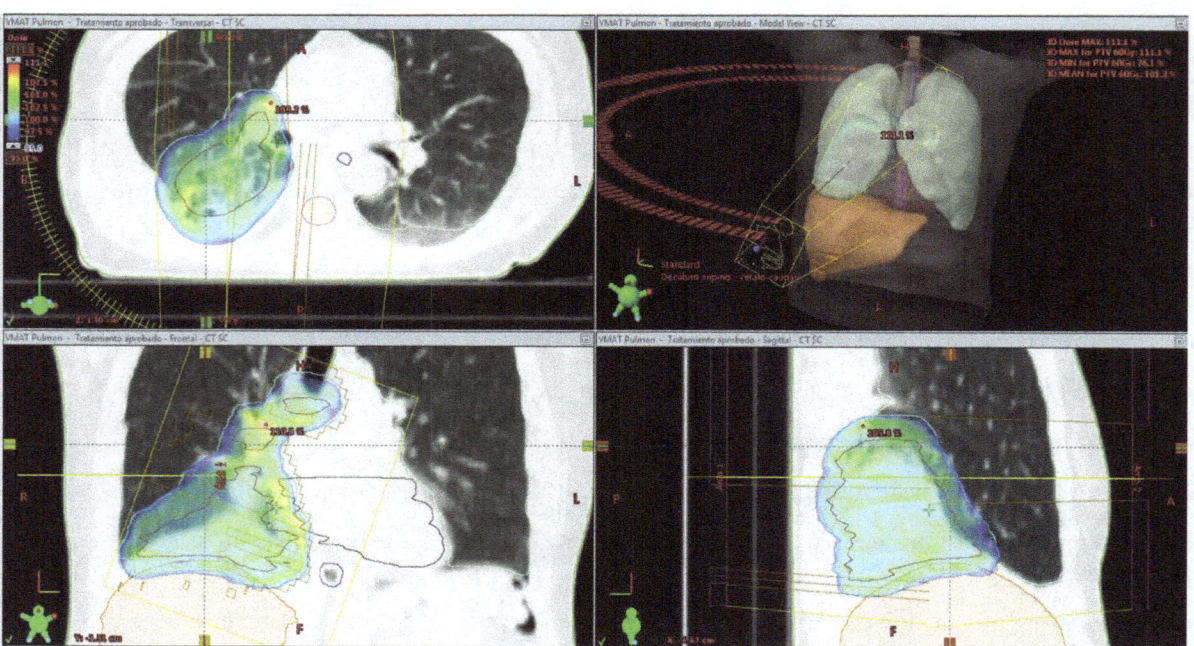

Figure 3. IMRT. Volumes of treatment with IMRT-VMAT on a patient with lung cancer diagnosis T3 N1 M.

In this respect, on a recent study on the protocol of the dose escalation for RTOG 0617, where patients treated with IMRT and 3DCRT are included, it can be concluded that, although the patients treated with IMRT had a PTV (Planning Treatment Volume) of 15% more and a higher percentage of stage IIIB tumors, the G3 pneumonitis rate was cut from 7.9 to 3.5%. Moreover, the group treated with IMRT presented a larger number of patients who were able to receive consolidated chemotherapy and reported lower cases of impaired quality of life [67]. This paper shows as well that patients treated on larger centers, where IMRT is used more frequently on treatments, have a higher 2-year survival rate (10% more).

Currently, a group of investigators is analyzing the possibility of delivering a higher dose on zones that are most metabolically active, detected by the PET-CT with [18] fluorodeoxy-glucose, with IMRT techniques. These protocols that are based on the metabolic activity are positively correlated with areas where developing a recurrence or lack of control is more frequent [66].

5. Strategies for the handling of breathing movements

5.1. 4DCT

An important challenge for lung cancer radiotherapy treatment is the management of the physiological movements related to breathing. The lung tumors move during the breathing, especially those closer to the diaphragmatic cupolas. Usually, to ensure the adequate dose delivery to the tumor, a margin is left around it. For tumors that move, this procedure presents some particular characteristics. For example, caudal skull movement is higher than latero-lateral and anteroposterior movement.

Four-dimensional computed tomography (4DCT) is a technique that allows the user to characterize and quantify the injury's movement during breathing (**Figures 4** and **5**). It is essential for more sophisticated radiotherapy techniques such as SBRT, IMRT, or VMAT, where great precision is needed, as it allows to reduce the geographical miss (parts of the injury remains outside the treatment's range) and the volume of the healthy tissue surrounding the tumor [71].

With images obtained by 4DCT and the precise knowledge of the tumor's movement, we could make advances in many senses [72]:

1. Determine a margin around the tumor according to the movement, usually denominated ITV (internal tumor volume).

2. Operate instruments that attempt to reduce the breathing movement (abdominal compressor).

3. Use techniques that allow to perform the treatment during breathing, at a certain stage called gating.

4. Operate radiotherapy robotic equipment that moves synchronized with breathing, "real time tumor tracking" (CyberKnife).

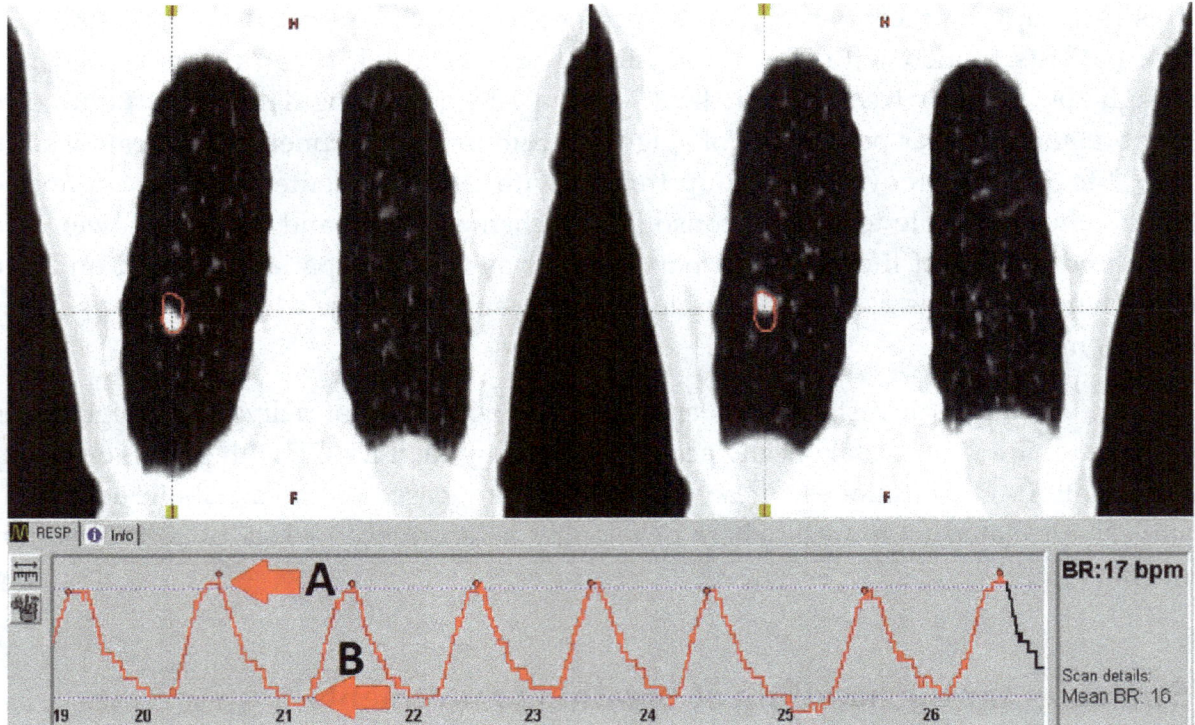

Figure 4. A 4DCT, appreciated on synchronized reconstructions with breathing signal (red curve on the bottom edge). The top left image corresponds to movement of the tumor at inhalation (reconstruction of the images on point A of the breathing signal). The top right image corresponds to the movement of the tumor at exhalation (reconstruction of images on point B of the breathing signal).

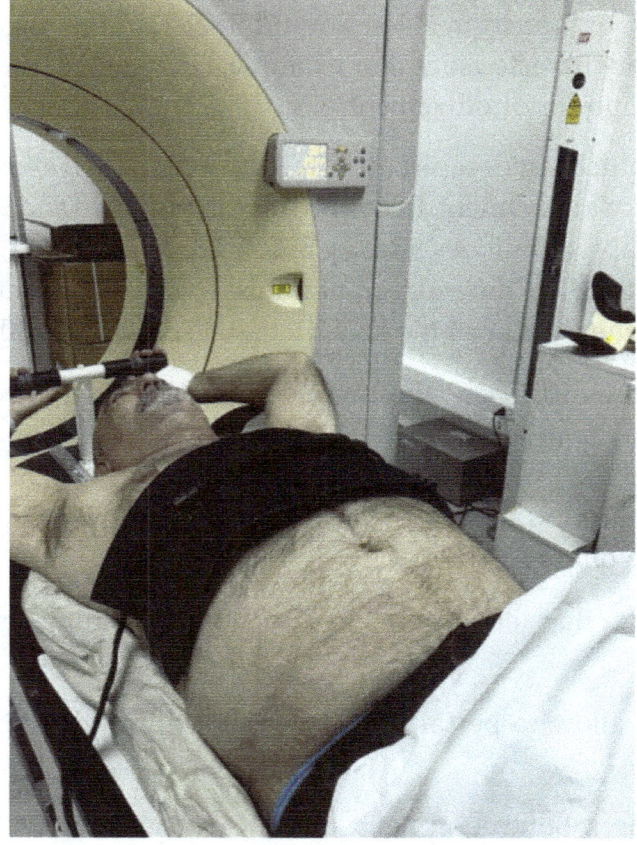

Figure 5. Device used to quantify the breathing movement on 4D scanner.

5.2. Gating

On this technique, radiotherapy is practiced on a specific stage of the breathing cycle, usually exhalation, and stops irradiating at the next stage, leaving the tumor out of the irradiation area. It requires the adequate technology, collaboration from the patient, and training, so that the cycle remains harmonious and stable [73, 74]. The election of one or another method depends on each case's preference and access.

6. Stereotactic radiotherapy on brain metastasis and hippocampus protection

Approximately 20% of non-small cell lung cancer patients develop brain metastasis, and as in small cell lung cancer, prophylactic cerebral irradiation is sometimes recommended [75]. This percentage increases as staging studies are performed on asymptomatic patients, also when the systematic disease's control is increased with new therapeutic means, such as chemotherapy or targeted drugs. Brain metastasis' prognosis varies based on the patient's age, overall health, the size and number of the metastasis, and the systematic control (or not) of the disease [76, 77]. The standard treatment for patients with multiple metastases used to be, until recently, whole brain radiotherapy, which achieved an average of 4- to 8-month survival.

On a group of patients with good prognosis, a limited number of injuries, young, overall healthy, and with a relatively controlled systematic disease, the most aggressive metastasis treatment, either surgery or radiosurgery, obtains an improvement on the survival rate as well as on the quality of life [78, 79].

Radiosurgery for patients with brain metastasis must only be considered for those whose injuries are not bigger than 3 cm. It consists of delivering only one fraction of radiation with high doses and highest precision (1 mm). To date, there are no randomized studies that compare radiosurgery to surgery, although it is believed that the second should be saved for bigger injuries, while radiosurgery is recommended when the metastases are multiple.

Even though the addition of whole brain radiotherapy benefits the raise of neurocognitive alterations, it is not clear if it also improves the local disease control on patients undergoing radiosurgery [80, 81].

Despite what was discussed before, for some patients who present a larger number of metastasis, whole brain treatment cannot be avoided. Some preclinical studies proposed that the neurocognitive deleterious effects are partly caused by the irradiation of the neuronal stem cells, located on the lateral ventricles' subventricular zone and also on the hippocampus and the dentate gyrus (both related to memory). These structures can be protected with the implementation of IMRT, which has proved to decrease the decay of memory to 7%, compared to a previous 30% [82, 83].

7. Radiotherapy on oligometastasis

As we mentioned before, a large number of patients present metastasis at the time of their diagnosis or during the evolution of the disease [84]. They receive a poor prognosis; however, those who present a limited number of injuries (for some authors up to six), seem to have a less aggressive behavior and a better prognosis [85]. This group of patients suffers from oligo-metastasis and could be benefitted from a more aggressive local treatment [9]. Just as a group of patients with hepatic metastases from colorectal cancer has been established, there is also a group of lung cancer patients who are benefited from a local control of the metastasis. In this sense, SBRT, as previously mentioned, is a noninvasive treatment with little undesirable effects. It has been successfully practiced, having controlled an 80% of the metastasis [86].

Recently, Iyengar et al. published the results of a randomized study that compares radiother-apy on the primary tumor and metastasis (less than six) to combined chemotherapy against only chemotherapy. These prove there is a difference in the progression-free survival (PFS) of 9.7 against 3.5 months, respectively ($p < 0.01$). This difference is also extremely higher than that found on different chemotherapy schedules [87].

Other authors have also proved that the use of targeted drugs (erlotinib) added to SBRT for patients with oligometastasis raises the PFS and the survival rate in relation to controls [88].

Certainly, big changes are occurring on the traditional concepts regarding this field and patients with metastasis. In the near future, enormous advances are expected to be underway on the field of combining radiotherapy with immunotherapy.

8. Radioimmunotherapy

For many years, radiotherapy has been known to be related to tumor immunotherapy, even the abscopal effect, also known as bystander, was descripted 30 years ago. This effect refers to the radiation's impact outside the irradiated area, when a tumor injury is treated with radio-therapy and another injury outside the irradiated area is reduced or disappears [89–91]. Ten years ago, Formetti et al. related the bystander effect to immunity [92].

Nowadays it is known that the traditional paradigm that stated that the damage caused by radiation was exclusively due to the effects on the irradiated cells' DNA has become more complex. Radiation causes a series of effects on the cells (tumors or not): inflammation, chain activation, and complex metabolic steps [93]. A bigger number of inhibitors, signal transduc-tion, related to DNA's damage reparation have been described. These present a tremendous opportunity to be used as interesting targets in new forms of treatments.

Recently, it has been proven that high doses of radiation, like those used on SBRT, cause various immunomodulating effects, similar to those on vaccines [93]. It has been established, for example, that performing a combination of radiotherapy and antibodies to treat some antigens associated with T cytotoxic lymphocytes like CTLA-4 (which suppresses its activity) results on a regression of the tumors that are not included in the volumes of radiation, pro-ducing the bystander effect [94].

The basic mechanisms used on radiotherapy to interact with the immune system are extremely complex and only partially known. The damage produced by radiotherapy when used on high doses, like SBRT, happens on the intra-tumor blood vessels. Changes on the membrane-spanning molecule and the release of soluble mediators have been discovered, so that the dendritic cells are stimulated, which also causes the stimulation of the T lymphocytes [92]. Radiotherapy induces multiple immunological changes, such as the tumor cell's death, thanks to the ionizing radiation, the overregulation of immunogenic surface markers like MHC-1, and discharge of danger signals or cytokine such as TNF-alfa. It also induces immunological death via calreticulin and other reticulins, simultaneously to the tumor DNA's exit and ATP, just as HMGB1 (high mobility group box 1 protein). These proteins are associated with chromatin and seem to have a big impact on the triggering of immune response through the incentive of dendritic cells. It has also been described the arrival of immunocompetent cells like cytotoxic T lymphocytes or the raise of tumor antigens from dendritic cells, the transformation of macrophages activated by M1 or M2, and the overregulation of surface antigen such as PD-L1 and other endless events [95] (**Figure 6**).

However, these effects get complex when the usual effects on traditional radiotherapy treatment are studied, when low doses are used on big volumes. The effects may be different on these treatments and also counterproductive from an immunological perspective, because of the possible implementation of other mediators (e.g., TGF-β), added to the phenotypic alteration of macrophages that are infiltrative tumors (M2 to M1). These would explain the nonstimulation of immunological effects contemplated on high doses and small volumes, which is clearly evidenced on immunosuppressive effects of radiotherapy on low doses and small volumes.

Therefore, this interaction of radiotherapy with different immunomodulating molecules is being thoroughly studied. Various teams are working on the combination of SBRT and immunotherapy, which is one of the most advantageous treatments for different tumors, lung cancer among them [96–99].

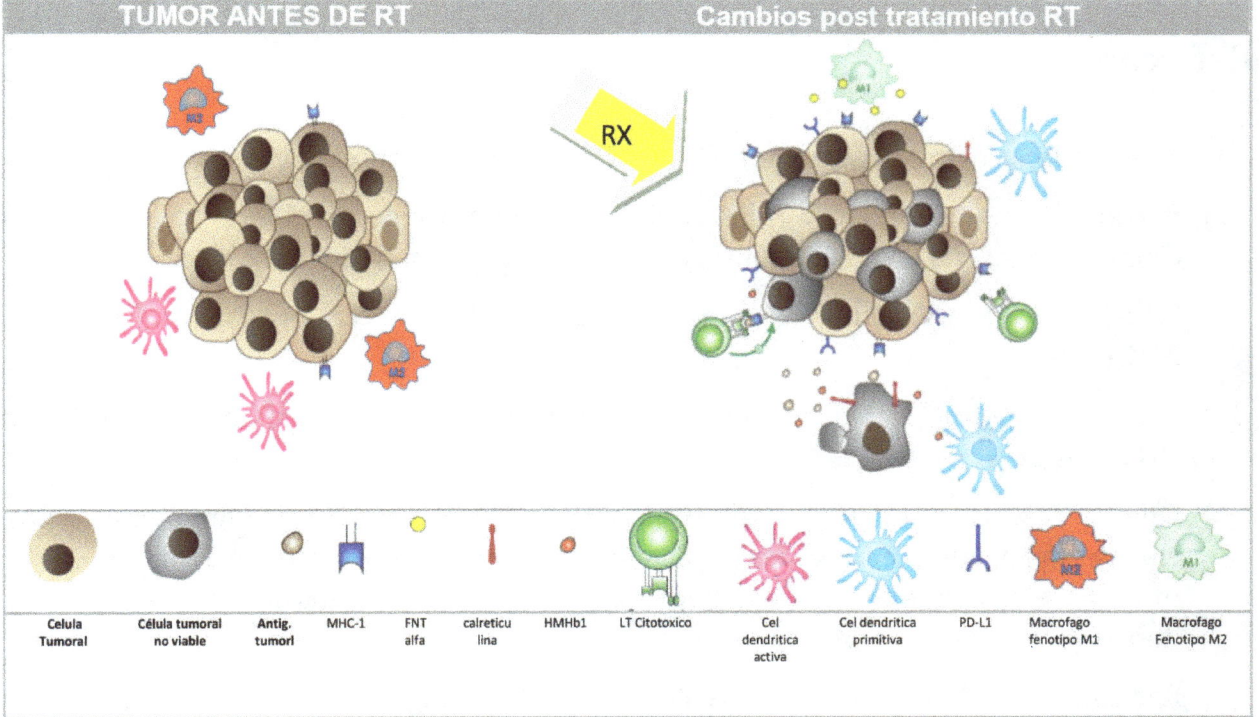

Figure 6. Molecular and cell effects that occur after the application of high doses of radiotherapy.

9. Conclusion

Certainly, radiotherapy still plays an important role on lung cancer treatment. In recent years, new sophisticated techniques have been developed and propelled themselves into different stages of the treatment. SBRT is a valid mean for treating patients with located tumors, as it presents surprising results and minimal side effects. This technique has been implemented on groups of patients suffering from oligometastasis and has showed great improvements on the survival rate. As previously mentioned, Iyengar et al. presented on the last ASTRO congress, September of 2017, an even higher survival rate of 3.5–9.7 with the addition of SBRT on patients suffering from oligometastasis. This kind of improvement has hardly been found on other new drugs for chemotherapy.

Lastly, we have begun to understand the molecular mechanisms triggered by radiotherapy with high doses, as the involved molecules are more familiar. These studies are the beginning of a new treatment, the combination of SBRT and immunotherapy.

Author details

Alejandro Santini Blasco*, Cristian Valdez Cortes, Veronica Sepúlveda Arcuch, Ricardo Baeza Letelier and Sergio Bustos Caprio

*Address all correspondence to: alejandro.santini@gmail.com

Centro Oncologico Antofagasta, Antofagasta, Chile

References

[1] Canceratlas.cancer.org Copyright © 2014 The American Cancer Society, Inc

[2] Barrios E, Musetti C et al. V Atlas de Mortalidad por cáncer en el Uruguay, 2009-2013 Comsio Honoraria de Lucha Contra el Cáncer. Registro nacional del cáncer

[3] Siegel R, Miller K, Jemal A. Cancer statistics 2017. Cancer Journal for Clinicians. 2017;**67**:7-30

[4] Sause W. The role of radiotherapy in non-small cell lung cancer. Chest. 1999;**116**(6); 504s-508s

[5] Diwanji T, Mohindra P, Vyfhuis M, et al. Advances in radiotherapy techniques an delivery for non-small cell lung cancer: Benefits of intensity-modulated radiation therapy, proton therapy, and stereotactic body radiation therapy. Translational Lung Cancer Research. 2017;**6**(2):131-147

[6] Rami-Porta R, Asamura H, Travis W, Rusch VW. Lung cancer-major changes in the American Joint Committee on cancer eighth edition cancer staging manual. CA: A Cancer Journal for Clinicians. 2017;**67**:138-155

[7] Detterbeck F, Boffa D, Kim A, et al. The eighth edition lung cancer stage classification. Chest. 2017;**151**(1):193-203

[8] Fernandez IP, Quero A, Cueto Ladron de Guevara A: Tratamiento quirurgico del CNCP etapas I y II. Revista Española de Patología Torácica. 2017;**21**(2, Suppl I):79-84

[9] National Comprehensive Cancer Network. NCCN clinical practice guidelines in oncology—Non-small-cell lung cancer. Fort Washington, org/professionals/physician_gls/pdf/nscl.pdf [Accessed: 21 September 2017]

[10] Macbeth F, Abratt R, Cho K, et al. Lung cancer management in limited resource settings: Guideline for appropriate good care. IAEA clinical Guideline. Radiotherapy and Oncology. 2007;**82**:123-131

[11] Janes S, Takrar R, Singer J, et al. London Cancer. Radiotherapy Guideline for Treatment of Lung Cancer. London Cancer, North and East. June 2014

[12] Bezjak A, Temin S, Franlin G, et al. Definitive and adjuvant radiotherapy in locally advanced non-small cell lung cancer. American Society of Clinical Oncology. Clinical Practice Guideline Endorsement of the American Society for Radiation Oncology Evidence-based Clinical Practice Guideline. Journal of Clinical Oncology. 2015;**33**(18):2100-2105

[13] Diwanji T, Mohindra P, Vyfhuis M, et al. Advances in radiotherapy techniques and delivery for non-small cell lung cancer: Benefits of intensity-modulated radiation therapy, proton therapy and stereotactic body radiation therapy. Translational Lung Cancer Research. 2017;**6**(2):13

[14] Blomegreen H, Lax I, Näslund Svansröm R. Stereotactic high dose fraction radiation therapy for extracranial tumors using an accelerator. Clinical experience of the first thirty-one patients. Acta Oncologica. 1995;**34**(6):861-870

[15] Santini A, Vandez C, Sepulveda V, et al. Radioterapia esterotaxica en cáncer de pulmón. Hacia un tratamiento conservador. Revista de Oncología Médica. 2016:34-44

[16] Chen H, Loule A. Stereotactic ablative radiotherapy and surgery: Two gold standard for early-stage non-small cell lung cancer? Annals of Translational Medicine. 2015;**3**(9):113-116

[17] Valle LE, Jagsi R, Robiak SN, Zornosa C, et al. Variation in definitive therapy for localized non-small cell lung cancer among National Comprehensive Cancer Network Institution. International Journal of Radiation Oncology, Biology, Physics. 2016;**94**(2):360-367

[18] Aberle DR, Adams AM, Berg CD, et al. National lung screening trial research team, reduced lung cancer mortality with low dose computed tomographic screening. The New England Journal of Medicine. 2011;**365**(5):395-409

[19] Wender R, Fontman E, Barrera E, et al. American cancer society lung cancer screening guideline. CA: A Cancer Journal for Clinicians. 2013;**63**(2):1-10

[20] Senan S, Paul M, Lagerwaard F. Treatment of early-stage lung cancer detected by screening: Surgery or stereotactic ablative radiotherapy? The Lancet Oncology. 2013;**14**:e270-e274

[21] Kang KH, Okoye CC, Patel RB, et al. Complication from stereotactic body radiotherapy for lung cancer. Cancers (Basel). 2015;**7**(2):981-1004

[22] Ricardi U, Badelino S, Filippi AR, et al. Stereotactic radiotherapy for early stage non-small cell lung cancer. Radiation Oncology Journal. 2015;**33**(2):57-65

[23] Simone CB, Dorsey JF. Additional data in the debate on stage I none-small cell lung cancer: Surgery versus stereotactic ablative radiotherapy. Annals of Translational Medicine. 2015;**3**(13):172-178

[24] Palma D, Visser O, Lagerwaard FJ, et al. Impacts of introducing stereotactic lung radiotherapy for elderly patients with stage I none-small cell lung cancer: A population-based time-trend analysis. Journal of Clinical Oncology. 2010;**28**(35):5153-5159

[25] Brown WT, Wu X, Fayad F, Amendola BE, et al. CyberKnife radiosurgery for stage I lung cancer: Results at 36 months. Clinical Lung Cancer. 2007;**8**(8):488-492

[26] Nagata Y, Hiraoka M, Shibata T, et al. Stereotactic body radiation therapy for T1 N0 M0 non-small cell lung cancer. First reports for inoperable populations of a phase II trial by Japan clinical oncology group (JCOG 0403). International Journal of Radiation Oncology, Biology, Physics. 2012;**84**(suppl):s46

[27] Onishi H, Shirato H, Nagata Y, et al. Hypofractionated stereotactic radiotherapy for stage I non-small cell lung cancer. Updated results of 257 patients in a Japanese multi-institutional study. Journal of Thoracic Oncology. 2007;**2**(7 suppl 3):S94-S100

[28] Senthi S, Lagerward FJ, Haasbeek CJ, et al. Patterns of disease recurrence after stereotactic ablative radiotherapy for early stage non-small cell lung cancer: A retrospective analysis. The Lancet Oncology. 2012;**12**:802-809

[29] Van der Voort VZ, Prevost JB, Hogerman MS, et al. Stereotactic radiotherapy with real-time tumor tracking for non-small cell lung cancer: Clinical outcome. Radiation Oncology. 2009;**91**:296-300

[30] Yu J, Soulos P, Crammer L, et al. Comparative effectiveness of surgery and radiosurgery for stage I none-small cell lung cancer. Cancer. 2015;**121**:2341-2349

[31] Timmerman R, McGarry R, Yiannoutsos C, et al. Excessive toxicity when treating central tumors in a phase II study of stereotactic body radiation therapy for medically inoperable early-stage lung cancer. Journal of Clinical Oncology. 2006;**24**(30):4833-4839

[32] Fakiris AJ, McGarry R, Yiannnoutsos C, et al. Stereotactic body radiotherapy for early stage non-small cell carcinoma: Four year results of a prospective phase II study. International Journal of Radiation Oncology, Biology, Physics. 2009;**75**(3):677-682

[33] Bral S, Gevaert T, Linthout N, et al. Prospective risk-adapted strategy of stereotactic body radiotherapy for early stage non-small cell lung cancer. Results of phase II trial. International Journal of Radiation Oncology, Biology, Physics. 2011;**80**(5):1343-1349

[34] Chang J, Shirvani S, Loo B, et al. Primary lung cancer. In: Lo S, The B, Lu J. Stereotactic Body Radiation Therapy. Berlin: Springer Verlag; 2012

[35] McGarry RC, Papiez L, Williams MY, et al. Stereotactic body radiation therapy of early-stage non-small cell lung cancer: Phase I study. International Journal of Radiation Oncology, Biology, Physics. 2005;**64**(4):1010-1015

[36] Timmerman R, Papiez L, Mcgarry R, et al. Extracranial stereotactic radioablation: Results of phase I study in medically inoperable stage I no-small cell lung cancer. Chest. 2003;**124**(5):1946-1955

[37] JY C, Balter PA, Dong L, et al. Stereotactic body radiation therapy in centrally and superiorly located stage I or isolated recurrent non-cell lung cancer. International Journal of Radiation Oncology, Biology, Physics. 2008;**7284**:967-971

[38] Milano MT, Chen Y, Katz AW, et al. Central thoracic lesions treated with hypofractionated stereotactic body radiotherapy. Radiotherapy and Oncology. 2009;**91**(3):301-306

[39] Haasbeek CJ, Lagerwaard FJ, Slotman BJ, et al. Outcome of stereotactic ablative radiotherapy for centrally located early-stage lung cancer. Journal of Thoracic Oncology. 2011;**6**(12):2036-2043

[40] Rowe BP, Boffa DJ, WLD, et al. Stereotactic body radiotherapy for central lung tumors. Journal of Thoracic Oncology. 2012;**7**(9):1394-1399

[41] Oshiro Y, Aruga T, Tsuboi K, et al. Stereotactic body radiotherapy for lung tumors at the pulmonary hilum. Strahlentherapie und Onkologie. 2010;**186**(5):274-279

[42] Unger K, Ju A, Oermann E, et al. CyberKnife for hilar lung tumors: Report of clinical response and toxicity. Journal of Hematology & Oncology. 2010;**3**:39

[43] Baba F, Shibamoto Y, Ogino H, et al. Clinical outcomes of stereotactic body radiotherapy for stage I non-small cell lung cancer using different doses depending on tumor size. Radiation Oncology. 2010;**5**:81-88

[44] Mahmood S, Bilal H, Faivre-Finn C, et al. Is stereotactic ablative radiotherapy equivalent to sublobar resection in high-risk surgical patients with stage I non-small cell lung cancer? Interactive Cardiovascular and Thoracic Surgery. 2013;**17**(5):845-853

[45] Onishi H, Shirato H, Nagata Y, et al. Stereotactic body radiotherapy (SBRT) for operable stage I non-small cell lung cancer: Can SRBT be comparable to surgery. International Journal of Radiation Oncology, Biology, Physics. 2011;**81**(5):1352-1358

[46] Palma D, Visser D, Lagenward FJ, et al. Treatment of stage I NSCLC in elderly patients: A population-based matched-pair comparison of stereotactic radiotherapy versus surgery. Radiotherapy and Oncology. 2011;**101**(2):2404

[47] Lagenward FJ, Veretegen NE, Haasbeek CJ, et al. Outcome of stereotactic ablative radiotherapy in patients with potentially operative stage I non-small cell lung cancer. International Journal of Radiation Oncology, Biology, Physics. 2012;**83**(1):384-353

[48] Zenng X, Schipper M, Kidwel K, et al. Survival outcome after stereotactic body radiation therapy and surgery for stage I non-small cell lung cancer: A meta-analysis. International Journal of Radiation Oncology, Biology, Physics. 2014;**9083**:603-611

[49] Clinical/Trials.gov (Internet). Bethesda (MD): National Library of medicine (US), 2013 Apr 5—Identifier NCT00840749. Randomized Study to compare CyberKnife to Surgical resection in stage I Non-small cell lung cancer (STARS) 2209 Feb 7 (Edited 2015 Apr 13). Available from: https://clinicaltrials.gov/ct2/show/NCT00940749

[50] Clinical/Trials.gov (Internet). Bethesda (MD): National Library of medicine (US) 2015 jun 2 –Identifier NCT00687986. Trial of Either surgery or Stereotactic Radiotherapy for early Stage (IA) Lung Cancer (ROSEL): 2008 May 28. Available from: https://clinicaltrials.gov/ct2/show/NCT00687986

[51] Chong J, Senan S, Paul M, et al. Stereotactic ablative radiotherapy versus lobectomy for operable stage I non-small-cell lung cancer: A pooled analysis of two randomized trials. The Lancet. 2015;**16**:630-3757

[52] Nieder C, Andratsche N, Guckenberger M. A pooled analysis of ablative radiotherapy versus lobectomy for operable stage I non-small cell lung cancer: Is failure to recruit patients into randomized trials also an answer to the research question? Annals of Thoracic Medicine. 2015;**3**(11):148

[53] Rusthoven C, Kavanagh BD, Karam S. Improved survival with stereotactic ablative radiotherapy (SRABT) over lobectomy for early stage non-small cell lung cancer (NSCLC): Addressing the fallout of disruptive randomized data. Annals of Thoracic Medicine. 2015;**3**(11):149

[54] Santini A, Bruna M. Cáncer localizado e próstata, la visión del radioterapeuta. Tendencias en medicina. 2010: Noviembre 1-9

[55] Radiation Therapy Oncology Group [Internet]. Philadelphia: RTOG. 2015 Jun 8—RTOG 0813 Protocol Information, Seamless Phase I/II Study of Stereotactic Lung Radiotherapy (SBRT) for Early Stage, Centrally Located, Non-Small Cell Lung Cancer (NSCLC) in Medically Inoperable Patients; 2013 Sep 5 [cited 2015 Apr 13]; [about 10 screens]. Available from: https://www.rtog.org/ClinicalTrials/ProtocolTable/StudyDetails.aspx?study=0813

[56] Radiation Therapy Oncology Group [Internet]. Philadelphia: RTOG. 2014 Mar 6—RTOG 0915 Protocol Information, A Randomized Phase II Study Comparing 2 Stereotactic

[57] Gold MK, Donington J, Lynch WR, et al. Evaluation of individuals with pulmonary nodules when is it lung cancer? Diagnosis and management of lung cancer. 3ed ed. American College of chest Physician evidence based clinical practice guideline. Chest. 2013;**143**(5 Suppl):e935-e1205

[58] Hiraki Y, Mimura H, Gobara H, et al. CT fluoroscopy guided biopsy of 1000 pulmonary lesions performed with 20-gauge coaxial cutting needle diagnostic yield and risk factors for diagnostic failure. Chest. 2009;**136**(6):1612-1617

[59] Guckenberger M, Allgäuer M, Appold S, et al. Safety and efficacy of stereotactic body radiotherapy for stage I non-small cell lung cancer in routine clinical practice: A patterns of care and outcome analysis. Journal of Thoracic Oncology. 2013;**8**(8):1050-1058

[60] Loui A, Senan S, Patel P, et al. When is biopsy-proven diagnosis necessary before stereotactic ablative radiotherapy for lung cancer? Chest. 2014;**146**(4):1021-1028

[61] Auperin A, Le Pechoux C, Rolland E, et al. Meta-analysis of concomitant versus sequential radiochemotherapy in locally advanced non-small cell lung cancer. Journal of Clinical Oncology. 2010;**28**(13):2181-2190

[62] Cancer Council Australia Lung Cancer. Guideline Working Party. Clinical Practice Guideline for the treatment of lung cáncer. Sydney: Cancer Council Australia; 2015. Disponible en: http//Wiki.cancer.org.au/australia/Guideline:Lung_Cancer/Treatment/ Non_small-Cell/summary_ofrecomentadion (Revisado 21 de Septiembre 2017)

[63] Villar Alvarez F, Muguruza Trueba I, Belda Sanchis J, et al. Recomendaciones de SEPAR de diagnostico y tratamiento del cáncer de pulmón de células no pequeñas, Archivos de Bronconeumología. 2016;**52**(Supl 1):2-62

[64] Garrido P, Olmedo MªE. State of the art of radiotherapy. Transl Lung Cancer Res. 2013;**2**(3): 189-199

[65] Senan S. Treatment of stage IIIA non-small cell lung cancer: Charting the next step. Journal of Oncology Practice/American Society of Clinical Oncology. 2016:12609-12610

[66] Baker S, Dahele M, Lagerwaaard F, et al. A critical review of recent developments in radiotherapy for non-small cell lung cancer. Radiation Oncology. 2016;**11**:115-121

[67] Chun SG, Hu C, Choy H, et al. Comparison of 3-D conformal and intensity modulated radiation therapy outcomes for locally advanced none-small cell lung cancer. In NRG oncology/RTOG 0617. International Journal of Radiation Oncology, Biology, Physics. 2015;**93**(suppl 3):s1-2

[68] Mursshed H, Liu HH, Liao Z, et al. Dose and volume reduction for normally lung used intensity modulated radiotherapy for advanced-stage non-small cell lung cancer. International Journal of Radiation Oncology, Biology, Physics. 2004;**58**:1258-1267

[69] Sher DI, Koshy M, Liptay ML, et al. Influence of conformal radiotherapy technique on survival after chemoradiotherapy for patients with stage III non-small cell lung cancer in the national cancer data base. Cancer. 2014;**120**:260-268

[70] Jegadesh N, Liu Y, Gillespie T, et al. Evaluating intensity modulated radiation therapy in locally advanced non-small cell lung cancer, results from the national cancer data base. Clinical Lung Cancer. 2016;**17**(5):398-405. DOI: 10.1016/j.cllc.2016.01.007

[71] Slotman BJ, Lagerward FJ, Senan S. 4D imaging for target definition in stereotactic radiotherapy for lung cancer. Acta Oncologica. 2006;**45**(7):966-972

[72] Nuyttens J. Stereotactic radiotherapy for lung tumors. In: Gaya A, Mahadevan. Stereotactic Body Radiotherapy, a Practical Guide. London: Springer-Verlag; 2015

[73] Keall P. 4-dimensional computed tomography imaging and treatment planning. Seminars in Radiation Oncology. 2004;**14**(1):81-90

[74] Maciejcyk A, Skrzypczynska I, Janiszewska M, et al. Lung cancer. Radiotherapy in Lung cancer: Actual methods and future trends. Reports of Practical Oncology and Radiotherapy. 1014;**19**(6):353-360

[75] Gore EM, Bae K, Wing SJ, et al. Phase III comparison of prophylactic cranial irradiation versus observation in patients with locally advanced non-small cell lung cancer. Primary analysis of radiation therapy oncology group study RTOG 0214. Journal of Clinical Oncology. 2011;**29**(3):272-278

[76] Speruto PW, Kased N, Roberge D, et al. Summary report on the graded prognostic assessment: An accurate and facile diagnosis-specific tool to estimate survival for patients with brain metastases. Journal of Clinical Oncology. 2012;**30**(4):419-425

[77] Gaspar L, Scott C, Rotman M, et al. Recursive portioning analysis (RPA) of prognosis factors in three radiation therapy oncology group (RTOG) brain metastases trials. International Journal of Radiation Oncology, Biology, Physics. 1997;**37**(4):745-751

[78] Andrews DW, Scott CB, Sperduto PE, et al. Whole brain radiation therapy with or without stereotactic radiosurgery boost for patients with one to tree brain metastases. Phase III results of the RTOG 9508 randomized trial. Lancet. 2004;**363**(9422):1665-1672

[79] Ampil F, Ellika S, Nanda A, et al. Long-term survival after stereotactic radiosurgery of brain metastases: A case series with 10 year follow-up. Anticancer Research. 2017;**37**(9):5113-5115

[80] Pinkham MB, Sanghera P, Wall GK, et al. Neurocognitive effects following cranial irradiation for brain metastases. Clinical Oncology (Royal College of Radiologists). 2015;**27**(11):630-639

[81] Soffietti R, Kocher M, Abacioglu UM, et al. A European Organization for research and Treatment of Cancer phase III trial of adjuvant Whole-brain radiotherapy versus observation in patients with one to tree brain metastases from solid tumors after surgical resection or radiosurgery: Quality-of-life results. Journal of Clinical Oncology. 2013;**31**(1):65-72

[82] Gondini V, Pugh SL, Tome WA, et al. Preservation of the memory with conformal avoidance of the hippocampal neural stem-cell component during whole-brain radiotherapy for brain metastases (RTOG 0933): A phase II multi-institutional trial. Journal of Clinical Oncology. 2014;**32**(34):3810-3816

[83] Gondi V, Tome WA, Mehta MP, et al. Why avoid the hippocampus? A Comprehensive review. Radiotherapy and Oncology. 2010;**97**(3):370-376

[84] Wei J, Moran T, Zou Z, et al. Customized chemotherapy in metastatic non-small cell lung cancer. In: Damico et al. Lung Cancer First Edition. AME Publishing Company; 2016

[85] Folket M, Timmerman R. Review of treatment options for Oligometastatic non-small cell lung cancer. Clinical Advances in Hematology & Oncology. 2015;**13**(3):186-193

[86] Tree AC, Khoo VS, Eeles RA, et al. Stereotactic body radiotherapy for oligometastases. The Lancet Oncology. 2013;**14**(1):e28-e37

[87] Iyengar P, Wardak Z, Gerber DE, et al. Consolidative radiotherapy for limited metastatic non-small-cell lung cancer. A Phase 2 randomized clinical trial. JAMA Oncology. 2018;**4**(1): e173501

[88] Iyengar P, Kavanagh BD, Wardak Z, et al. Phase II trial of esterotáxica body radiation therapy combined with erlotinib for patients with limited but progressive metastatic no-small cell lung cancer. Journal of Clinical Oncology. 2014;**32**(34):3824-3830

[89] Marconi R, Strolin S, Bosi G, et al. A meta-analysis of the abscopal effects in preclinical models: Is the biologically effective dose relevant physical trigger? PLoS ONE. 2017;**21**:1-6

[90] Demaria S, Fomenti S. Can abscopal effects of local radiotherapy be predicted by modeling T cell trafficking? Journal for ImmunoTherapy of Cancer. 2016;**4**:29-31

[91] Widel M. Radiation induced Bystander effects: From in vivo studies to clinical application. International Journal of Medical Physics, Clinical Engineering and Radiation Oncology. 2016;(5):1-17

[92] Formenti SC, Demaria S. Systemic effects of local radiotherapy. The Lancet Oncology. 2009;**10**(7):718-26

[93] Longo D. Recent developments in radiotherapy. The New England Journal of Medicine. 2017;**14**:1065-1075

[94] Hinker SM, Chen DS, Reddy A, et al. A systemic complete response of metastatic melanoma to local radiation and immunotherapy. Translational Oncology. 2012;**5**:404-407

[95] Spiroto M, Fu YX, Weichselaun R. The interaction of radiotherapy an immunotherapy mechanisms an clinical implication. Science Immunology. 2016;**1**:1-12

[96] Zeng J, Baik C, Bhatia A, et al. Combination of stereotactic ablative body radiation therapy with targeted therapies. The Lancet Oncology. 2014;**15**:e426-e434

[97] Formenti S, Demaria S. Combining radiotherapy and cancer Immunotherapy: A paradigm Shift. Journal of the National Cancer Institute. 2013;**105**(4):256-265

[98] Daly M, Monjazeb A, Kelly K. Clinical trials integrating immunotherapy and radiation for non-small cell lung cancer. Journal of Thoracic Oncology. 2015;**10**:1685-1693

[99] Crittenden M, Kohrt H, Levy R, et al. Current clinical trials testing combinations of immunotherapy and radiation. Seminars in Radiation Oncology. 2015;**25**:54-64

5

Management of Brain Metastases from Solid Tumors

Roman Liubota, Roman Vereshchako,
Mykola Anikusko and Iryna Liubota

Abstract

Brain metastases (BM) are most common intracranial tumors in adults. Recently, significant progress has been shown in diagnosing, prognosis, and treating patients with BM of various malignant tumors. The treatment decisions must be based on the disease prognosis and include radiation therapy, surgery, systemic antitumor therapy, or a combination thereof. Systemic therapy capable of preventing BM or which affects both intracranial and extracranial disease is of paramount importance in the treatment of BM patients. The purpose of this chapter is to consider important prognostic factors that can determine treatment decisions, review the role of blood–brain barrier (BBB), and systemic anticancer treatment to manage BM from solid tumors.

Keywords: brain metastases, solid tumors, prognostic scores, blood–brain barrier, systemic anticancer treatment

1. Introduction

Brain tumors constitute for 85–90% of all tumors of the central nervous system (CNS) [1]. Brain metastases (BM) are ten times more prevalent than primary tumors of the central nervous system (CNS) and are diagnosed in 10–20% of all cancer patients. The frequency of detection of BM is steadily increasing, which can be explained by such causes. First, this may be due to the increased availability and improvement of diagnostic methods for brain tumors. Second, the use of screening brain examinations of patients with tumors has a high incidence of the CNS metastases. Third, the improved effectiveness of anticancer treatment leads to increased overall survival rates of patients and increased risk of developing BM [2]. All malignant tumors have the potential to provide distant metastasis to the brain. Approximately 75% of all cases of brain metastases are due to patients with lung cancer (40–50%), breast cancer (15–25%), and melanoma (5–20%) [1]. Among the remaining 25%, BM is more predominant in patients with renal cell cancer (4–17%) and gastrointestinal cancer (0.6–3%) [3, 4]. At autopsy, BM are found to be 1.5–3 times more frequent and are detected in more than 65% of patients with lung cancer, 30–40% of patients with malignant melanoma (MM), and 30% of patients with breast cancer (BC). About 85% of metastatic lesions are located in the brain hemispheres, 15% in the cerebellum, and 5% in the brain stem [5].

The aim of this review is to consider important prognostic factors that can determine the treatment decisions and to review the role of blood–brain barrier (BBB) and systemic anticancer treatment (SAT) to manage BM from solid tumors.

2. Determination of prognosis of patients with brain metastases

The BM patients have significantly worsened the prognosis because the median overall survival (OS) in BM cases varies from 2.79 to 25.3 months. The disease prognosis depends on a number of factors that must be taken into account when determining the treatment algorithm of patients with BM. **Table 1** presents prognostic scales assessment of the prognosis in patients with cerebral metastases [6].

Table 1 presents the assessment scales of the overall survival prognosis of brain metastases patients have a number of limitations who restrict their use in routine clinical practice and clinical trials. The Recursive partitioning analysis (RPA) scale can be used only if the patient is shown to be carrying out the whole brain radiotherapy (WBRT). RPA cannot be used on patients who underwent palliative surgery, stereotactic radiosurgery (SRS), and/or systemic anticancer therapy, but this treatment option has significant effect on BM patient's survival. Another limiting factor of the RPA score system is that it does not take into account the size and number of BM. The drawbacks of the Rotterdam score system are the lack of consideration of the patient's age, number, and size of BM. The most complete predictive system is the Score

Prognostic factors	RPA	Rotterdam score	SIR	BSBM	GPA	DS-GPA
Age	+	−	+	−	+	+
Performance status	KPS	ECOG	KPS	KPS	KPS	KPS
Extracranial metastases	+	+	+	+	+	+
Control of primary tumor	+	−	+	+	−	−
Number of BM	−	−	+	−	+	+
Volume of BM	−	−	+	−	−	−
Response to steroids	−	+	−	−	−	−
Number of classes	3	3	3	4	4	4

RPA: Recursive partitioning analysis; SIR: Score Index for Radiosurgery; BSBM: Basic Score for Brain Metastases; GPA: Graded Prognostic Assessment; DS-GPA: Disease specific Graded Prognostic Assessment; KPS: Karnofsky performance status; ECOG: Eastern Cooperative Oncology Group Score.

Table 1. Prognostic scores for brain metastasis patients.

Index for Radiosurgery (SIR) scale, but it has not been widely used in clinical practice since it does not take into account systemic influence to disease. The Basic Score for Brain Metastases (BSBM) scale is an analogue of RPA scale and takes into account the impact of SRS on the survival of BM patients, but it does not take into account the patient's age and the effectiveness of systemic drug therapy. In 2007, the Graded Prognostic Assessment (GPA) scoring system was proposed, which took into account four factors: age, Karnofsky performance status (KPS), availability of extracranial metastases, and the number of BM. A number of studies have proved the prognostic significance of these indicators, and the GPA scale is recognized as the most objective and most commonly used scoring system for survival prognosis of BM patients. However, GPA system does not consider the influence of primary tumor type for prognosis of BM, which has different sensitivity to the drug and radiation therapy. To account the influence of the prognostic value of the histological and molecular type of the primary tumor, a Disease Specific Graded Prognostic Assessment (DS-GPA) system was developed. **Table 2** presents the factors and prognosis of overall survival rates of patients with BM from lung cancer, MM, BC, renal cell (RCC), and gastrointestinal cancer (GI) [7].

Prognostic factor	GPA scale score					Total score	Median of overall survival, months (95% CI)	
	0	0.5	1.0	—	—			
Lung cancer								
Age (years)	>60	50–60	<50	—	—		NSCLC	SCLC
KPS	<70	70–80	90–100	—	—	0–1	3.02 (2.63–3.84)	2.79 (1.83–3.12)
Extracranial metastases	Yes	n/a	No	—	—	1.5–2.0	5.49 (4.83–6.40)	4.90 (4.04–6.51)
				—	—	2.5–3.0	9.43 (8.38–10.80)	7.67 (6.27–9.13)
Number of BM	>3	2–3	1	—	—	3.5–4.0	14.78 (11.80–18.80)	17.05 (4.70–27.43)
Malignant melanoma								
Prognostic factor	GPA scale score					Total score	Median of overall survival, months (95% CI)	
	0	1.0	2.0	—	—			
KPS	<70	70–80	90–100	—	—	0–1	3.38 (2.53–4.27)	
Number of BM	>3	2–3	1	—	—	1.5–2.0	4.7 (4.07–5.39)	
						2.5–3.0	8.77 (6.74–10.77)	
						3.5–4.0	13.23 (9.13–15.64)	
Breast cancer								
Prognostic factor	GPA scale score					Total score	Median of overall survival, months (95% CI)	
	0	0.5	1.0	1.5	2.0			
Age (years)	≥60	<60	—	—	—	0–1	3.35 (3.13–3.78)	

Prognostic factor	GPA scale score					Total score	Median of overall survival, months (95% CI)
	0	0.5	1.0	—	—		
KPS	≤ 50	60	70–80	90–100	—	1.5–2.0	7.70 (5.62–8.74)
Molecular type	Triple negative	—	Lum A	HER2-type	Lum B	2.5–3.0	15.07 (12.94–15.87)
						3.5–4.0	25.30 (23.10–26.51)

Renal cell cancer

Prognostic factor	GPA scale score					Total score	Median of overall survival, months (95% CI)
	0	1.0	2.0	—	—		
KPS	<70	70–80	90–100			0–1	3.27 (2.04–5.10)
Number of BM	>3	2–3	1			1.5–2.0	7.29 (3.73–10.91)
						2.5–3.0	11.27 (8.80–14.80)
						3.5–4.0	14.77 (9.73–19.79)

Gastrointestinal cancer

Prognostic factor	GPA scale score					Total score	Median of overall survival, months (95% CI)
	0	1.0	2.0	3.0	4.0		
KPS	< 70	70	80	90	100	0–1	3.13 (2.37–4.57)
						1.5–2.0	4.40 (3.37–6.53)
						2.5–3.0	6.87 (4.86–11.63)
						3.5–4.0	13.54 (9.76–27.12)

NSCLC: non-small cell lung cancer; SCLC: small cell lung cancer; KPS: Karnofsky performance status; n/a: not applicable; ER: estrogen receptors; PR: progesterone receptors; Her2/neu (ErbB2): human epidermal growth factor receptor 2; Triple negative: ER-negative, PR-negative, Her2/neu-negative; Lum A: ER-positive and/or PR-positive, Her2/neu-negative; HER2-type: ER-negative, PR-negative, Her2/neu-overexpression/amplification; Lum B: ER-positive and/or PR-positive, Her2/neu-overexpression/amplification.

Table 2. Median of overall patient survival with BM from solid tumors according to the DS-GPA scale prognosis indices.

Prognostic scores are very important to take decisions on the most appropriate treatment options for patients with BM in each case. The need for palliative treatment for patients with poor prognosis is controversial, but patients with good prognosis must receive multidisciplinary palliative therapy to increase overall survival rates [8]. Moreover, prognostic score systems can be used to increase the applicability, objectivity, and validity of the clinical trial results that investigate the effectiveness of treatment in patients with BM from various malignant tumors.

3. Role of the blood-brain barrier in the formation of brain metastases

The blood-brain barrier (BBB) plays a prominent role in the brain colonization by malignant tumor cells and determines the effectiveness of drug therapy. BBB is a natural obstacle for the penetration of malignant tumor cells within the brain parenchyma. Endothelial cells of brain vessels serve as a mechanical barrier, and astrocytes and microglia are capable of destroying tumor cells. However, after brain colonization, the cerebral endothelial cells, astrocytes, and microglia provide crucial support in the growth and proliferation of tumor cells, and BBB protects cancer cells from influencing the immune system and most anticancer drugs [9].

The penetration of the BBB depends on its functional condition, as well as on the morphological, molecular, and genetic characteristics of tumor cells, that may explain the opportunity of some malignant cells to easily overcome this highly selective barrier relatively. For example, the compound density reduction of the cerebral endothelial cells, which increase the permeability of BBB, was detected in severe CNS diseases such as Alzheimer's disease, multiple sclerosis, and primary and metastatic brain tumors [10]. The expression CDH2 (N-cadherin), KIFC1, and FALZ genes in a primary tumor in lung cancer patients with BM determine the high cerebral metastatic potential of lung cancer cells. The CDH2 gene encoded N-cadherin (cadherin-2 or neural cadherin (NCAD)) is involved in tumor progression, such as migration and invasion of tumor cells, including in the CNS. Also, in non-small cell lung cancer, patients' expression of DCUN1D1 squamous cell carcinoma-associated oncogene may promote the tumor cell migration through the BBB and development of BM. High KLF6-SV1 expression in prostate cancer cells associated with poor patient's survival predict a high risk of lymph nodes, brain, and bones metastasis [11]. Several factors have been identified in breast cancer cells that promote the BC cell migration through the BBB, such as cyclooxygenase-2 (COX2), heparin-binding epidermal growth factor-like growth factor (HB-EGF), and ST6GALNAC5 ((alpha-N-acetyl-neuraminyl-2,3-beta-galactosyl-1,3)-N-acetylgalactosaminide-alpha-2,6-sialyltransferase 5 ST6). The ST6GALNAC5 gene expression is recognized as a tumor cells BBB migration specific marker because COX2 and HB-EGF are associated with the brain and lung metastases. In vitro studies of melanoma cells were shown to increase the BBB permeability by reduce transendothelial electrical resistance of endothelial cells. Expression of melanotransferrin (MELTF, CD228, MAP97, MTF1, MTf, MFI2) and signal transducer and transcriptional activator 3 (STAT3) can serve as potential markers of cerebral metastases in patients with melanoma. The availability of MELTF on the melanoma cell membrane determines their ability to penetrate through the BBB. High levels of STAT3 in melanoma BM compared to primary tumor cells indicate a relationship between STAT3 expression and tumor cell migration to the brain [9]. Thus, the identification of tumor cells specific markers of penetration through the BBB can be a basis for the development of specific methods for the prevention of BM. The main factor of the BM treatment resistance is BBB efflux transporters which prevent the drug's penetration into the brain parenchyma. **Table 3** shows the main drug efflux transporters of the BBB and their substrates and inhibitors [12].

P-glycoprotein (Pgp, gp170) is a protein encoded by the gene MDR1 (multidrug resistance 1) whose main function is the active removal of many different substances, including some drugs, from the cell cytoplasm to the intercellular environment. Pgp molecules are found in the proximity of the apical membrane of the choroid plexus secretory cells and at the luminal membrane of the brain capillary, which allows transferring most of the Pgp substrates from the endothelium and parenchyma of the BM to the cerebrospinal fluid and blood. The role of Pgp in the maintenance of BBB was investigated through in vivo studies. Studies conducted on MDR1 gene knockout mice revealed an increased effect on brain parenchyma of parenterally administered P-glycoprotein substrates compared with wild-type mice. The use

Efflux transporter	Substrates	Inhibitors
P-glycoprotein	Doxorubicin, daunorubicin, docetaxel, paclitaxel, epirubicin, idarubicin, vinblastine, vincristine, etoposide	Verapamil, cyclosporine A, quinidine, valspodar, elacridar, biricodar, zosuquidar, tariquidar
MRP1	Etoposide, teniposide, daunorubicin, doxorubicin, epirubicin, melphalan, vincristine, vinblastine	Probenecid, sulfinpyrazone, MK-571, cyclosporin A, verapamil, valspodar
MRP2		Probenecid, MK-571, leukotriene C4
MRP3		Sulfinpyrazone, indomethacin, probenecid
MRP4	Methotrexate, 6-mercaptopurine, thioguanine	Probenecid
MRP5	6-Mercaptopurine, thioguanine	Probenecid, sildenafil
MRP6	Actinomycin D, cisplatin, daunorubicin, doxorubicin, etoposide	Probenecid, indomethacin
BCRP	Mitoxantrone, methotrexate, SN-38, topotecan, imatinib, erlotinib, gefitinib	Elacridar, fumitremorgin C

Table 3. Substrates and inhibitors of the main drug efflux transporters of the BBB.

of Pgp-inhibitors in wild-type animals was accompanied by an increase in the brain penetration of Pgp substrates including anticancer drugs (vincristine, paclitaxel, daunorubicin, etc.). Similar results were obtained on using P-glycoprotein inhibitors (verapamil and cyclosporin A) to increase the BBB penetration [7].

Multidrug resistance-associated proteins (MRP) are the ABCC family of transporter (ATP-binding cassette subfamily C) proteins, which are an important component determining the selective permeability of the BBB for different drugs [13]. In vivo studies performed on mice with knockout of the MRP1 gene were found to have higher accumulation of MRP1 substrates, including etoposide versus wild-type mice. And after the use of the inhibitor MRP1 (probenecid), a double increase in the concentration of fluorescein in the brain was observed [7].

Breast cancer-resistant protein (BCRP, ABCG2). ABCG2 (ATP-binding cassette subfamily G member 2) is an efflux transporter called the breast cancer resistance protein, since it was first detected in the drug-resistant MCF-7 human breast cancer cells [14]. BCRP is an important component in determining BBB permeability, and its concentration in the CNS endothelium is greater than the P-glycoprotein and MRP1 concentrations. In mice with BCRP1 gene knockout, the imatinib concentration in the brain parenchyma was increased 2.5-fold in knockout versus control mice. The administration of a BCRP inhibitor (elacridar) in wild-type mice results in an increase in the penetration of imatinib 4.2 times, while in knockout MDR1 gene mice, elacridar increases cerebral cells absorption of BCRP substrates such as prazosin and mitoxantrone [15].

The structure of BBB in brain metastatic tumors has some features. In contrast to the normal cerebral vascular network, the brain metastases have an increased perivascular space, number, and activity of pinocytotic vacuoles in endothelial cells; these features are more typical for tumor vessels than for the CNS vessels. Thus, metastatic tumor BBB is more permeable than in the normal CNS parenchyma and is more likely to be a capillary barrier than a performed BBB [7].

3.1. Influence of radiation therapy on the BBB permeability

Brain radiotherapy is the standard of palliative care as per the guidelines of clinical practice for patients with BM. In several in vivo studies in rats after brain radiation were such changes observed: dilation and thickening of the blood vessel wall, increase of endothelial cell nuclei, astrocyte hypertrophy, and 60% decrease the P- glycoprotein concentration [7]. These changes in the brain of rats were a prerequisite for a hypothesis about influence of radiation to the BBB permeability and increase in the clinical effectiveness of chemotherapy in patients with BM, because radiation could raise the penetration of anticancer drugs into the brain parenchyma. Murrell D.H., et al. (2016) did not found changes in BBB permeability at the 1st and 11th days after radiation in mice after WBRT therapeutically relevant doses to human equivalent doses. The results of clinical studies have not revealed an increase in clinical effectiveness in the concurrent use of radiation and chemotherapy [16]. The BBB permeability modification under the influence of radiation on the BM at the moment is controversial and needs further study.

3.2. Increasing of drug's penetrations through the BBB

The ideal compound to treat BM must have the following physicochemical properties such as low molecular weight, lipophilicity, and absence of ionization at physiological pH. Physicochemical properties of most anticancer drugs not match the above specifications, that limit BBB permeability of drugs, and was a basis for developing ways to deliver drugs to the brain. There are several ways to improve the delivery of substances to the central nervous system, for example, the BBB opening under conditions of temporary osmotic shock, the use of chemical vectors (transporters), increasing the dose and the frequency of drug administration, the use of implants from biodegradable materials, and so on. All methods of increasing drug delivery to the CNS can be attributed to one or more of the three main approaches: change in the chemical structure and/or physicochemical properties, and/or drug dose (concentration), increasing the BBB permeability, and using alternative routes of administration. The low efficiency of most approaches, with the need for performing technically complex manipulations that are accompanied by pronounced side effects and complications, limits their use in everyday clinical practice [17].

The most available methods for improving the drug delivery to BM in routine clinical practice are the use of nanoparticles and efflux transporters inhibitors (**Table 3**). Application of nanoparticles for targeted drug delivery has several advantages: overcoming chemoresistance, increasing the drug bioavailability and specificity, dose reduction without loss of efficacy, and reduction in adverse reactions. The clinical studies performed on the effectiveness of the nanoparticle application with anticancer drugs served as a basis for the use of these drugs as standard therapy for BM patients. **Table 4** shows chemotherapeutic drugs with nanoparticles, the use of which has been approved by the US Food and Drug Administration (FDA) for the treatment BM patients [18].

The clinical trial results of the efficacy of anticancer nanomedicines and efflux transporter inhibitors in BM patients are encouraging, but further trials are needed to study biodistribution, pharmacokinetics, toxicity, and side effects for inclusion of this drug practice guidelines for the management of CNS tumors.

Name	Description	Indication
DaunoXome	Liposomal daunorubicin	First-line therapy against advanced Kaposi's sarcoma associated with HIV
DepoCyt	Liposomal cytarabine	Lymphomatous meningitis
Oncaspar	L-asparaginase conjugated with monomethoxypolyethylene glycol (mPEG)	Acute lymphoblastic leukemia
Abraxane	Albumin-bound paclitaxel nanospheres	Pancreatic cancer, NSCLC, breast cancer
Myocet	Liposomal doxorubicin	Breast cancer
Marqibo	Liposomal vincristine	Acute lymphoblastic leukemia
Genexol	Paclitaxel-loaded polymeric micelle	Breast cancer, NSCLC, ovarian cancer
Onivyde	Liposomal irinotecan	Pancreatic cancer

Table 4. Anticancer nanomedicines approved by the FDA.

4. Decision-making of palliative care options of BM patients

The decision-making of BM patient's treatment must rely on some factors such as: the patient Karnofsky performance status; the number, size, and location of BM; the primary tumor type; and the presence and control of extracranial metastases. **Table 5** presents palliative treatment options of BM patients depending on the set of predictive factors listed above [7].

Type of palliative treatment	Indications
Systemic anticancer therapy	- BM from systemic anticancer therapy-sensitive primary tumor;
	- Asymptomatic BM, detected during planning of systemic anticancer therapy;
	- BM from PT with identified molecular alteration amenable to targeted therapy;
	- Poor effect of other treatment options in case presence of potentially effective systemic anticancer agents.
Whole brain radiotherapy	- Multiple MGM (> 3–10), especially if the primary tumor is sensitive to radiation therapy;
	- Large (4 cm) BM;
	- After surgical resection of a dominant large metastatic tumor and the presence of multiple BM (> 3–10);
	- BM disease progression during systemic drug therapy;
	- Salvage therapy for recurrent BM after SRS or WBRT failure.
SRS	- Oligo-BM or multi-BM (≤3), especially if primary tumor is known to be radiotherapy resistant;
	- After surgical resection of a single BM if it diameter > 3 cm and/or BM localized in the posterior cranial fossa;
	- Local recurrence after surgical resection of a single BM;
	- Salvage therapy for recurrent oligo-BM or multi-BM (≤ 3) after WBRT failure.

Type of palliative treatment	Indications
Surgical resection	- BM localized (or most of it) in the brain critical structures (eyes, optical tracts, brainstem, etc.); - Oligo-BM (1–2), especially when associated with extensive brain swelling; - If morphological examination of CNS lesions is necessary.
Supportive care alone	- Systemic disease progression after several types of palliative therapy in patients with poor performance status.

SACT: systemic anticancer therapy, WBRT: whole brain radiotherapy, SRS: stereotactic radiosurgery.

Table 5. Decision-making of palliative treatment options of BM patients.

According to **Table 5**, patients with brain metastases are not receiving anticancer therapy only if they have progression of the disease after receiving several types of anticancer therapy and them performance status stay poor after adequate supportive care [19].

5. Systemic anticancer therapy for BM patients

The evidence of the effectiveness of systemic anticancer therapy in patients with BM is contradictory. Nevertheless, SACT may be an effective treatment option for patients with BM, because it prolongs overall survival, especially in patients with metastatic lesions in other organs, since the progression of extracranial metastases is a common cause of death of most patients [20]. The BBB is a natural barrier for most anticancer drugs, and it is the primary mechanism responsible for BM resistance to systemic therapy. Several retrospective clinical studies determined that the chemotherapy was effective in 4–38% of patients with BM having various solid tumors [21]. Results are found to be limited on randomized trials on the effectiveness of anticancer drugs, which hinder the development of a generally accepted strategy for effective SACT of BM, especially in patients without extracranial metastases and/or progression after BM local therapy (surgery, radiotherapy). **Table 6** presents the effectiveness of chemotherapy in patients with brain metastases from NSCLC, melanoma, and breast cancer.

In a study performed by Franciosi et al. (1999), 107 patients with BM received a combination of cisplatin 100 mg/m^2 (IV day 1) + etoposide 100 mg/m^2 (IV on days 1, 3, and 5 or on days 4, 6, and 8) every 21 days, was continued to a maximum of 6 cycles. The distribution according to the primary tumor site was non-small cell lung cancer in 43 (40%) patients, breast cancer in 56 patients (52%), and malignant melanoma in 8 (8%). Among the 107 patients with BM, 7 BC patients achieved complete response (CR) (13%), 3 NSCLC patients achieved CR (7%), and none of the 8 MM patients achieved an objective response. The objective response rate (ORR) of the chemotherapy (CR + partial response (PR)) was recorded in 37.5% of patients with BC and in 30% of patients with NSCLC. The median survival was 7.5 months (range 0–91.5+ months) for patients with NSCLC, 7.2 months (range 0–67 months) for patients with BC, and 4.0 months (range 0.5–11.2 months) for patients with MM. This chemotherapy regime is effective for patients with BM from BC and NSCLC [22].

Chemotherapy regimen	Primary tumor type	Number of patients	Response rate	Median overall survival (months)
Cisplatin + etoposide	NSCLC, breast cancer, melanoma	Total 107 (100%): NSCLC–43(40%), BC–56 (52%), MM–8 (8%)	Total 34 (32%): NSCLC–13 (30%), BC–21 (37.5%), MM–0	NSCLC–7.5 (0–91,5+), BC–7.2 (0–67), MM–4.0 (0,5–11.2)
Etirinotecan pegol	BC	32	5 (15.6%)	All molecular types - 10 (7,8–15.7); Triple negative – 7,6; Lum A and B–12.2; HER2-type–16.1.
Temozolomide	NSCLC, breast cancer, melanoma	Total 157 (100%): NSCLC–53(34%), BC–51 (32%), MM–53 (34%)	Total 10 (6%): NSCLC–3 (6%), BC–2 (4%), MM–5 (9%)	NSCLC–5.7; BC–n/a, MM–3.3.
Gemcitabine + carboplatin	NSCLC	66	56 (29%)	7.6 (6.3–10.1)
Gemcitabine + paclitaxel		64		8.2 (4.6–10.5)
Carboplatin + paclitaxel		64		7.7 (6.1–10.2)
Cisplatin + gemcitabine	BC	30	16 (53.3%)	10
		18	All molecular types: 6 (33.4%); Triple negative: 66.6%, Lum A and B: 25%, HER2-type: 12.5%	Median PFS: All molecular types – 5.6 (2.4–8.8); Triple negative – 7.4 (2.4–12.3); Luml A and B: –3.6; HER2-type: 5.
Carmustine + methotrexate	BC	48	11 (23%)	All molecular types: 6.9 (4.2–10.7); Her2/neu: overexpression/amplification ($n = 8$): 14,1; Her2/neu-negative: 5.9 (3,9–8.2).
Pemetrexed	NSCLC	39	15 (38.4%)	10

Chemotherapy regimen	Primary tumor type	Number of patients	Response rate	Median overall survival (months)
Pemetrexed + cisplatin	NSCLC	43	18 (41.9%)	7.4 (5.8–9.6)
Capecitabine + lapatinib	BC with Her2/neu: overexpression/amplification	799	29.2% (18.5–42.7)	11.2 (8.9–14.1)

NSCLC: non-small cell lung cancer, BC: breast cancer, MM: malignant melanoma, Triple negative: ER-negative, PR-negative, Her2/neu-negative; Lum A: ER-positive and/or PR-positive, Her2/neu-negative; HER2-type: ER-negative, PR-negative, Her2/neu-overexpression/amplification; Lum B: ER-positive and/or PR-positive, Her2/neu-overexpression/amplification, n/a: not applicable.

Table 6. The efficacy of systemic chemotherapy in patients with brain metastases.

In open-label, multicentre, randomised phase 3 study (BEACON; BrEAst Cancer Outcomes with NKTR-102), was study the effectiveness of etirinotecan pegol 145 mg/m² (IV day 1 every 3 weeks) monotherapy in 32 BC patients with BM previously treated with an anthracyclines, a taxanes, and capecitabine. In this study, there were no recorded cases of CR, partial response was detected only in 5 (15.6%), and 14 (43.8%) patients had disease progression. With a median follow-up of 21.1 months, the progression-free survival (PFS) for 32 patients was 3.1 months (range 1.8–4.0 months), and the median OS 10 months (range 7.8–15.7 months). The efficacy of etirinotecan pegol in BM patients depended on the BC molecular type and median OS was: 16.1 months in HER2-type, 12.2 months in luminal A and B types, and 7.6 months in patients with triple negative BC. The results of the BEACON study recommend the etirinotecan pegol for treatment in BM patients with HER2-type and luminal breast cancer types [23].

Siena and co-workers (2010) reported on a nonrandomized multicenter phase II study of 157 patients with cerebral metastases of NSCLC 53 (34%), BC 51 (32%), and melanoma 53 (34%) who received temozolomide 150 mg/m² per day (oral administration for 1–7 and 15–21 days every 28 or 35 days). The BM complete response was recorded in one (<1%) patient with NSCLC. Among 157 patients, 9 (6%) had PR, and stabilization of disease (SD) was detected in 31 (20%) of 157 patients. The PFS was 66, 58, and 56 days for NSCLC, breast cancer, and melanoma BM patients, respectively. The median OS for patients with NSCLC was 172 days, melanoma was 100 days, and was not applicable in the breast cancer group. The results of this study indicate a low effectiveness of high dose-dense temozolomide regimen for the treatment of brain metastases from NSCLC, BC, and melanoma [24].

At randomized phase 3 clinical trial comparing 3 chemotherapy regimens in 194 patients with clinically stable BM from NSCLC, all patients were randomized into 3 groups: group 1 ($n = 66$) received the gemcitabine 1000 mg/m² (on days 1 and 8) + carboplatin AUC 5.5 (on day 1), group 2 ($n = 64$) received gemcitabine 1000 mg/m² (on days 1 and 8) + paclitaxel 200 mg/m² (on day 1), and group 3 ($n = 64$) received carboplatin AUC 5.5 (on day 1) + paclitaxel 225 mg/m² (on day 1) IV every 3 weeks, was continued to a maximum of 6 cycles. The study results showed the same clinical efficacy for all three regimens. Median OS was 7.6 months (range 6.3–10.1 months) for patients from group 1, 8.2 months (range 4.6–10.5 months) for group 2, and 7.7 months (range 6.1–10.2 months) for group 3 [25].

Two studies evaluated the efficacy of BM patients from BC treatment with cisplatin + gemcitabine chemotherapy regimen. Naskhletashvili and colleagues reported results of treatment in 30 patients with BC brain metastases who received cisplatin 50 mg/m² (on days 1 and 8) + gemcitabine 1000 mg/m² (on days 1 and 8) IV every 3–4 weeks. ORR for chemotherapy was recorded in 6 (53.3%) patients, and the median OS was 10 months [26]. Similar results were obtained by Erten et al. [27]. In this study, 18 BC patients with BM who were treated with cisplatin 30 mg/m² (on days 1 and 8) + gemcitabine 1000 mg/m² (on days 1 and 8) IV every 21 days. The ORR depended on the primary tumor molecular type and was 33.4% for all BC molecular types, 66.6% for triple-negative BC, 25% for luminal types, and 12.5% for patients with HER2- type. The overall survival rates of these study patients have not been reported. Median PFS also depended on the type of breast cancer and was greatest in patients with triple-negative breast cancer at 7.4 months (range 2.4–12.3 months); in patients with HER2-type at 5 months, with luminal types at 3.6 and 5.6 months (range 2.6–8.8 months) for all breast cancer molecular types [27].

Jacot and co-workers reported on 48 breast cancer patients treated with carmustine 100 mg/m^2 (on day 1) + methotrexate 600 mg/m^2 (on days 1 and 15) IV of a 28-day cycle. Patients with Her2/neu overexpression and/or amplification received trastuzumab 4 mg/kg (on days 1 and 15) IV during each cycle of chemotherapy. The ORR was detected in 11 (23%) patients. The PFS was 4.2 months (range 2.8–5.3 months), and the median OS at 6.9 months (range 4.2–10.7 months) for all BC molecular type. The median OS was different in patients with the Her2/neu overexpression and/or amplification tumors (14.1 months) and without Her2/neu overexpression and/or amplification BC (5.9 months) [28].

The efficacy of pemetrexed in NSCLC patients with BM was evaluated in several studies. Bearz et al. (2009) reported about clinically significant efficacy monotherapy of pemetrexed 500 mg/m^2 IV (on day 1) every 3 weeks as a 2- or 3-line chemotherapy. ORR was detected in 15 (38.4%) from 39 patients with BM from NSCLC, and median OS was 10 months. Barlesi et al. (2011) evaluated the efficacy of the regimen pemetrexed 500 mg/m^2 + cisplatin 75 mg/m^2 (IV on day 1) every 3 weeks for 6 cycles. The ORR was recorded in 18 (41.9%) of 43 patients with BM from NSCLC, and the median OS was 7.4 months (range 5.8–9.6 months). The concurrent administration of WBRT with chemotherapy pemetrexed + cisplatin significantly increases the treatment effectiveness according to the results obtained by Dinglin et al. (2013). The ORR of the pemetrexed + cisplatin + WBRT regimen was detected in 28 (68.3%) of 41 NSCLC patients with BM, and median OS was 12.6 months [29].

The efficacy of combination capecitabine and lapatinib for the treatment of Her2/neu overexpression on BC patients with BM has been investigated in several studies. A systematic review and meta-analysis of 12 studies, for total 799 patients with BM from Her2/neu-positive breast cancer, was show revealed ORR was 21.4% (range 11.7-35.9). After excluding from the analysis patients who received lapatinib alone, the ORR was 29.2% (range 18.5–42.7). The median OS of patients with BM from Her2/neu-positive BC was 11.2 months (range 8.9–14.1 months), and PFS was 4.1 months (range 3.1–6.7 months) [30].

The targeted therapies and immunotherapies that have the significant efficacy for treatment on patients with BM from various malignant tumors are presented in **Table 7**.

Iuchi et al. [31] reported on 41 patients with BM from epidermal growth factor receptors (EGFR) mutant lung adenocarcinoma treated with gefitinib. Patients were assigned gefitinib 250 mg/day until the disease progression or development of unacceptable toxicity. The ORR was 87.8%, and the median OS and PFR were 21.9 months (range 18.5–30.3 months) 14.5 months (range 10.2–18.3 months), respectively [31].

Gerber and associates [32] presented the results of treatment on 110 patients with BM EGFR-mutated lung adenocarcinoma. Depending on the treatment regimen, all patients were divided into 3 groups: group 1 (n = 63) patients who received erlotinib day until the disease progression or development of unacceptable toxicity, group 2 (n = 32) was treated only WBRT, group 3 (n = 15) was treated only SRS. The median OS of all 110 patients was 33 months: 26 months in group 1 and 35 and 63 months in groups 2 and 3, respectively [32].

An open-label, single-arm, phase 2, multicenter study was performed to investigate the efficacy of vemurafenib in 146 patients with BM from BRAFV600-mutated melanoma. Patients were divided into two cohorts: cohort 1 (n = 90) patients who had not previously received BM

Name	Primary tumor type	Number of patients	Response rate	Median overall survival (months)
Gefitinib	NSCLC	41	36 (87.8%)	21.9 (18.5–30.3)
Erlotinib		63	n/a	26
Vemurafenib	MM	cohort 1–90	16 (18%)	8.9 (0.6–34.5)
		cohort 2–56	10 (18%)	9.6 (0.7–34.3)
Dabrafenib		cohort 1–89	cohort 1	cohort 1
		cohort 2–83	V600E–39%	V600E–7.6;
			V600 K–31%	V600K–3.7;
			cohort 2	cohort 2
			V600E–7%	V600E–7.2;
			V600 K–22%	V600 K–5.0;
Crizotinib	NSCLC	20	3 (15%)	10.3
Ceritinib	NSCLC	124 (ASCEND-1)	10* (36%)	n/a
		140 (ASCEND-2)	54 (38.6%)	n/a
		50 (ASCEND-3)	29 (58%)	n/a
Alectinib	NSCLC	136 (100%)	32* (64%)	n/a
		50* (37%)	37** (43%)	
		86** (63%)		
Bevacizumab + carboplatin + paclitaxel		67	42 (62.7%)	16
Trastuzumab	BC	56	n/a	10.5 (8.3–17.7)
Lapatinib		30	n/a	21.4 (12.5–27.1)
Trastuzumab + lapatinib		28	n/a	25.9 (18.5–30.1)
Ipilimumab	MM	cohort A–51	cohort A	cohort A
		cohort B–21	9 (18%)	7 (4.1–10.8)
			cohort B	cohort B
			1 (5%)	3.7 (1.6–7.3)
Ipilimumab + fotemustine	MM	20	1 (5%)	12.7 (2.7–22.7)
Pembrolizumab	NSCLC, MM	18	6 (33%)	7.7
		18	4 (22%)	n/a

n/a, not applicable. *Patients with measurable target brain lesions.
**Patients without measurable target brain lesions.

Table 7. The efficacy targeted therapy and immunotherapy in patients with brain metastasis.

local therapy (radiation therapy or surgery), and previous systemic therapy did not include BRAF or MEK inhibitors; cohort 2 (n = 6) patients with progression of melanoma BM after previous local therapy. ORR was 18% in both cohorts (16 and 10 patients in cohort 1 and 2, respectively). The PFS was 3.7 months (range 0.03–33.4 months) in cohort 1 and 4.0 months (range 0.3–27.4 months) in cohort 2. The median OS was 8.9 months (range 0.6–34.5 months) and 9.6 months (range 0.7–34.3 months) in cohort 1 and 2, respectively [33].

An open-label, phase 2, multicenter study (BREAK-MB) was evaluated to observe the effectiveness of oral administration of dabrafenib 150 mg twice daily in 172 patients with brain parenchyma metastases from melanoma with a mutation of BRAF V600E (139 patients) and V600E (33 patients). Patients were divided into two cohorts: cohort 1 (n = 89) patients who had not previously received BM local therapy (radiotherapy or surgery), cohort 2 (n = 83) patients with intracranial progression of melanoma after previous BM local therapy. The ORR in cohort 1 was 39% and 31% in patients with mutations V600E and V600K, respectively, and in cohort 2 in 7% of patients with mutation V600E and 22% with mutation V600K. The median OS in patients with the V600E mutation was 7.6 and 7.2 months, and 3.7 and 5.0 months in patients with V600K mutation in cohort 1 and 2, respectively. The PFS was 3.7 months in patients with mutations BRAF V600E and V600K in cohort 1 and 2, respectively, and 1.8 months in patients with BRAF V600K mutation in cohort 1, and 3.8 months in patients with BRAF V600K mutation in cohort 2 [34]. Xing P. and associates (2016) presented the results of crizotinib treatment on 20 advanced ALK-rearranged NSCLC patients with baseline brain metastases in Chinese population. The median OS of patients was 10,3 months and PFS was 21,2 months [35].

The efficacy of ceritinib for the treatment of BM in patients with ALK-positive NSCLC was evaluated in the ASCEND-1, ASCEND-2, and ASCEND-3 trials. In the ASCEND-1 study, 124 patients with ALK-positive NSCLC were diagnosed with BM, 98 of the 124 patients had previously received ALK (crizotinib) inhibitor therapy prior to progression, and 26 patients without previously ALK inhibitors treatment. Only 14 patients (10 patients had received crizotinib before and 4 had not received ALK inhibitors before) had investigator-assessed brain lesions selected as target lesions at baseline. In seven of them (four patients after previous therapy with ALK inhibitors and three without previous therapy) was detected PR and in three patients discovered SD (all after previous crizotinib therapy). The PFS was 6.9 months (range 5.4–8.4 months) for all patients or 6.7 months (range 4.9–8.4 months) for patients previously treated with ALK inhibitors and 8.3 months (range 4.6–not applicable) for patients who have not previously received ALK inhibitors [36] .

Crino and co-workers [37] reported a single-arm, open-label, multicenter, phase 2 study of ceritinib in a heavily pretreated patient population with ALK-rearranged NSCLC (ASCEND-2) in 140 patients who received at least two lines of therapy including platinum-based chemotherapy and crizotinib. The ORR was 38.6% (range 30.5%–47.2). The median of follow-up time 8.8 months (range, 0.1–19.4 months) and the median PFS was 5.7 months (range 5.4–7.6 months) [37].

In ASCEND-3 trial, efficacy of ceritinib was investigated in 124 ALK-positive NSCLC patients who had not previously received therapy with ALK inhibitors. Among 124 patients included in this study, 50 patients (40%) had BM, and radiation was performed on 27 (54%) patients for brain metastatic lesions. The median PFS was 10.8 months (range 7.3–not available), and ORR was detected in 27 (54%) patients [38].

Gadgeel and assistants analyzed the results of two studies (NP28761 and NP28673) to investigate the efficacy and safety of the use of alectinib for treating patients with BM from ALK-positive NSCLC with disease progression after previous treatment with crizotinib. Measurable target brain lesions were detected in 50 (37%) patients and in 86 (63%)—without measurable target brain lesions. The disease control rate (DCR) was detected in 32 (64%) patients with measurable target brain lesions (PR = 22%) and in 37 (43%) patients without measurable target brain lesions (PR = 27%). In patients who underwent radiation therapy of BM ($n = 95$) before started alectinib therapy intracranial response rate (ICRR) was 35.8% versus 58.5% in patients ($n = 41$) who did not receive previously radiation therapy [39].

At phase II prospective, noncomparative BRAIN study investigated efficacy and safety of combination bevacizumab (15 mg/kg) + carboplatin (AUC 6) + paclitaxel (200 mg/m^2) IV every 3 weeks as the first line of treatment of non-squamous NSCLC patients ($n = 67$) with asymptomatic, previously untreated BM. PR and SD of intracranial metastases was recorded in 42 (62.7%) and 18 (26.9%), respectively. Median PFS was 6.7 months. (5.7–7.1), and the median OS was 16 months [40].

In the retrospective multicenter study, Yap and co-workers [41] evaluated the efficacy of anti-Her2/neu therapy in patients with BM from Her2/neu overexpression BC. Among 280 patients with BM Her2/neu-positive BC, 260 (92.9%) patients underwent radiation therapy, 160 (57.1%) patients underwent chemotherapy, and 114 (40.7%) anti-Her2/neu therapy. Of the 114 patients receiving anti-Her2/neu therapy, 56 (49.1%) patients receive trastuzumab, 30 (26.3%)—lapatinib and 28 (24.6%) trastuzumab plus lapatinib combination. The median OS was significantly higher in patients receiving combined anti-Her2/neu therapy and was 10.5 months (range 8.3–17.7 months) in the trastuzumab group, 21.4 months (range 12.5–27.1 months) in the lapatinib group, and 25.9 months (range 18.5–30.1 months) in patients from the trastuzumab + lapatinib group [41].

An open-label, phase 2 trial investigated efficacy of ipilimumab for the treatment of patients with BM from melanoma. A total of 72 melanoma patients with BM were divided into 2 cohorts: cohort A ($n = 51$)—patients with asymptomatic BM, cohort B ($n = 21$)—patients with symptomatic BM and received glucocorticoids. All patients received ipilimumab at 10 mg/kg IV every 3 weeks for a total of 4 cycles. The DCR was 18% in cohort A and 5% in cohort B. Overall survival for 1 year was 31% and 19% with a median OS 7 months (range 4.1–10.8 months) and 3.7 months (range 1.6–7.3 months) in the cohort A and B, respectively [42].

In the NIBIT-M1 study Di Giacomo and co-workers [43] reported on 20 patients with asymptomatic BM from melanoma who received combined systemic therapy of ipilimumab (10 mg/kg IV every 3 weeks for a total of 4 injections) and fotemustine (100 mg/m^2 IV weekly total 3 injections). Maintenance therapy was carried out according to the regiment: fotemustine every 3 weeks from 9 weeks of therapy and ipilimumab every 12 weeks from 24 weeks from the onset of systemic therapy to disease progression or patient failure, or to the occurrence of excessive toxicity. Maintenance therapy was carried out according to the regiment: fotemustine every 3 weeks from 9 weeks of therapy and ipilimumab every 12 weeks from 24 weeks from the onset of systemic therapy to disease progression or patient failure, or to the occurrence of excessive toxicity. Seven patients (35%) before systemic treatment were radiotherapy.

The ORR was 5% at an immunological response rate was 50%. With median follow-up of 39.9 months, the 3-year OS was 27.8%, and the median OS was 12.7 months.

Goldberg et al. [44] in non-randomized, open-label, phase 2 trial was investigated effectiveness of pembolizumab in 36 patients with asymptomatic BM from NSCLC (n = 18) and melanoma (n = 18). The PD-L1 expression in primary tumor was detected in patients with NSCLC only. All patients received pembolizumab 10 mg/kg IV every 2 weeks before disease progression. The ICRR was 33% for NSCLC and 22% for melanoma. The median follow-up was 11.6 months (range 8.5–13.9 months) and median OS was not achieved (NA) in the patients with melanoma BM. The median follow-up was 6.8 months (range 3.1–7.8 months) and median OS was 7.7 months (range 3,5–ND) in the NSCLC patients with BM [44].

6. Conclusions

In recent decades, significant progress has been made in diagnosing, predicting, and treatment of patients with BM of various malignant tumors. Nevertheless, the successes achieved are not sufficient, since the overall survival rates of patients remain low. Further studies of the mechanisms of metastasis of malignant tumors in the brain can serve as a basis for the development of methods for the prevention of BM, and the study of the role of BBB in the development of resistance to systemic therapy will help develop methods that overcome this natural barrier and increase the effectiveness of antitumor drugs. Applying a multidisciplinary approach to developing patient treatment, tactics using the current flow forecast scales will lead to a more valid appointment of radiation therapy, surgery, systemic antitumor and symptomatic therapy to preserve the neurological and neurocognitive function, and the quality of life of patients.

Author details

Roman Liubota[1]*, Roman Vereshchako[1], Mykola Anikusko[2] and Iryna Liubota[2]

*Address all correspondence to: lyubota@ukr.net

1 Department of Oncology, National Medical University named after O.O Bogomolets, Kyiv, Ukraine

2 Municipal City Clinical Oncological Centre, Kyiv, Ukraine

References

[1] Mehta M, Vogelbaum MA, Chang S, et al. Neoplasms of the central nervous system. In: DeVita VT Jr, Lawrence TS, Rosenberg SA, editors. Cancer: Principles and Practice of Oncology. 9th ed. Philadelphia, PA: Lippincott Williams & Wilkins; 2011. pp. 1700-1749

[2] Villano JL, Durbin EB, Normandeau C, Thakkar JP, Moirangthem V, Davis FG. Incidence of brain metastasis at initial presentation of lung cancer. Neuro-Oncology. 2015;17(1):122-128. DOI: 10.1093/neuonc/nou099

[3] Ippen FM, Mahadevan A, Wong ET, Uhlmann EJ, Sengupta S, Kasper EM. Stereotactic radiosurgery for renal cancer brain metastasis: Prognostic factors and the role of whole-brain radiation and surgical resection. Journal of Oncology. 2015:636918. DOI: 10.1155/2015/636918, 0.44

[4] Christensen TD, Spindler KL, Palshof JA, Nielsen DL. Systematic review: Brain metastases from colorectal cancer—Incidence and patient characteristics. BMC Cancer. 2016;16:260. DOI: 10.1186/s12885-016-2290-5

[5] Wilhelm I, Molnar J, Fazakas C, Hasko J, Krizbai IA. Role of the blood-brain barrier in the formation of brain metastases. International Journal of Molecular Sciences. 2013;14:1383-1411. DOI: 10.3390/ijms14011383

[6] Vernur VA, Ahluwalia MS. Prognostic scores for brain metastasis patients: Use in clinical practice and trial design. Chinese Clinical Oncology. 2015;4(2):18. DOI: 10.3978/j.issn.2304-3865.2015.06.01

[7] Lin X, DeAngelis LM. Treatment of brain metastases. Journal of Clinical Oncology. 2015; 33(30):3475-3484. DOI: 10.1200/JCO.2015.60.9503

[8] Liubota R, Cheshuk V, Vereshchako R, Zotov O, Zaychuk V, Anikusko N, Liubota I. The impact of locoregional treatment on survival of patients with primary metastatic breast cancer. Experimental Oncology. 2017;39(1):75-77

[9] Wrobel JK, Toborek M. Blood-brain barrier remodeling during brain metastasis formation. Molecular Medicine. 2016;22:32-40. DOI: 10.2119/molmed.2015.00207

[10] Abbott NJ, Ronnback L, Hansson E. Astrocyte-endothelial interactions at the blood-brain barrier. Nature Reviews. Neuroscience. 2006;7(1):41-48. DOI: 10.1038/nrn1824

[11] Rahmathulla G, Toms SA, Weil RJ. The molecular biology of brain metastasis. Journal of Oncology. 2012;2012:723541. DOI: 10.1155/2012/723541

[12] Deeken JF, Löscher W. The blood-brain barrier and cancer: Transporters, treatment, and Trojan horses. Clinical Cancer Research. 2007;13:1663-1674. DOI: 10.1158/1078-0432.CCR-06-2854

[13] Mahringer A, Fricker G. ABC transporters at the blood–brain barrier. Expert Opinion on Drug Metabolism & Toxicology. 2016;12:499-508. DOI: 10.1517/17425255.2016.1168804

[14] Horsey AJ, Cox MH, Sarwat S, Kerr ID. The multidrug transporter ABCG2: Still more questions than answers. Biochemical Society Transactions. 2016;44:824-830. DOI: 10.1042/BST20160014

[15] Agarwal S, Uchida Y, Mittapalli RK, Sane R, Terasaki T, Elmquist WF. Quantitative proteomics of transporter expression in brain capillary endothelial cells isolated from P-glycoprotein (P-gp), breast cancer resistance protein (Bcrp), and P-gp/Bcrp knockout

mice. Drug Metabolism and Disposition: The Biological Fate of Chemicals. 2012;**40**:1164-1169. DOI: 10.1124/dmd.112.044719

[16] Murrell DH, Zarghami N, Jensen MD, Chambers AF, Wong E, Foster PJ. Evaluating changes to blood-brain barrier integrity in brain metastasis over time and after radiation treatment. Translational Oncology. 2016;**9**(3):219-227. DOI: 10.1016/j.tranon.2016.04.006

[17] Sandipan R. Strategic drug delivery targeted to the brain: A review. Der Pharmacia Sinica. 2012;**3**(1):76-92

[18] Cerna T, Stiborova M, Adam V, Kizek R, Eckschlager T. Nanocarrier drugs in the treatment of brain tumors. Journal of Cancer Metastasis and Treatment. 2016;**2**:407-416. DOI: 10.20517/2394-4722.2015.95

[19] Mulvenna P, Nankivell M, Barton R, Barton R, Faivre-Finn C, Wilson P, McColl E, Moore B, Brisbane I, Ardron D, Holt T, Morgan S, Lee C, Waite K, Bayman N, Pugh C, Sydes B, Stephens R, Parmar MK, Langley RE. Dexamethasone and supportive care with or without whole brain radiotherapy in treating patients with non-small cell lung cancer with brain metastases unsuitable for resection or stereotactic radiotherapy (QUARTZ): Results from a phase 3, non-inferiority, randomised trial. Lancet. 2016;**388**(10055):2004-2014. DOI: 10.1016/S0140-6736(16)30825-X

[20] Ahluwalia MS, Vogelbaum MV, Chao ST, Mehta MM. Brain metastasis and treatment. F1000Prime Reports. 2014;**6**:114. DOI: 10.12703/P6-114

[21] Lombardi G, Di Stefano AL, Farina P, Zagonel V, Tabouret E. Systemic treatments for brain metastases from breast cancer, non-small cell lung cancer, melanoma and renal cell carcinoma: An overview of the literature. Cancer Treatment Reviews. 2014;**40**:951-959. DOI: 10.1016/j.ctrv.2014.05.007

[22] Brastianos HC, Cahill DP, Brastianos PK. Systemic therapy of brain metastases. Current Neurology and Neuroscience Reports. 2015;**15**:518. DOI: 10.1007/s11910-014-0518-9

[23] Cortés J, Rugo HS, Awada A, Twelves C, Perez EA, Im S-A, et al. Prolonged survival in patients with breast cancer and a history of brain metastases: Results of a preplanned subgroup analysis from the randomized phase III BEACON trial. Breast Cancer Research and Treatment. 2017;**165**(2):329-341. DOI: 10.1007/s10549-017-4304-7

[24] Chamberlain MC, Baik CS, Gadi VK, Bhatia S, Chow L. Systemic therapy of brain metastases: Non–small cell lung cancer, breast cancer, and melanoma. Neuro-Oncology. 2017;**19**(1):i1-i24. DOI: 10.1093/neuonc/now197

[25] Metro G, Chiari R, Ricciuti B, et al. Pharmacotherapeutic options for treating brain metastases in non-small cell lung cancer. Expert Opinion on Pharmacotherapy. 2015;**16**:2601-2613. DOI: 10.1517/14656566.2015.1094056

[26] Naskhletashvili DR, Gorbunova VA, Bychkov MB, Chmutin GE, Karahan VB, Aloshin VA, Moskvina EA. Gemcitabine plus cisplatin in patients with heavily pretreated breast cancer with brain metastases. Journal of Clinical Oncology. 2010;**28**(suppl; abstr):1125

[27] Erten C, Demir L, Somali I, Alacacioglu A, Kucukzeybek Y, Akyol M, Can A, Dirican A, Bayoglu V, Tarhan MO. Cisplatin plus gemcitabine for treatment of breast cancer patients with brain metastases; a preferential option for triple negative patients? Asian Pacific Journal of Cancer Prevention. 2013;14(6):3711-3717. DOI: 10.7314/APJCP.2013.14.6.3711

[28] Jacot W, Gerlotto-Borne MC, Thezenas S, Pouderoux S, Poujol S, About M, Romieu G. Carmustine and methotrexate in combination after whole brain radiation therapy in breast cancer patients presenting with brain metastases: A retrospective study. BMC Cancer. 2010;10:257. DOI: 10.1186/1471-2407-10-257

[29] Inno A, Di Noia V, D'Argento E, Modena A, Gori S. State of the art of chemotherapy for the treatment of central nervous system metastases from non-small cell lung cancer. Translational Lung Cancer Research. 2016;5:599-609. DOI: 10.21037/tlcr.2016.11.01

[30] Petrelli F, Ghidini M, Lonati V, Tomasello G, Borgonovo K, Ghilardi M, Cabiddu M, Barni S. The efficacy of lapatinib and capecitabine in HER-2 positive breast cancer with brain metastases: A systematic review and pooled analysis. European Journal of Cancer 201784:141-148. DOI: 10.1016/j.ejca.2017.07.024

[31] Iuchi T, Shingyoji M, Sakaida T, Hatano K, Nagano O, Itakura M, Kageyama H, Yokoi S, Hasegawa Y, Kawasaki K, Iizasa T. Phase II trial of gefitinib alone without radiation therapy for Japanese patients with brain metastases from EGFR-mutant lung adenocarcinoma. Lung Cancer. 2013;82(2):282-287. DOI: 10.1016/j.lungcan.2013.08.016

[32] Gerber NK, Yamada Y, Rimner A, Shi W, Riely GJ, Beal K, Yu HA, Chan TA, Zhang Z, Wu AJ. Erlotinib versus radiation therapy for brain metastases in patients with EGFR-mutant lung adenocarcinoma. International Journal of Radiation Oncology, Biology, Physics. 2014;89:322-329. DOI: 10.1016/j.ijrobp.2014.02.022

[33] McArthur GA, Maio M, Arance A, Nathan P, Blank C, Avril MF, Garbe C, Hauschild A, Schadendorf D, Hamid O, Fluck M, Thebeau M, Schachter J, Kefford R, Chamberlain M, Makrutzki M, Robson S, Gonzalez R, Margolin K. Vemurafenib in metastatic melanoma patients with brain metastases: An open-label, single-arm, phase 2, multicentre study. Annals of Oncology. 2017;28:634-641. DOI: 10.1093/annonc/mdw641

[34] Azer MW, Menzies AM, Haydu LE, Kefford RF, Long GV. Patterns of response and progression in patients with BRAF-mutant melanoma metastatic to the brain who were treated with dabrafenib. Cancer. 2014;120:530-536. DOI: 10.1002/cncr.28445

[35] Xing P, Wang S, Hao X, Zhang T, Li J. Clinical data from the real world: Efficacy of crizotinib in Chinese patients with advanced ALK-rearranged non-small cell lung cancer and brain metastases. Oncotarget. 2016;7:84666-84674. DOI: 10.18632/oncotarget.13179

[36] Shaw A, Mehra R, Tan DSW, Felip E, Chow LQM, Camidge DR, Vansteenkiste J, Sharma S, De Pas T, Riely GJ, Solomon BJ, Wolf J, Thomas M, Schuler M, Liu G, Santoro A, Geraldes M, Sen P, Boral AJ, Yovine A, Kim DW. Ceritinib (LDK378) for the treatment of patients with ALK-rearranged (ALK+) non-small cell lung cancer (NSCLC) and brain metastasis (BM) in the ascend-1 trial. Neuro-Oncology. 2014;16(suppl 5):39. DOI: 10.1093/neuonc/nou240.32

[37] Crino L, Ahn MJ, De Marinis F, Groen HJM, Wakelee H, Hida T, Mok T, Spigel D, Felip E, Nishio M, Scagliotti G, Branle F, Emeremni C, Quadrigli M, Zhang J, Shaw AT. Multicenter phase II study of whole-body and intracranial activity with ceritinib in patients with ALK-rearranged non-small-cell lung cancer previously treated with chemotherapy and crizotinib: Results from ASCEND-2. Journal of Clinical Oncology. 2016;**34**:2866-2873. DOI: 10.1200/JCO.2015.65.5936

[38] Felip E, Orlov S, Park K, Yu CJ, Tsai CM, Nishio M, Dols MC, McKeage MJ, Su WC, Mok T, Scagliotti GV, Spigel D, Branle F, Emeremni C, Quadrigli M, Shaw AT. ASCEND-3: A single-arm, open-label, multicenter phase ii study of ceritinib in alki-naive adult patients (pts) with ALK- rearranged (ALK+) non-small cell lung cancer (NSCLC) [abstract 8060]. Journal of Clinical Oncology. 2015;**33**:16

[39] Gadgeel SM, Shaw AT, Govindan R, Gandhi L, Socinski MA, Camidge DR, et al. Pooled analysis of CNS response to alectinib in two studies of pretreated patients with ALK-positive non-small-cell lung cancer. Journal of Clinical Oncology. 2016;**34**:4079-4085. DOI: 10.1200/jco.2016.68.4639

[40] Besse B, Le Moulec S, Mazières J, Senellart H, Barlesi F, Chouaid C, Dansin E, Berard H, Falchero L, Gervais R, Robinet G, Ruppert AM, Schott R, Lena H, Clement-Duchene C, Quantin X, Souquet PJ, Trédaniel J, Moro-Sibilot D, Perol M, Madroszyk AC, Soria JC. Bevacizumab in patients with nonsquamous non-small cell lung cancer and asymptomatic, untreated BRAIN metastases (BRAIN): A nonrandomized, phase II study. Clinical Cancer Research. 2015;**21**:1896-1903. DOI: 10.1158/1078-0432.CCR-14-2082

[41] Yap YS, Cornelio GH, Devi BC. Brain metastases in Asian HER2-positive breast cancer patients: Anti-HER2 treatments and their impact on survival. British Journal of Cancer. 2012;**107**:1075-1082. DOI: 10.1038/bjc.2012.346

[42] Margolin K, Ernstoff MS, Hamid O, Lawrence D, McDermott D, Puzanov I, et al. Ipilimumab in patients with melanoma and brain metastases: An open-label, phase 2 trial. The Lancet Oncology. 2012;**13**:459-465. DOI: 10.1016/S1470-2045(12)70090-6

[43] Di Giacomo AM, Ascierto PA, Queirolo P, Pilla L, Ridolfi R, Santinami M, Testori A, Simeone E, Guidoboni M, Maurichi A, Orgiano L, Spadola G, Del Vecchio M, et al. Three-year follow-up of advanced melanoma patients who received ipilimumab plus fotemustine in the Italian network for tumor biotherapy (NIBIT)-M1 phase II study. Annals of Oncology. 2015;**26**:798-803. DOI: 10.1093/annonc/mdu577

[44] Goldberg SB, Gettinger SN, Mahajan A, Chiang AC, Herbst RS, Sznol M, et al. Pembrolizumab for patients with melanoma or non-small-cell lung cancer and untreated brain metastases: Early analysis of a non-randomised, open-label, phase 2 trial. The Lancet Oncology. 2016;**17**:976-983. DOI: 10.1016/S1470-2045(16)30053-5

6

Breast and Axilla Treatment in Ductal Carcinoma In Situ

Ambrogio P. Londero, Serena Bertozzi,
Roberta Di Vora, Fabrizio De Biasio, Luca Seriau,
Pier Camillo Parodi, Lorenza Driul, Andrea Risaliti,
Laura Mariuzzi and Carla Cedolini

Abstract

Ductal carcinoma in situ (DCIS) represents a challenge for the breast unit team, beginning from its difficult radiological detection and continuing with its controversial multimodal treatment and management. With the introduction of the mammographic screening, DCIS has become a common diagnosis. In fact, today DCIS is mostly identified by mammography or magnetic resonance imaging (MRI). The increased prevalence of DCIS diagnosis, in the past, raised the problem of the therapeutic management. In this chapter, the breast and axillary surgery in case of DCIS and the most controversial aspects regarding DCIS management are reviewed based on international guidelines and on the current literature.

Keywords: ductal carcinoma in situ, ductal intraepithelial neoplasia, breast-conserving surgery, sentinel lymph node biopsy, breast cancer, breast surgery

1. Introduction

Ductal carcinoma in situ (DCIS) represents a current challenge for the breast specialists, beginning from its difficult radiological detection and continuing with its controversial surgical and nonsurgical management. In this chapter, breast surgery and axillary surgery in case of DCIS are reviewed, as well as some aspects of its preoperative evaluation, based on the more recent international guidelines, and the controversial issues are discussed.

2. Histopathological aspects

The breast gland contains a ductal system that, with successive branches, ends distally in the terminal ductal-lobular units. Ducts and lobules are coated with two types of cells: luminal epithelial cells and myoepithelial cells. The myoepithelial cells contain myofilaments, have contractile capacity, and form a network structure located on the basal membrane. Histologically, the retention of the myoepithelial cell layer helps to distinguish in situ forms from invasive ones.

DCIS is a neoplastic breast lesion, characterized by the presence in the ductal-lobular terminal unit of a malignant epithelial cell clone that does not exceed the basal membrane. DCIS includes a spectrum of different lesions from the histological point of view, with different architecture, nuclear morphology, degree, and the eventual presence of necrosis and calcifications.

DCIS has been historically divided into five histological subtypes, based on the tumor cell growth modality: comedogenic, solid, cribriform, papillary, and micropapillary; however, in most cases the appearance is composite.

Comedogenic DCIS is characterized by a solid proliferation of large pleomorphic cells, with abundant eosinophilic cytoplasm and high-grade hyperchromatic nuclei. A peculiar aspect of this DCIS is the presence of central necrosis which may give place to dystrophic calcifications, which are usually detected by mammography as clustered microcalcifications. Frequently, these lesions contain periductal fibrosis, due to the fibroblast response in the surrounding stroma, and a chronic inflammation component which may sometimes make these lesions clinically palpable.

Noncomedogenic DCIS consists of a population of smaller and monomorphic neoplastic cells, with variable nuclear grading. Necrosis is minimal or absent and the periductal fibrosis is unfrequent. In the cribriform subtype, neoformed glandular spaces are uniformly distributed and have a regular shape. In the solid DCIS, neoplastic cells completely fill in the interested tissue. The papillary subtype grows, giving rise to papillary formations with the fibrovascular axis missing in the micropapillary DCIS, also characterized by interstitial papillary protrusions.

The importance of this morphological classification has been downsized in recent years since this distinction does not take into account important prognostic factors such as nuclear grading, necrosis, and architecture [1, 2]. However, a distinction between comedogenic and noncomedogenic DCIS remains very significant, because of the poorer prognosis of the comedogenic type, which is at higher risk of evolution toward invasive carcinoma and of local recurrence [3].

Several classifications were subsequently proposed [1], taking into consideration nuclear grading, presence of necrosis, histological architecture and pattern, lesion size, number of involved ducts, cell polarization, and positivity for some receptors. The most used classification systems are those endowed with prognostic power.

2.1. Natural history

Several recent studies have shown that invasive breast cancer results from a progression of in situ cancer that proliferates and increases to overcome the basal membrane of the ductal epithelium, thus becoming infiltrating. However, the probability that all invasive carcinomas originate from in situ forms is difficult to demonstrate, despite the many studies that have tried different approaches to achieve this. In particular, some studies focused on women with untreated DCIS, and some others used animals, as well as genomic studies of expression of cellular markers.

DCIS greatly differs from benign proliferative breast lesions for its biological and clinical features. Alterations in the normal number of chromosomes occur in the evolution of breast lesions from benign hyperplasia to preinvasive malignant forms [4]. Heterozygosis lost occurs in more than 70% of high-grade DCIS, in 35–40% of atypical ductal hyperplasia, and in 0% of normal mammary tissue samples [5–7]. The p53 oncosuppressor gene is mutated in 25% of DCIS and only rarely in benign breast lesions [8]. Genomic analyses identified some genetic alterations related to the nuclear grading of DCIS [9]: loss of genetic material in the chromosome 16q resulted associated with well or moderately differentiated DCIS, while DNA amplifications were related to a poorer differentiation. Thereafter, the genetic characteristics of DCIS were also compared with those of the adjacent invasive cell carcinomas, showing almost identical patterns.

Several other studies reported genetic similarities between invasive carcinoma and DCIS, especially high-grade DCIS, supporting the hypothesis that invasive carcinomas derive from the progression of preexisting DCIS [4, 10, 11]. The first step might be the abnormal response to growth factors, for example, mediated by estrogen receptors, which let the benign cells lose their ability to respond to normal apoptosis signals. Then, there would be the loss of function of some oncosuppressor genes as p53, the acquisition of some genetic instability with the loss of heterozygosity, and the onset of abnormal oncogenes such as HER2/neu. Finally, also changes in the surrounding stroma and neoangiogenesis occur, so that the preinvasive lesion becomes capable of invading the surrounding tissues for an imbalance between the gain of function by malignant cells and loss of function by the surrounding normal cells.

Many of the typical molecular characteristics of invasive lesions are already present in DCIS, such as genetic mutations, oncogenic expression, and loss of normal cell cycle regulation ability. The expression of molecular markers seems to have many points in common between in situ and invasive ductal carcinoma, supporting again the evolution of invasive carcinoma from DCIS. In the following section, these markers are discussed.

2.2. Biomolecular markers

The estrogen receptor is expressed in about 60% of DCIS [1] especially in those that exhibit less aggressive histological features such as low grading of differentiation and necrosis. The progesterone receptor expression seems to be consensual to that of the estrogen receptor.

HER2/neu is a member of the epidermal growth factor receptor (EGFR) family and is routinely studied in invasive carcinomas. It seems to be expressed by more than 40% of DCIS, especially by high-grade or comedogenic ones [12], so it would appear to be expressed in these lesions with a much higher frequency than that of invasive forms.

The expression of markers differs according to the nuclear grading of DCIS. In fact, considering only low-grade DCIS, some studies showed that in over 90% of cases it expresses the estrogen receptor, while in less than 20% of cases, it overexpresses HER2/neu or presents p53 mutations. In contrast, HER2/neu overexpression and p53 mutations are found in two thirds of high-grade DCIS, which expresses the estrogen receptor in only the 25% of cases.

2.3. Multifocal and multicentric disease

For its ability to spread within the ductal system, DCIS frequently presents with multiple outbreaks within the same quadrant (multifocality) or in different quadrants (multicentricity). Multifocality occurs in two thirds of patients with low- or intermediate-grade DCIS, characterized by a discontinuous growth. On the other hand, high-grade lesions tend to be continuous, with neoplastic cell outbreaks usually not farer than 5 mm [4, 13, 14]. Other reports, albeit with lower incidence, show a higher frequency of multifocality and multicentricity in DCIS, and many authors highlighted how mammography is less sensitive than magnetic resonance imaging in such cases and underestimates the extent of the disease [4, 15].

In a very old study, Lagios and colleagues found that the incidence of multicentricity increases with the lesion size [16]. In addition, DCIS can spread through the ducts within the ductal system to reach the nipple, without ever overcoming the basal membrane. This mode of growth characterizes Paget's disease of the nipple, a rare manifestation of breast cancer that occurs with crusty and pruriginous nipple erythema.

3. Diagnosis and imaging

In the past, DCIS was clinically identified by objective examination by the presence of nipple discharge, Paget's disease, or a palpable mass. Today, clinical finding is rare, and DCIS is mostly identified by mammography or magnetic resonance imaging.

3.1. Mammography

The sensitivity of mammography in detecting DCIS varies in the literature between 87 and 95% [17–19]. In a comparative study of mammographic and anatomopathological findings, the number of high-grade lesions not detected in mammography was significantly low [18]. Microcalcifications are the expression of cellular debris and calcified secretions within the intraductal lumen; can be extremely variable in size, shape, and appearance; and account for about 60–75% of all mammographic abnormalities in case of DCIS [20–25].

The diagnostic approach to breast microcalcifications is the analysis of morphology, distribution, and eventual modifications over time. According to the terminology of BI-RADS, the morphology can be classified as "pleomorphic," "linear," "branched linear," "amorphous," or "indistinct." The distribution of calcifications can be widespread or scattered throughout the breast, regional or distributed within a large volume of breast tissue (>2 cc), clustered if there are at least five calcifications in a small breast volume, segmental in the case where calcific deposits lie in ducts or branches of a lobe or breast segment.

Considering the changes in microcalcifications over time, in the presence of doubtful but probably benign mammographic findings, the absence of modifications after a certain period of time is reassuring. On the other hand, as underlined in a retrospective study, in the case of suspicious microcalcifications, the morphological aspect stability is not enough to exclude malignancy [26]. In this study, 25% of patients with malignancy finding at biopsy had microcalcifications with a stable appearance for 8–63 months. It is thus evident that morphology and distribution of microcalcifications are much more relevant in the decision-making process of clinicians.

Several studies attempted to correlate the appearance of microcalcifications and other DCIS mammographic findings with the biology of these lesions [13, 20, 21, 26–34]. The layout of calcifications reflects the localization of DCIS in the ductal system. Calcifications in a subareolar major duct may appear as a bundle of calcifications oriented toward the nipple. Calcifications in smaller ducts may have a branched appearance that reflects the extralobular endpoints, where most of the carcinomas originate. A branched radial pattern of calcifications means that intralobular endpoints are involved [21].

In several studies, most DCIS presented with granular microcalcifications [20, 27–31], but a radio-pathological correlation study showed that the histological type of DCIS cannot be accurately determined on the basis of the morphological aspect of microcalcifications found in mammography [31]. However, in this study, almost 80% of linear microcalcifications were associated with the comedogenic subtype, while granular microcalcifications were associated with non-comedogenic DCIS subtypes in more than half cases [31]. Fine pleomorphic or linear-branching calcifications were significantly associated with high-grade DCIS and necrosis [25, 31], whereas round calcifications were significantly associated with low-grade DCIS [25]. Similarly, other mammographic studies showed that linear calcifications are most frequently expression of high-grade DCIS, while fine granular ones are more typical of well-differentiated DCIS [32–35].

Although microcalcifications are the most frequent mammographic finding in the diagnosis of DCIS, this may assume less commonly other radiological aspects. Various studies in the literature report more than 10% of DCIS presenting with solid mass aspect, usually with well-defined margins [20, 21, 25]. This percentage rises if narrowing the survey to low-grade DCIS [17]. A mass-like aspect of DCIS may be the direct manifestation of a soft tissue mass or may be the result of periductal fibrosis, causing in this latter case an irregular or a bulging aspect of the mass [36].

Further mammographic manifestations include architectural distortion and focal asymmetries. Architectural distortion may also be determined by the sclerosis of the interstitial tissue surrounding the DCIS [21] or the tumor invasion of Cooper's ligament [37]. Many low-grade DCIS appear to be mammographic masses or asymmetries [25] and, as a result, appear more frequently to be noncalcific lesions [34, 36]. Finally, Tabar et al. reported that the survival of women with masses or linear and linear-branching calcifications is considerably worse than women with other types of microcalcifications [38].

3.2. Magnetic resonance imaging

The use of magnetic resonance imaging (MRI) in the diagnosis of DCIS remains still an argument of great debate. The interest in using this tool for DCIS has grown following the brilliant results of its use in the invasive carcinoma. Initially, due to the different appearance of the two pathologies, this instrument was not considered adequate alone for the study of in situ lesions. A fundamental factor which led MRI to become an important tool in the preoperative diagnosis and evaluation of DCIS was the transition from high time resolution to high spatial resolution [39]. Another important factor is that MRI was used to study patients who had already been diagnosed with cancer by mammography, and only when MRI began to be used as a tool for screening on high-risk patients allowed more data to be compared about the accuracy of the two different diagnostic tools.

Several studies have been conducted to find out the multiple manifestations of DCIS by MRI and to correlate these with the biological characteristics of the disease. The superiority of MRI in the diagnosis of DCIS has been demonstrated in numerous studies with sensitivity ranging from 86 to 92% [15, 40–43]. MRI sensitivity is higher for high-grade lesions, regardless of whether or not there is necrosis, which instead affects the sensitivity of mammography in identifying high-grade DCIS [41, 42, 44, 45]. The pattern of breast lesion enhancement correlates with the biological profile of DCIS [46], because the diagnosis is based on tissue enhancement after administration of a contrast medium and to the hyperdensity of neoplastic lesions due to vascular permeability [47].

Angiogenesis in DCIS may be partly due to the destruction of the cellular myoepithelial cell surrounding the ducts [48]. Myoepithelial cells tend to be more preserved in low-grade DCIS while being lost or significantly absent in high-grade DCIS or with comedic necrosis. Recent studies also show that focal damage to the myoepithelial layer could trigger tumor invasion. The tumor cells adjacent to the point of damage tend to be more frequently associated with genetic and phenotypic alterations, such as loss of estrogen receptors, reduced expression of oncosuppressors, and increased expression of genes related to the cell cycle, angiogenesis, and invasive capacity [49].

The terminology of BI-RADS includes three types of responses to breast MRI: "mass-like enhancement" defined as a three-dimensional injury occupying a generally rounded area of oval or irregular shape, "focal enhancement" defined as a small enhancement spot <5 mm that does not allow a further morphological description, and "non-mass-like enhancement" described as enhancement of an area without forming a mass. This last manifestation is most common in DCIS, present in 60–80% of cases [15, 24, 39, 41], while invasive or mixed ductal lesions appear in over 75% of cases as "mass-like enhancement" [41].

Non-mass-like enhancement lesions are distinguished on the basis of the distribution pattern as segmental, linear, ductal, focal, regional, multiregional, and diffuse. Segmental means a triangular enhancement area with the apex toward the nipple suggesting the distribution of a duct and its branches. Linear is defined as an enhancement area that may not correspond to a duct, while ductal indicates a linear enhancement zone with ramifications like a duct. The regional pattern has a large volume of enhancement that cannot be assimilated to a duct, and the focal enhancement is confined to a smaller area than 25% of a quadrant. The segmental distribution is the most common non-mass-like DCIS presentation [15, 24, 41].

On the basis of the internal enhancement pattern, non-mass-like enhancement lesions are distinguished also as clumped, heterogeneous, and homogeneous. The internal enhancement pattern can be clumped if it takes a cobbled appearance with occasional confluence areas. It may be homogeneous or otherwise heterogeneous when it is or not uniform. The most common internal enhancement pattern is the clumped one (51.5%), followed by the heterogeneous (21%) and homogeneous ones (15%) [41].

Evaluation of kinetics in DCIS is less significant compared to invasive lesions, and in fact the extent of perfusion increases with the progression of lesions from benign to in situ and even more invasive lesions [47]. Based on the BI-RADS classification, the kinetic aspect of DCIS has been standardized, and two phases of the enhancement can be recognized: an initial phase, within the first 2 minutes after administration of the contrast medium, and a delayed phase after 2 minutes. The initial phase can be rapid, intermediate, or slow; the delayed phase can be classified as persistent (the signal continues to increase), plateau (the signal density does not change after the initial increase), or washout (the signal decreases after the initial climb). DCIS is usually characterized by the fast initial phase and a washout in the delayed phase [24, 50]. Moreover, there is no statistically significant difference in the kinetic characteristics between DCIS of different grading [24, 51].

Despite the superiority of MRI in terms of sensitivity, its role in the management of in situ disease remains still controversial. According to recent studies, the routine use of MRI in DCIS does not change the clinical management in 99% of patients and lead to more unnecessary reexamination and longer time interval before surgery [52]. In a recent meta-analysis, the proportion of patients who changed the treatment based on MRI findings results about 15% [53]. Available evidence suggests that the percentage of patients with noninvasive cancer who may benefit from a preoperative MRI assessment is not very high and should be weighed with the economic availability and the delay in definitive treatment resulting from the increase in preoperative investigations.

Patients undergoing MRI do not show a significant reduction in the re-intervention rate for positive margins after conservative surgery [53]. Several studies also show that the routine use of preoperative MRI is associated with a greater incidence of mastectomy for invasive carcinoma and the trend seems to be the same for DCIS [43, 53–56]. On the contrary, conservative surgery rates are higher among women who do not undergo preoperative MRI [53], and this probably reflects the MRI ability to detect multifocal and multicentric disease and results in a greater number of women who are not candidates for conservative surgery.

The identification of a subgroup of patients with DCIS that could benefit from preoperative MRI needs further studies on DCIS biology, in particular on its potential to progress and recur. In fact, as outlined in the literature, only 30–50% of cases of DCIS evolve to invasive disease if untreated [57, 58], and consequently many patients who undergo mastectomy for DCIS would receive an overtreatment; whether preoperative MRI results an advantage in terms of local control of disease and survival in patients with DCIS is still unclear.

However, many agree that there is definitely an improvement of surgical outcomes [52–54, 59], and a study on DCIS and early invasive breast cancer does not reveal, after 4.6 years of median follow-up, significant differences in terms of recurrence, metastasis occurrence, mortality, or contralateral lesions rate between patients undergoing or not preoperative MRI [60]. The use of MRI in addition to mammography could help in defining the exact extension of DCIS, although MRI often overestimates the size of the primitive tumor [59].

3.3. Screening

Mammography is considered to be the most effective screening test for the detection of early breast cancer. In Italy, biennial mammography is recommended in women aged between 50 and 69 [61, 62]. In women aged between 40 and 49, it should be performed only based on the familiar history, individual risk, and breast density, possibly accompanied by an ultrasound examination. In women aged over 70, there is no evidence of the effectiveness of mammographic screening, but the possibility of extending it to 75 years is considered. The relative reduction in mortality for breast cancer is 14% in women aged between 50 and 59 and 32% in the 60–69 range, reflecting the direct correlation of mammography sensitivity with age, related to the reduction in breast density [63].

MRI is not recommended as a screening survey in the general population [64] due to its low specificity and hence its higher number of false positives. The use of MRI as a screening method, in addition to mammography and clinical examination, is justified in high- and moderate-risk women, who include women with BRCA1 or BRCA2 mutations; previous chest wall radiotherapy between 10 and 30 years of age; Li-Fraumeni, Cowden, or Bannayan-Riley-Ruvalcaba syndrome; personal history of DCIS; atypical ductal hyperplasia; and lobular intraepithelial neoplasia.

Tomosynthesis, which combines conventional, two-dimensional images with three-dimensional, multilayer images, appears to be particularly effective in case of dense breasts, where the volumetric overlap of traditional mammography images prevents some lesions from being identified. In a study of 9672 women, the combination of mammography and tomosynthesis increased not only the cancer detection rate but also the number of false positives [65].

The incidence of screen-detected DCIS varies between 15 and 30% [66–70]. It is greater in women aged between 40 and 49 (28.2%) than in older women (16–20.5%). The age-adjusted incidence rate increased from 2.4 to 27.7 per 100,000 women between 1981 and 2001 [36]. In line with these data, some studies reported an estimated annual DCIS incidence of 32.5 per 100,000 women [71]. The overall screen-detected DCIS rate results 0.78 per 1000 mammograms, indicating that one DCIS is approximately identified every 1300 screening mammograms [66].

The mammographic screening resulted in a mortality reduction of about 20–30% [72–74], but screening value remains uncertain in the case of DCIS. Some authors argue that it prevents the incidence of a large number of invasive tumors and contributes substantially to survival improvement. Others claim that this type of injury does not always progress to invasive cancer and in those cases it would not lead to death, and indeed, its response to screening would be a source of overdiagnosis, resulting in more harm than good [75]. The epidemiological definition of overdiagnosis is the difference between observed and expected incidences [70].

A study estimated that, of the 141 screened deaths, 17 were determined by the progression of DCIS to invasive carcinoma and therefore concluded that the detection of DCIS at screening prevented 12% of the overall avoided deaths with screening [75]. Another interesting evidence is that the majority of screen-detected DCIS are of high-grade and have a more pronounced tendency to present necrosis, suggesting that screen-detected lesions have a higher risk of progression [76].

The main objection to the screen detection of DCIS comes from the observation that misdiagnosed DCIS is much less likely than invasive tumors to become clinically evident [66]. In fact, it is evident that there are breast cancers that will never become lethal and that many women receive systemic therapies without knowing who will benefit from it, but the risk of overdiagnosis is lower than the benefits [70]. From a clinical point of view, the best and most prudent way to deal with DCIS is to consider it as a potential future invasive carcinoma [71].

4. Surgical treatment

The uncertainty about the natural history of DCIS and the impossibility to determine predictive factors for which lesions will progress to invasive forms make the therapeutic choice extremely difficult. Initially, standard therapy was the simple mastectomy in 98–99% of patients [77]. Subsequently, with the introduction of always more conservative treatments for invasive carcinomas, the breast-conserving surgery (BCS) became progressively the most frequently used surgery for DCIS. There are, however, no randomized studies comparing outcomes after mastectomy and BCS [12, 64].

The currently recommended therapeutic options of the National Comprehensive Cancer Network (NCCN) include mastectomy and lumpectomy with or without radiotherapy and with the possible addition of tamoxifen in the case of hormone-positive DCIS. Randomized trials indicate that lumpectomy associated with radiotherapy results in the lowest recurrence rate but does not show any difference in overall and disease-free survival [78].

According to a recent article by Worni and colleagues, among 121,080 women with DCIS diagnosed from 1991 to 2010, most patients received radiotherapy (43%) after lumpectomy, followed by lumpectomy alone (26.5%), unilateral mastectomy (23.8%), bilateral mastectomy (4.5%), and ultimately no treatment (2.3%) [78]. In the 20 years of study, trends in the treatment choice have changed, with a considerable increase in lumpectomy with radiotherapy (100% increase). Also, the significant increase in the number of bilateral mastectomies, a trend that seems to be driven more by the choice of bilateral prophylactic mastectomy than by the need to treat bilateral disease, is interesting.

4.1. Conservative breast surgery

Breast-conserving surgery (BCS) in the treatment of invasive breast cancer has gone affirming over the years, thanks to studies that demonstrated no significant difference in survival rates compared to mastectomy. However, this evidence has not yet been reached in the case of DCIS, and to date there are no randomized comparisons of mastectomy and BCS in women with DCIS. However, retrospective studies did not show any difference in the overall and disease-free survival between the two strategies [79, 80].

Several studies have been conducted in the attempt to determine the magnitude of the recurrence risk in patients with DCIS, in order to use this information to improve the therapeutic approach, but there are no definitive results on the effectiveness of BCS without radiotherapy, which, according to Worni et al., is still used today in about a quarter of cases [78].

BCS consists in the excision of the lesion surrounded by about 1 centimeter of macroscopically health tissue. It may be a simple wide excision of breast parenchyma, also called lumpectomy, or a cylindrical excision of breast tissue including the overlying skin and the underlying muscle fascia, also known as quadrantectomy [81]. In case of nonpalpable breast lesions, many different techniques can be used in order to intraoperatively guide the surgical resection, such as the preoperative placement of a wire hook or a radioactive tracer [82].

The specimen is then oriented with some stitched in order to facilitate the margin evaluation by the pathologist [83]. In particular, a negative margin greater than 2 mm represents nowadays the adequate margin for DCIS [84]. Moreover, in some cases also a cavity shaving may be performed, although there is no evidence that this procedure will significantly reduce re-interventions for margin positivity.

4.2. Mastectomy

Mastectomy consists in the complete mammary gland excision together with the overlying skin and the nipple-areola complex, as well as the underlying muscle fascia. Nowadays, even more conservative techniques have been developed, so that it is possible to spare the skin with or without the nipple-areola complex by performing the so-called nipple-sparing mastectomy or skin-sparing mastectomy [85–91].

For what concerns these two last procedures, there are still controversies about the long-term oncological results, as, for example, the nipple includes the terminal portion of the breast ducts and may then represent a place at risk of recurrence. However, the esthetic results are undiscussed, and these kinds of techniques result in an essential improvement in the psychophysical wellness of women undergoing breast demolition.

Mastectomy is a healing process in 98–99% of patients with DCIS. The relapses after this intervention may be in situ but also invasive and can occur both as a local recurrence and a distant metastasis [77]. After mastectomy, the reported recurrence rate is less than 1.5% in most studies [92, 93]. The use of skin-sparing mastectomy does not correlate with a significant increase in local recurrences [93].

Recurrence after mastectomy for DCIS could be due to the lack of sampling or recognition of an invasive component or incomplete removal of the involved breast tissue. However, the fact that the majority of recurrences after mastectomy occur in the first 5 years suggests that most of these are due to the lack of recognition of an invasive carcinoma rather than the malignant transformation of the residual breast tissue [77].

Finally, mastectomy is an effective treatment for DCIS, but its use should be carefully evaluated in the light of a pathology that does not present the risk of remote metastasis, typical of infiltrating forms, which will not necessarily become invasive.

5. Adjuvant treatments

Although DCIS is a local disease, the use of both local and systemic adjuvant therapies is widespread. In particular, adjuvant radiotherapy after BCS and the use of tamoxifen or aromatase inhibitors are considered, while no evidence supports the use of adjuvant chemotherapy in the treatment of DCIS [64].

5.1. Radiation therapy

With the introduction of adjuvant radiotherapy after BCS for invasive breast carcinoma, the interest in radiotherapy application for DCIS has also greatly increased. A lot of studies in the literature evaluated the efficacy of this treatment in DCIS patients, and according to the current guidelines, radiotherapy after BCS results is strongly recommended in patients with DCIS [64].

Breast irradiation usually includes all the residual breast (whole breast irradiation), is classically performed within 6 months after surgery, and usually consists in 25 sessions, even if also shorter hypofractionated protocols are described. Anyway, radiation therapy may be also limited to the area surrounding the tumor (partial breast irradiation) and be performed intraoperatively immediately after the tumor excision, as happens for the intraoperative radiotherapy (IORT) [94].

A recent meta-analysis of the Early Breast Cancer Trialists' Collaborative Group (EBCTCG) on individual data from four randomized studies showed that adjuvant radiotherapy reduces 15.2% of the absolute risk of 10-year ipsilateral invasive relapse after surgery for DCIS, anyway without any significant effect on survival [95]. These data confirm the findings of previous international randomized trials that generally showed a reduction by about 50–60% in ipsilateral breast recurrences in patients who received radiotherapy after BCS compared to BCS alone [96–99].

Recurrences after BCS for DCIS are usually half invasive and half in situ. With the addition of radiotherapy to BCS, the annual invasive recurrence rate results about 0.5–1%. The possible benefits of this therapeutic choice on survival would be the reduction of invasive recurrences and the consequent reduction of mortality [77, 98].

According to recent reports, most patients are subjected to lumpectomy followed by radiotherapy, and this therapeutic option raised from the 25% of treatments in 1991 to the 50% in 2010 [78]. Patients who refuse radiotherapy after BCS should be properly informed of the potential for greater local recurrence risk, although a survival benefit may not yet be evidenced by studies due to the insufficient number of patients examined and to the very low mortality rate for this disease [71].

5.2. Hormonal therapy

Given the important role of the estrogenic pathway in the pathogenesis of breast carcinomas, many strategies have been developed which can control estrogen-sensible tissues. The first experimented drug was tamoxifen, a selective estrogen receptor modulator (SERM), which has the ability to act as an estrogenic agonist in certain tissues such as bone and endometrium, while it acts as a powerful estrogenic antagonist in others including the breast. For these properties it is widely used in the treatment of invasive breast cancer, where it has been shown to reduce the risk of relapse and death after surgical treatment [100].

The role of adjuvant therapy with tamoxifen for DCIS was analyzed in two major randomized trials. The NSABP B-24 study randomized 1804 women with DCIS between BCS followed by radiotherapy and tamoxifen for 5 years versus BCS followed by radiotherapy and placebo for 5 years [101]. This study demonstrated a significant reduction of events after 5 years in the tamoxifen group compared to the placebo one. In particular, a reduction was observed in the risk of invasive relapse in both the ipsilateral and the contralateral breasts. However, for what concerns noninvasive relapses, the addition of tamoxifen was not proven to be significant.

The benefit in women treated with tamoxifen was also significant after 163 months of follow-up [95], and over 15 years of follow-up, adjuvant tamoxifen reduced the risk of recurrence of ipsilateral breast cancer by 31% [99]. A retrospective analysis, conducted on 41% of the original study population, evaluated the relationship between estrogen receptor expression and tamoxifen benefit. It has been shown that treatment with tamoxifen significantly reduced the risk of subsequent breast cancer at 10 and 14.5 years, while in patients without expression of estrogen receptors, no benefit was observed. Finally, there were no differences in survival between the two arms of the NSABP B-24 trial.

The randomized phase II trial UK/ANZ DCIS93 evaluated the role of radiotherapy and tamoxifen in the treatment of patients undergoing BCS for DCIS, enrolling 1701 patients [102]. It analyzed the following therapeutic approaches: surgery alone, surgery followed by radiotherapy, surgery followed by tamoxifen for 5 years, and surgery followed by both radiotherapy and tamoxifen for 5 years. As for the use of tamoxifen, at 12 years of median follow-up, the study showed a reduction of ipsilateral in situ relapses, while there seemed to be no effect on the invasive ipsilateral recurrence.

Considering these two trials as a whole, it emerges that adjuvant tamoxifen, associated with radiotherapy, reduces the risk of in situ ipsilateral recurrences in the case of DCIS which expresses hormonal receptor, independently by the patient's age [48, 64]. Thereafter, the decision whether to propose tamoxifen as adjuvant treatment should be based on the evaluation of its side effects and potential benefits.

In postmenopausal women with invasive breast cancer, the aromatase inhibitors have been shown to be more effective than tamoxifen in reducing recurrences and preventing new contralateral cancers after surgery [100]. The second International Breast Cancer Intervention Study (IBIS-II) had the aim of studying the role of aromatase inhibitors in both primary prevention and adjuvant therapy in women with DCIS [102]. The NSABP B-35 study had similar objectives and compared tamoxifen with anastrozole for 5 years in 3000 postmenopausal women who underwent surgery and radiotherapy for DCIS, and, at a median follow-up of 8.6 years of treatment, anastrozole significantly improved the disease-free survival [103].

5.3. Other medical therapies

HER-2/neu is overexpressed in a variable number of DCIS [100] and appears to be related to an increase in local recurrences [104]. A retrospective analysis of 10,853 women enrolled in the EORTC trial showed that, of the 31 local relapses occurring in patients with DCIS, 24 were associated with in situ lesions that overexpressed HER-2/neu. The real meaning of HER-2/neu overexpression in DCIS is currently the object of the study, given its importance as a prognostic and predictive factor in the invasive cancer. The use of trastuzumab, a monoclonal antibody targeting HER-2/neu, is interesting given the relative frequency of its presence in the DCIS and the lack of effective medical therapies for DCIS which does not express estrogen receptors. These considerations have led to the development of two studies on the role of trastuzumab in DCIS. The first study, conducted by Gonzalez et al. with not yet conclusive results, evaluated the benefit of neoadjuvant trastuzumab in DCIS of less than 1 cm. The second one, conducted from the NSBP, has not yet been completed.

6. The microinvasive component

In agreement with the American Joint Committee on Cancer, microinvasive breast cancer is defined as a DCIS where the invasive component is microscopic and does not exceed the size of 1 mm [105]. In the current literature, microinvasive cancer prevalence accounts for about 10–20% of DCIS cases, and it does not represent more than 1% of all breast cancers [1, 106–110].

The natural history of these lesions is unclear; however, DCIS with microinvasion could be an intermediate stage in the invasive evolution. As a proof of this, the microinvasive carcinoma is often associated with DCIS, particularly large and with comedonecrosis [1, 64], and may be formed by small foci of tumor cells that, after crossing the basal membrane, infiltrate the surrounding stroma [64]. The age of presentation does not seem to be significantly different from that of invasive or in situ forms [106].

Almost all DCIS with microinvasion are identified by the presence of microcalcifications at mammography [111]. Occasionally, the microinvasive carcinoma appears as a palpable mass with serum or blood vessel secretions from the nipple or as Paget's disease [112–114]. Microinvasive lesions tend to be larger in size and therefore more often palpable than purely in situ lesions. The detection of a microinvasion within a DCIS can be extremely difficult for the pathologist because of the many patterns with which the lesion can invade the stroma [77]. Usually, the microinvasion foci tend to be accompanied by a stromal response characterized by inflammatory cells scattered in one neoformed connective matrix [115]. Moreover, the use of immunohistochemical markers specific for the basal membrane or myoepithelial cells can help identify microinvasion in doubtful cases [115].

Concerning the therapeutic implications, data is not uniform. Surgical treatment can be both conservative and radical. According to recent reports, the use of mastectomy is significantly less frequent for this type of lesion than for invasive carcinomas, and the same happens for adjuvant therapies, generally reserved only for patients with triple-negative carcinomas, HER2-positive breast cancer, or with lymph node involvement [106]. The use of adjuvant radiotherapy is even higher in the group of microinvasive carcinoma than in that of invasive one, possibly due to the higher prevalence of conservative surgery.

According to the AIOM guidelines, mastectomy is indicated in these tumors in the presence of large intraductal component, particularly unfavorable histological characteristics (high-grade and comedonecrosis), or when it is not possible to obtain an adequate resection margin with a conservative resection [64]. BCS is also contraindicated after previous chest wall irradiation, during pregnancy, or in the case of multicentric lesions or diffused microcalcifications [110].

Regarding the use of adjuvant systemic treatments, endocrine therapies may be administered in the case of hormone receptor expression, while chemotherapy is not indicated, except in patients with axillary lymph node metastases [64, 106]. There are currently no prospective randomized studies comparing BCS followed by radiotherapy with mastectomy in the subset of patients with microinvasive carcinoma [105].

Prior to the spread of the sentinel lymph node technique, due to its significant morbidity and poor clinical benefits, axillary dissection was not recommended in the management of noninvasive or microinvasive lesions [109]. With the introduction of the sentinel lymph node biopsy, burdened with much minor complications, axillary surgery has extended also to DCIS in the case of mastectomy, as the technique would not be reliable in the second time if needed [116, 117]. However, in the literature there is insufficient evidence of the efficacy of the sentinel lymph node biopsy for the microinvasive cancer, mainly because the studies are mostly retrospective and based on small sample sizes.

The detection of microinvasive foci at the definitive histological examination of specimen of women initially diagnosed with DCIS is quite frequent. In particular, the upstaging rate to invasive carcinoma varies in the literature about 10–20% of in situ or microinvasive lesions [118]. In the case of unexpected microinvasive carcinoma, the sentinel lymph node biopsy can be performed both in conjunction with the primary lesion excision and later on.

In the literature, the sentinel lymph node metastasis rates reported in the case of microinvasive carcinomas are about 6–10%, and about half of these are micrometastasis [77]. In a recent meta-analysis, Gojon et al. studied the role of the lymph node biopsy in 968 patients with microinvasive carcinoma [116]. It emerged that the macrometastasis rate in the sentinel lymph nodes was 3.2% (CI (95%): 2.1–4.6%) without significant differences between the data of the various considered studies. Patients with macrometastatic sentinel nodes would have a risk of almost 30% of having more non-sentinel lymph node metastases, but, due to the rarity of nodal macrometastases, the global incidence of non-sentinel metastases in microinvasive carcinoma resulted less than 1%. Thereafter, given the low rates of nodal positivity, this meta-analysis does not justify the routine use of sentinel lymph node biopsy in patients with microinvasive carcinoma.

Several studies have tried to identify predictive factors for lymph node involvement but with contrasting results [116]. In addition, many studies have reported excellent prognosis in patients with microinvasive carcinoma, irrespective of the eventual asynchronous lymph node involvement [116]. Some authors reported a similar local or distant recurrence risk in patients with in situ or microinvasive carcinomas and positivity for sentinel lymph biopsy [119]. Then, despite the absence of clear scientific evidence, in the case of microinvasive cancer, the use of the sentinel lymph node biopsy is still recommended, especially given the low morbidity of this practice [77].

The survival of patients with microinvasive carcinoma seems to be a halfway between that of pure DCIS and that of early invasive carcinoma [77]. Some dated studies reported no recurrence after average follow-up of 57 and 47 months, respectively [112, 113]. Kinne et al. reported a disease-free survival of about 94% at a median follow-up of 11.5 years [120]. Solin et al. compared the outcomes of invasive carcinoma with those of DCIS and microinvasive carcinoma treated in the same period [114] and found that patients with microinvasive cancer had a higher local recurrence rate than those with pure DCIS, as well as an intermediate survival rate between in situ and frankly invasive carcinomas. In contrast, Silverstein and Lagios did not detect differences between patients with microinvasive carcinoma and DCIS in terms of overall and disease-free survival [121].

In a review of Adamovich and Simmons, the median time of appearance of a local relapse resulted in 42 months, most of the local recurrences of microinvasive carcinoma were invasive recurrences, and only the 7% were distant ones [110]. A study by Parikh et al. on 393 women with breast cancer treated with BCS and radiotherapy suggested that microinvasion is not predictive of a significant worsening of local recurrence and distant metastasis-free survival, overall survival, and disease-free survival [122]. This study concluded that, despite the greater aggressiveness in treating patients with microinvasion, clinical and pathological characteristics and outcome did not differ for DCIS with and without microinvasion. Even more recent data emerging from Fang et al.'s work confirmed that disease-free survival of over 2 years in patients with microinvasive carcinoma was significantly worse than that of pure DCIS and similar to that of invasive carcinoma smaller than 5 mm [106].

In conclusion, clinical and pathological features and outcomes do not significantly differ between DCIS with and without microinvasion [106]. Overall survival do not differ significantly in the two groups, which altogether have a good prognosis overall. The prevalence of lymph node metastases in the microinvasive carcinomas is low and does not associate with a prognosis worsening, as it does not lead to an increased risk of recurrence, either local or distant [119]. According with the ASCO guidelines published in 2016, a 6-month clinical follow-up together with annual instrumental examinations should be recommended [123].

7. The role of sentinel lymph node biopsy

Complete axillary dissection was the only possible approach in surgery until the early 1990s of the last century. Nowadays, the sentinel lymph node biopsy represents the standard in most centers that deal with mammary surgery [64, 82, 124–127] and significantly reduced the complications associated with axillary surgery [128] while providing high levels of accuracy in the staging [129–131]. The multicentric NSABP B-32 trial randomized 5611 women with clinically negative axillary nodes to the sentinel lymph node biopsy alone or followed by axillary dissection [131]. No significant differences in disease-free and overall survival and locoregional recurrences were observed between the two groups at a median follow-up of 96 months.

The concept of sentinel lymph node was born in the 1970s and completely developed 20 years later, based on the principle that tumors are drained from a lymphatic channel through the first sentinel node of that region. In 1991 Giuliano and colleagues first applied the method of sentinel lymph node biopsy at the John Wayne Cancer Institute in the context of breast surgery. They reached 100% accuracy in predicting axillary nodal status in a few years [125, 132, 133], opening the way to the spread of the method.

In a recent work, analyzing data from the Surveillance, Epidemiology, and End Results (SEER) registers, Worni and colleagues reported that in 2010 the sentinel lymph node biopsy was performed in over 70% of mastectomies for DCIS and in at least 20% of lumpectomies. The indications of the sentinel lymph node biopsy for DCIS are not always supported by scientific evidence and are sometimes the result of a consensus of experts, leading to a significant variability among the various centers dealing with breast surgery.

8. Local recurrences

The local recurrence rate after surgery for DCIS, associated or not with subsequent radiotherapy, ranges from 0 to 10% at 5 years and from 8 to 23% at 10 years [77]. A study on a large number of patients undergoing conservative surgical excision and radiotherapy, conducted by an international group, described a recurrence rate at 5, 10, and 15 years of, respectively, 6, 11, and 16% [134]. The cumulative annual local recurrence rate found in this study was approximately 1% and was thus lower than that reported by the NSABP trial, which is 1.8%. This value is similar to that found for invasive carcinoma treated in the same way [77].

Many prognostic factors of local recurrence have been hypothesized in patients with DCIS treated with BCS, associated or not with complementary radiation therapy. In almost all studies, the margin involvement was correlated with a higher local recurrence rate. On the other hand, the local recurrence rate is lower after radical excision with negative margins. However, the adequate distance of the excision margin from the lesion is not precisely defined [77].

In some studies, negative margins of 0 mm (also defined "no ink on tumor") were compared with negative margins up to 10 mm from the lesion, concluding that wider margins give more protection against recurrences [135]. In a meta-analysis conducted by Dunne et al., considering the effect of the state of margins after BCS and radiotherapy, the highest recurrence rate was observed among women with excision margins of less than 2 mm, whereas for margins greater than 2 mm, no further benefits were observed in comparison to margins of 5 mm or more [136]. Therefore, these data imply that for women receiving BCS and radiotherapy, 2 mm margins can be considered adequate to reduce as much as possible the risk of recurrences.

However, without the addition of radiotherapy, conservative surgery with margins lower than 10 mm results in a greater recurrence risk (of more than fivefold), while with the addition of radiation therapy, there seems to be no additional benefit for larger margins [137]. Anyway, no successful study has been performed to compare women with greater or lesser margins, which may conclude for a benefit of a certain margin distance [71].

Young patients show a consistently higher risk of local recurrence than older patients. The reasons for this difference are not clear, but a study found that younger patients tend to have smaller excision volumes, higher prevalence of high-grade tumors, and higher frequency of necrosis [138, 139]. On the other hand, another study did not confirm these differences in terms of pathological characteristics between the two groups of patients and identified in younger women a higher rate of HER2/neu overexpression [140].

Histological features have been evaluated in several studies with different results. From the EORTC87 trial, the local recurrence rate at 5.4 years of follow-up proportionally increased together with the increase of high-grade tumor (8, 14, and 18%, respectively, for low-, intermediate-, and high-grade lesions). This data is confirmed by the NSABP B-17.89 trial, which also revealed a difference between low-grade tumors with or without necrosis in terms of local recurrences. Between groups of patients with tumors of different grading, but both involving necrosis, recurrence rates did not seem to substantially differ. Moreover, necrosis has been identified as a risk factor for recurrence in many other studies, and comedonecrosis is strongly associated with worse outcome and increased risk of invasive recurrences [98, 140, 141].

The size of DCIS was evaluated in several studies but without definitive responses, also due to the difficulty and lack of uniformity in measuring this kind of lesions [77]. In general, larger tumors have been associated with higher rates of recurrence, both in situ and invasive [93, 142].

A further step forward in the prediction of relapse could be the evaluation of the biomolecular profile, through the study of molecular marker expression. In fact, the positivity for the estrogen receptor has been reported to be associated with a reduction in the risk of recurrence, while the HER2/neu overexpression seems to be associated with an increased incidence of local recurrences [143]. The frequency of expression of HER2/neu in DCIS in some reports exceeds the 40%.

In an attempt to summarize all these predictive factors of recurrence, Silverstein and colleagues developed the Van Nuys Prognostic Index that considers four important variables, each of which is assigned a score from 1 to 3, generating a total score ranging from a score of 4 (predicting the best prognosis) to 12 (predicting the worst prognosis) [144, 145]. The analyzed variables are the size of the lesion, the margin amplitude, the pathological classification including the nuclear grading and the eventual presence of comedonecrosis, and the patient age. The prognostic utility of this score was confirmed by NSABP B-17 trial, and, since half of the local recurrences after BCS were invasive carcinomas, it is very important to evaluate the outcome of the rescue treatment in these patients [146].

Solin et al. studied 41 cases of local relapse in 422 women with DCIS treated with BCS followed by radiotherapy [134]. The median time to local relapse was 4.8 years. In 22 of these 41 patients, the relapse was invasive. Among these lasts, after 4 years from the local recurrence, in 19% of cases, a distant metastasis occurred, and 13% died as a consequence. On the other hand, none of the patients with a noninvasive local relapse experienced metastasis or died due to cancer.

Another study presented similar data, with a 15% of distance metastasis rate after 12 years from invasive local relapse and a 12% mortality rate in this group of women [92]. These studies show how important it is, in the field of BCS, to minimize the risk of invasive local recurrence and consequently the risk of distant metastasis, which are associated with a significantly higher risk of death for cancer-related causes.

Acknowledgements

The authors would like to thank the whole collaborating staff of the Universitât dal Friûl and the support from the Ennergi Research, nonprofit association.

Author details

Ambrogio P. Londero[1,†*], Serena Bertozzi[2,†], Roberta Di Vora[2], Fabrizio De Biasio[3], Luca Seriau[2], Pier Camillo Parodi[3], Lorenza Driul[4], Andrea Risaliti[2], Laura Mariuzzi[5] and Carla Cedolini[2]

*Address all correspondence to: ambrogio.londero@gmail.com

1 Unit of Obstetrics and Gynecology, S. Polo Hospital, Monfalcone, GO, Italy

2 Clinic of Surgery, University of Udine, Italy

3 Clinic of Plastic Surgery, University of Udine, Italy

4 Clinic of Obstetrics and Gynecology, University of Udine, Italy

5 Institute of Pathologic Anatomy, University of Udine, Italy

† These two authors contributed equally to this work.

References

[1] Leonard GD, Swain SM. Ductal carcinoma in situ, complexities and challenges. Journal of the National Cancer Institute. 2004;**96**:906-920

[2] The Consensus Conference Committee. Consensus conference on the classification of ductal carcinoma in situ. The Consensus Conference Committee. Cancer. 1997;**80**:1798-1802

[3] Claus EB, Chu P, Howe CL, Davison TL, Stern DF, Carter D, et al. Pathobiologic findings in DCIS of the breast: Morphologic features, angiogenesis, HER-2/neu and hormone receptors. Experimental and Molecular Pathology. 2001;**70**:303-316. DOI: 10.1006/exmp.2001.2366

[4] Burstein HJ, Polyak K, Wong JS, Lester SC, Kaelin CM. Ductal carcinoma in situ of the breast. The New England Journal of Medicine. 2004;**350**:1430-1441. DOI: 10.1056/NEJMra031301

[5] O'Connell P, Pekkel V, Fuqua SA, Osborne CK, Clark GM, Allred DC. Analysis of loss of heterozygosity in 399 premalignant breast lesions at 15 genetic loci. Journal of the National Cancer Institute. 1998;**90**:697-703

[6] Aubele MM, Cummings MC, Mattis AE, Zitzelsberger HF, Walch AK, Kremer M, et al. Accumulation of chromosomal imbalances from intraductal proliferative lesions to adjacent in situ and invasive ductal breast cancer. Diagnostic Molecular Pathology: The American Journal of Surgical Pathology, Part B. 2000;**9**:14-19

[7] Farabegoli F, Champeme MH, Bieche I, Santini D, Ceccarelli C, Derenzini M, et al. Genetic pathways in the evolution of breast ductal carcinoma in situ. The Journal of Pathology. 2002;**196**:280-286. DOI: 10.1002/path.1048

[8] Rudas M, Neumayer R, Gnant MF, Mittelböck M, Jakesz R, Reiner A. p53 protein expression, cell proliferation and steroid hormone receptors in ductal and lobular in situ carcinomas of the breast. European Journal of Cancer (Oxford, England: 1990). 1997;**33**:39-44

[9] Buerger H, Otterbach F, Simon R, Poremba C, Diallo R, Decker T, et al. Comparative genomic hybridization of ductal carcinoma in situ of the breast-evidence of multiple genetic pathways. The Journal of Pathology. 1999;**187**:396-402. DOI: 10.1002/(SICI)1096-9896(199903)187:4<396::AID-PATH286>3.0.CO;2-L

[10] Buerger H, Otterbach F, Simon R, Schäfer KL, Poremba C, Diallo R, et al. Different genetic pathways in the evolution of invasive breast cancer are associated with distinct morphological subtypes. The Journal of Pathology. 1999;**189**:521-526. DOI: 10.1002/(SICI)1096-9896(199912)189:4<521::AID-PATH472>3.0.CO;2-B

[11] James LA, Mitchell EL, Menasce L, Varley JM. Comparative genomic hybridisation of ductal carcinoma in situ of the breast: Identification of regions of DNA amplification and deletion in common with invasive breast carcinoma. Oncogene. 1997;**14**:1059-1065. DOI: 10.1038/sj.onc.1200923

[12] Millis R, Bobrow L, Barnes D. Immunohistochemical evaluation of biological markers in mammary carcinoma in situ: Correlation with morphological features and recently proposed schemes for histological classification. The Breast. 1996;**5**:113-122. DOI: 10.1016/s0960-9776(96)90054-5

[13] Holland R, Hendriks JH, Vebeek AL, Mravunac M, Schuurmans Stekhoven JH. Extent, distribution, and mammographic/histological correlations of breast ductal carcinoma in situ. Lancet (London, England). 1990;**335**:519-522

[14] Faverly DR, Burgers L, Bult P, Holland R. Three dimensional imaging of mammary ductal carcinoma in situ: Clinical implications. Seminars in Diagnostic Pathology. 1994;**11**:193-198

[15] Menell JH, Morris EA, Dershaw DD, Abramson AF, Brogi E, Liberman L. Determination of the presence and extent of pure ductal carcinoma in situ by mammography and magnetic resonance imaging. The Breast Journal. 2005;**11**:382-390. DOI: 10.1111/j.1075-122X.2005.00121.x

[16] Lagios MD, Westdahl PR, Rose MR. The concept and implications of multicentricity in breast carcinoma. Pathology Annual. 1981;**16**:83-102

[17] Evans A, Pinder S, Wilson R, Sibbering M, Poller D, Elston C, et al. Ductal carcinoma in situ of the breast: Correlation between mammographic and pathologic findings. American Journal of Roentgenology. 1994;**162**:1307-1311. DOI: 10.2214/ajr.162.6.8191988

[18] Yang WT, Tse GMK. Sonographic, mammographic, and histopathologic correlation of symptomatic ductal carcinoma in situ. American Journal of Roentgenology. 2004;**182**:101-110. DOI: 10.2214/ajr.182.1.1820101

[19] Wright B, Shumak R. Part II. Medical imaging of ductal carcinoma in situ. Current Problems in Cancer. 2000;**24**:112-124

[20] Stomper PC, Connolly JL, Meyer JE, Harris JR. Clinically occult ductal carcinoma in situ detected with mammography: Analysis of 100 cases with radiologic-pathologic correlation. Radiology. 1989;**172**:235-241. DOI: 10.1148/radiology.172.1.2544922

[21] Ikeda DM, Andersson I. Ductal carcinoma in situ: Atypical mammographic appearances. Radiology. 1989;**172**:661-666. DOI: 10.1148/radiology.172.3.2549563

[22] Dershaw DD, Abramson A, Kinne DW. Ductal carcinoma in situ: Mammographic findings and clinical implications. Radiology. 1989;**170**:411-415. DOI: 10.1148/radiology.170.2.2536185

[23] Stomper PC, Margolin FR. Ductal carcinoma in situ: The mammographer's perspective. American Journal of Roentgenology. 1994;**162**:585-591. DOI: 10.2214/ajr.162.3.8109501

[24] Jansen SA, Newstead GM, Abe H, Shimauchi A, Schmidt RA, Karczmar GS. Pure ductal carcinoma in situ: Kinetic and morphologic MR characteristics compared with mammographic appearance and nuclear grade. Radiology. 2007;**245**:684-691. DOI: 10.1148/radiol.2453062061

[25] Barreau B, de Mascarel I, Feuga C, MacGrogan G, Dilhuydy MH, Picot V, et al. Mammography of ductal carcinoma in situ of the breast: Review of 909 cases with radiographic-pathologic correlations. European Journal of Radiology. 2005;**54**:55-61. DOI: 10.1016/j.ejrad.2004.11.019

[26] Lev-Toaff AS, Feig SA, Saitas VL, Finkel GC, Schwartz GF. Stability of malignant breast microcalcifications. Radiology. 1994;**192**:153-156. DOI: 10.1148/radiology.192.1.8208928

[27] Ahmed A. Calcification in human breast carcinomas: Ultrastructural observations. The Journal of Pathology. 1975;**117**:247-251. DOI: 10.1002/path.1711170407

[28] Levitan LH, Witten DM, Harrison EG. Calcification in breast disease mammographic-pathologic correlation. The American Journal of Roentgenology, Radium Therapy, and Nuclear Medicine. 1964;**92**:29-39

[29] Egan RL, McSweeney MB, Sewell CW. Intramammary calcifications without an associated mass in benign and malignant diseases. Radiology. 1980;**137**:1-7. DOI: 10.1148/radiology.137.1.7422830

[30] Fechner RE. Ductal carcinoma involving the lobule of the breast. A source of confusion with lobular carcinoma in situ. Cancer. 1971;**28**:274-281

[31] Stomper PC, Connolly JL. Ductal carcinoma in situ of the breast: Correlation between mammographic calcification and tumor subtype. American Journal of Roentgenology. 1992;**159**:483-485. DOI: 10.2214/ajr.159.3.1323923

[32] Knutzen AM, Gisvold JJ. Likelihood of malignant disease for various categories of mammographically detected, nonpalpable breast lesions. Mayo Clinic Proceedings. 1993;**68**:454-460

[33] Holland R, Hendriks JH. Microcalcifications associated with ductal carcinoma in situ: Mammographic-pathologic correlation. Seminars in Diagnostic Pathology. 1994;**11**:181-192

[34] Slanetz PJ, Giardino AA, Oyama T, Koerner FC, Halpern EF, Moore RH, et al. Mammographic appearance of ductal carcinoma in situ does not reliably predict histologic subtype. The Breast Journal. 2001;**7**:417-421

[35] Tabar L, Gad A, Parsons W, Neeland D. Mammographic appearances of in situ carcinomas. In: Ductal Carcinoma In Situ of the Breast. Baltimore: Williams and Wilkins; 1997. pp. 95-117

[36] Yamada T, Mori N, Watanabe M, Kimijima I, Okumoto T, Seiji K, et al. Radiologic-pathologic correlation of ductal carcinoma in situ. Radiographics: A Review Publication of the Radiological Society of North America, Inc. 2010;**30**:1183-1198. DOI: 10.1148/rg.305095073

[37] Sekine K, Tsunoda-Shimizu H, Kikuchi M, Saida Y, Kawasaki T, Suzuki K. DCIS showing architectural distortion on the screening mammogram – comparison of mammographic and pathological findings. Breast Cancer (Tokyo, Japan). 2007;**14**:281-284

[38] Tabar L, Tony Chen HH, Amy Yen MF, Tot T, Tung TH, Chen LS, et al. Mammographic tumor features can predict long-term outcomes reliably in women with 1-14-mm invasive breast carcinoma. Cancer. 2004;**101**:1745-1759. DOI: 10.1002/cncr.20582

[39] Lehman CD. Magnetic resonance imaging in the evaluation of ductal carcinoma in situ. Journal of the National Cancer Institute Monographs. 2010;**2010**:150-151. DOI: 10.1093/jncimonographs/lgq030

[40] Berg WA, Gutierrez L, NessAiver MS, Carter WB, Bhargavan M, Lewis RS, et al. Diagnostic accuracy of mammography, clinical examination, US, and MR imaging in preoperative assessment of breast cancer. Radiology. 2004;**233**:830-849. DOI: 10.1148/radiol.2333031484

[41] Rosen EL, Smith-Foley SA, DeMartini WB, Eby PR, Peacock S, Lehman CD. BI-RADS MRI enhancement characteristics of ductal carcinoma in situ. The Breast Journal. 2007;**13**:545-550. DOI: 10.1111/j.1524-4741.2007.00513.x

[42] Kuhl CK, Schrading S, Bieling HB, Wardelmann E, Leutner CC, Koenig R, et al. MRI for diagnosis of pure ductal carcinoma in situ: A prospective observational study. Lancet (London, England). 2007;**370**:485-492. DOI: 10.1016/S0140-6736(07)61232-X

[43] Del Frate C, Borghese L, Cedolini C, Bestagno A, Puglisi F, Isola M, et al. Role of presurgical breast MRI in the management of invasive breast carcinoma. Breast (Edinburgh, Scotland). 2007;**16**:469-481. DOI: 10.1016/j.breast.2007.02.004

[44] Ottinetti A, Sapino A. Morphometric evaluation of microvessels surrounding hyperplastic and neoplastic mammary lesions. Breast Cancer Research and Treatment. 1988;**11**:241-248

[45] Brown LF, Guidi AJ, Schnitt SJ, Van De Water L, Iruela-Arispe ML, Yeo TK, et al. Vascular stroma formation in carcinoma in situ, invasive carcinoma, and metastatic carcinoma of the breast. Clinical Cancer Research: An Official Journal of the American Association for Cancer Research. 1999;**5**:1041-1056

[46] Esserman LJ, Kumar AS, Herrera AF, Leung J, Au A, Chen YY, et al. Magnetic resonance imaging captures the biology of ductal carcinoma in situ. Journal of Clinical Oncology: Official Journal of the American Society of Clinical Oncology. 2006;**24**:4603-4610. DOI: 10.1200/JCO.2005.04.5518

[47] Furman-Haran E, Schechtman E, Kelcz F, Kirshenbaum K, Degani H. Magnetic resonance imaging reveals functional diversity of the vasculature in benign and malignant breast lesions. Cancer. 2005;**104**:708-718. DOI: 10.1002/cncr.21225

[48] Rosen. Rosen Breast Pathology 3E. Philadelphia: Wolters Kluwer/Lippincott Williams & Wilkins; 2009

[49] Man Y. Focal degeneration of aged or injured myoepithelial cells and the resultant auto-immunoreactions are trigger factors for breast tumor invasion. Medical Hypotheses. 2007;**69**:1340-1357. DOI: 10.1016/j.mehy.2007.02.031

[50] Raza S, Vallejo M, Chikarmane SA, Birdwell RL. Pure ductal carcinoma in situ: A range of MRI features. American Journal of Roentgenology. 2008;**191**:689-699. DOI: 10.2214/AJR.07.3779

[51] Viehweg P, Lampe D, Buchmann J, Heywang-Köbrunner SH. In situ and minimally invasive breast cancer: Morphologic and kinetic features on contrast-enhanced MR imaging. Magma (New York, NY). 2000;**11**:129-137

[52] Lallemand M, Barron M, Bingham J, Mosier A, Hardin M, Sohn V. The true impact of breast magnetic resonance imaging on the management of in situ disease: More is not better. American Journal of Surgery. 2017;**213**:127-131. DOI: 10.1016/j.amjsurg.2016.05.002

[53] Fancellu A, Turner RM, Dixon JM, Pinna A, Cottu P, Houssami N. Meta-analysis of the effect of preoperative breast MRI on the surgical management of ductal carcinoma in situ. The British Journal of Surgery. 2015;**102**:883-893. DOI: 10.1002/bjs.9797

[54] Davis KL, Barth RJ, Gui J, Dann E, Eisenberg B, Rosenkranz K. Use of MRI in preoperative planning for women with newly diagnosed DCIS: Risk or benefit? Annals of Surgical Oncology. 2012;**19**:3270-3274. DOI: 10.1245/s10434-012-2548-3

[55] Morrow M, Waters J, Morris E. MRI for breast cancer screening, diagnosis, and treatment. Lancet (London, England). 2011;**378**:1804-1811. DOI: 10.1016/S0140-6736(11)61350-0

[56] Houssami N, Turner R, Morrow M. Preoperative magnetic resonance imaging in breast cancer: Meta-analysis of surgical outcomes. Annals of Surgery. 2013;**257**:249-255. DOI: 10.1097/SLA.0b013e31827a8d17

[57] Erbas B, Provenzano E, Armes J, Gertig D. The natural history of ductal carcinoma in situ of the breast: A review. Breast Cancer Research and Treatment. 2006;**97**:135-144. DOI: 10.1007/s10549-005-9101-z

[58] Jansen SA. Ductal carcinoma in situ: Detection, diagnosis, and characterization with magnetic resonance imaging. Seminars in Ultrasound, CT, and MR. 2011;**32**:306-318. DOI: 10.1053/j.sult.2011.02.007

[59] Allen LR, Lago-Toro CE, Hughes JH, Careaga E, Brown AT, Chernick M, et al. Is there a role for MRI in the preoperative assessment of patients with DCIS? Annals of Surgical Oncology. 2010;17:2395-2400. DOI: 10.1245/s10434-010-1000-9

[60] Solin LJ, Orel SG, Hwang WT, Harris EE, Schnall MD. Relationship of breast magnetic resonance imaging to outcome after breast-conservation treatment with radiation for women with early-stage invasive breast carcinoma or ductal carcinoma in situ. Journal of Clinical Oncology: Official Journal of the American Society of Clinical Oncology. 2008;26:386-391. DOI: 10.1200/JCO.2006.09.5448

[61] Driul L, Bernardi S, Bertozzi S, Schiavon M, Londero AP, Petri R. New surgical trends in breast cancer treatment: Conservative interventions and oncoplastic breast surgery. Minerva Ginecologica. 2013;65:289-296

[62] Cedolini C, Bertozzi S, Londero AP, Bernardi S, Seriau L, Concina S, et al. Type of breast cancer diagnosis, screening, and survival. Clinical Breast Cancer. 2014;14:235-240. DOI: 10.1016/j.clbc.2014.02.004

[63] Nelson HD, Tyne K, Naik A, Bougatsos C, Chan B, Nygren P, et al. Screening for Breast Cancer: Systematic Evidence Review Update for the US Preventive Services Task Force. Report No: 10-05142-EF-1. 2009

[64] AIOM. Linee guida neoplasie della mammella. Techreport, AIOM. 2016

[65] Bernardi D, Macaskill P, Pellegrini M, Valentini M, Fantò C, Ostillio L, et al. Breast cancer screening with tomosynthesis (3D mammography) with acquired or synthetic 2D mammography compared with 2D mammography alone (STORM-2): A population-based prospective study. The Lancet Oncology. 2016;17:1105-1113. DOI: 10.1016/S1470-2045(16)30101-2

[66] Ernster VL, Ballard-Barbash R, Barlow WE, Zheng Y, Weaver DL, Cutter G, et al. Detection of ductal carcinoma in situ in women undergoing screening mammography. Journal of the National Cancer Institute. 2002;94:1546-1554

[67] Minister of Public Works and Government Services Canada. Organized Breast Cancer Screening Programs in Canada. Minister of Public Works and Government Services Canada. 1999. Cat. No. H1-9/13-1999. ISBN: 0-662-64516-2

[68] UK Trial of Early Detection of Breast Cancer Group. 16-year mortality from breast cancer in the UK trial of early detection of breast cancer. Lancet (London, England). 1999;353:1909-1914

[69] Fracheboud J, Groenewoud J, Boer R, Broeders M, Baan C, Verbeek A, et al. Landelijke evaluatie van bevolkingsonderzoek in Nederland (VIII), instituut Maatschappelijke Gezondheidszorg. Rotterdam: Erasmus Universiteit Rotterdam. 2000

[70] Kopans DB, Smith RA, Duffy SW. Mammographic screening and "overdiagnosis". Radiology. 2011;260:616-620

[71] Virnig BA, Tuttle TM, Shamliyan T, Kane RL. Ductal carcinoma in situ of the breast: A systematic review of incidence, treatment, and outcomes. Journal of the National Cancer Institute. 2010;**102**:170-178

[72] Tabar L, Fagerberg G, Chen HH, Duffy SW, Smart CR, Gad A, et al. Efficacy of breast cancer screening by age. New results swedish two-county trial. Cancer. 1995;**75**:2507-2517

[73] Nyström L, Andersson I, Bjurstam N, Frisell J, Nordenskjöld B, Rutqvist LE. Long-term effects of mammography screening: Updated overview of the Swedish randomised trials. The Lancet. 2002;**359**:909-919

[74] Hendrick RE, Smith RA, Rutledge III JH, Smart CR. Benefit of screening mammography in women aged 40-49: A new meta-analysis of randomized controlled trials. JNCI Monographs. 1997;**1997**:87-92

[75] Duffy S, Tabar L, Vitak B, Day N, Smith R, Chen H, et al. The relative contributions of screen-detected in situ and invasive breast carcinomas in reducing mortality from the disease. European Journal of Cancer. 2003;**39**:1755-1760

[76] Evans A, Pinder S, Ellis I, Wilson A. Screen detected ductal carcinoma in situ (DCIS): Overdiagnosis or an obligate precursor of invasive disease? Journal of Medical Screening. 2001;**8**:149-151

[77] Harris JR. Diseases of the Breast. Philadelphia, PA, USA: Lippincott Williams & Wilki; 2014

[78] Worni M, Akushevich I, Greenup R, Sarma D, Ryser MD, Myers ER, et al. Trends in treatment patterns and outcomes for ductal carcinoma in situ. Journal of the National Cancer Institute. 2015;**107**:djv263. DOI: 10.1093/jnci/djv263

[79] Silverstein MJ, Cohlan BF, Gierson ED, Furmanski M, Gamagami P, Colburn WJ, et al. Duct carcinoma in situ: 227 cases without microinvasion. European Journal of Cancer (Oxford England: 1990). 1992;**28**:630-634

[80] Vargas C, Kestin L, Go N, Krauss D, Chen P, Goldstein N, et al. Factors associated with local recurrence and cause-specific survival in patients with ductal carcinoma in situ of the breast treated with breast-conserving therapy or mastectomy. International Journal of Radiation Oncology, Biology, Physics. 2005;**63**:1514-1521. DOI: 10.1016/j.ijrobp.2005.04.045

[81] De Biasio F, Zingaretti N, Marchesi A, Vaienti L, Almesberger D, Parodi PC. A simple and effective technique of breast remodelling after conserving surgery for lower quadrants breast cancer. Aesthetic Plastic Surgery. 2016;**40**:887-895. DOI: 10.1007/s00266-016-0709-7

[82] Bernardi S, Bertozzi S, Londero AP, Gentile G, Giacomuzzi F, Carbone A. Incidence and risk factors of the intraoperative localization failure of nonpalpable breast lesions by radio-guided occult lesion localization: A retrospective analysis of 579 cases. World Journal of Surgery. 2012;**36**:1915-1921. DOI: 10.1007/s00268-012-1577-1

[83] Bernardi S, Bertozzi S, Londero AP, Gentile G, Angione V, Petri R. Influence of surgical margins on the outcome of breast cancer patients: A retrospective analysis. World Journal of Surgery. 2014;**38**:2279-2287. DOI: 10.1007/s00268-014-2596-x

[84] Curigliano G, Burstein HJ, Winer EP, Gnant M, Dubsky P, Loibl S, et al. De-escalating and escalating treatments for early-stage breast cancer: The St. Gallen international expert consensus conference on the primary therapy of early breast cancer 2017. Annals of Oncology: Official Journal of the European Society for Medical Oncology. 2017;28: 1700-1712. DOI: 10.1093/annonc/mdx308

[85] De Biasio F, Zingaretti N, De Lorenzi F, Riccio M, Vaienti L, Parodi PC. Reduction Mammaplasty for breast symmetrisation in implant-based reconstructions. Aesthetic Plastic Surgery. 2017;41:773-781. DOI: 10.1007/s00266-017-0867-2

[86] De Biasio F, Zingaretti N, Mura S, Fin A, Riccio M, Parodi PC. A new method of salvaging nipple projection after secondary nipple reconstruction using locoregional flap. Indian Journal of Plastic Surgery: Official Publication of the Association of Plastic Surgeons of India. 2017;50:107-108. DOI: 10.4103/ijps.IJPS_47_17

[87] Zingaretti N, De Lorenzi F, Dell'Antonia F, De Biasio F, Riccio M, Parodi PC. The use of "Precapsular space" in secondary breast reconstruction. Aesthetic Plastic Surgery. 2016;40:716-723. DOI: 10.1007/s00266-016-0683-0

[88] Semprini G, Cattin F, De Biasio F, Cedolini C, Parodi PC. The bovine pericardial patch in breast reconstruction: A case report. Il Giornale di chirurgia. 2012;33:392-394

[89] Germanò D, De Biasio F, Piedimonte A, Parodi PC. Nipple reconstruction using the fleur-de-lis flap technique. Aesthetic Plastic Surgery. 2006;30:399-402. DOI: 10.1007/s00266-005-0199-5

[90] De Biasio F, Nadalig B, Salemi S, Parodi PC. Re: Nipple reconstruction: The top hat technique. Annals of Plastic Surgery. 2006;56:224. DOI: 10.1097/01.sap.0000194946.92450.52

[91] Parodi PC, De Biasio F, Guarneri GF, Rampino Cordaro E, Panizzo N, Riberti C. Microsurgical latissimus dorsi flap in a case of breast aplasia caused by radiation therapy. Microsurgery. 2005;25:473-476. DOI: 10.1002/micr.20151

[92] Lee LA, Silverstein MJ, Chung CT, Macdonald H, Sanghavi P, Epstein M, et al. Breast cancer-specific mortality after invasive local recurrence in patients with ductal carcinoma-in-situ of the breast. American Journal of Surgery. 2006;192:416-419. DOI: 10.1016/j.amjsurg.2006.06.005

[93] Boyages J, Delaney G, Taylor R. Predictors of local recurrence after treatment of ductal carcinoma in situ: A meta-analysis. Cancer. 1999;85:616-628

[94] Cedolini C, Bertozzi S, Seriau L, Londero AP, Concina S, Moretti E, et al. Feasibility of conservative breast surgery and intraoperative radiation therapy for early breast cancer: A single-center, open, non-randomized, prospective pilot study. Oncology Reports 2014;31:1539-1546. doi:10.3892/or.2014.3018.

[95] Correa C, McGale P, Taylor C, Wang Y, Clarke M, et al. Overview of the randomized trials of radiotherapy in ductal carcinoma in situ of the breast. Journal of the National Cancer Institute Monographs. Early Breast Cancer Trialists' Collaborative Group (EBCTCG). 2010;2010:162-177. DOI: 10.1093/jncimonographs/lgq039

[96] Bijker N, Meijnen P, Peterse JL, Bogaerts J, Van Hoorebeeck I, et al. Breast-conserving treatment with or without radiotherapy in ductal carcinoma-in-situ: Ten-year results of European Organisation for Research and Treatment of Cancer randomized phase III trial 10853 – A study by the EORTC Breast Cancer Cooperative Group and EORTC Radiotherapy Group. Journal of Clinical Oncology: Official Journal of the American Society of Clinical Oncology.EORTC Breast Cancer Cooperative Group and EORTC Radiotherapy Group. 2006;**24**:3381-3387. DOI: 10.1200/JCO.2006.06.1366

[97] Emdin SO, Granstrand B, Ringberg A, Sandelin K, Arnesson LG, Nordgren H, et al. SweDCIS: Radiotherapy after sector resection for ductal carcinoma in situ of the breast. Results of a randomised trial in a population offered mammography screening. Acta Oncologica (Stockholm, Sweden). 2006;**45**:536-543. DOI: 10.1080/02841860600681569

[98] Fisher B, Land S, Mamounas E, Dignam J, Fisher ER, Wolmark N. Prevention of invasive breast cancer in women with ductal carcinoma in situ: An update of the National Surgical Adjuvant Breast and bowel project experience. Seminars in Oncology. 2001;**28**:400-418

[99] Houghton J, George WD, Cuzick J, Duggan C, Fentiman IS, Spittle M, et al. Radiotherapy and tamoxifen in women with completely excised ductal carcinoma in situ of the breast in the UK, Australia, and New Zealand: Randomised controlled trial. Lancet (London, England). 2003;**362**:95-102

[100] Schmale I, Liu S, Rayhanabad J, Russell CA, Sener SF. Ductal carcinoma in situ (DCIS) of the breast: Perspectives on biology and controversies in current management. Journal of Surgical Oncology. 2012;**105**:212-220. DOI: 10.1002/jso.22020

[101] Fisher B, Dignam J, Wolmark N, Wickerham DL, Fisher ER, Mamounas E, et al. Tamoxifen in treatment of intraductal breast cancer: National Surgical Adjuvant Breast and bowel project B-24 randomised controlled trial. Lancet (London, England). 1999;**353**:1993-2000. DOI: 10.1016/S0140-6736(99)05036-9

[102] Cuzick J, Sestak I, Pinder SE, Ellis IO, Forsyth S, Bundred NJ, et al. Effect of tamoxifen and radiotherapy in women with locally excised ductal carcinoma in situ: Long-term results from the UK/ANZ DCIS trial. The Lancet Oncology. 2011;**12**:21-29. DOI: 10.1016/S1470-2045(10)70266-7

[103] Vogel VG, Costantino JP, Wickerham DL, Cronin WM. National surgical adjuvant breast and bowel project update: Prevention trials and endocrine therapy of ductal carcinoma in situ. Clinical Cancer Research: An Official Journal of the American Association for Cancer Research. 2003;**9**:495S-501S

[104] Bijker N, Peterse JL, Duchateau L, Robanus-Maandag EC, Bosch CA, Duval C, et al. Histological type and marker expression of the primary tumour compared with its local recurrence after breast-conserving therapy for ductal carcinoma in situ. British Journal of Cancer. 2001;**84**:539-544. DOI: 10.1054/bjoc.2000.1618

[105] Edge S, Byrd D, Compton C, Fritz G, Greene F, Trotti A. AJCC Cancer Staging Manual. 7th ed. New York: Springer; 2009

[106] Fang Y, Wu J, Wang W, Fei X, Zong Y, Chen X, et al. Biologic behavior and long-term outcomes of breast ductal carcinoma in situ with microinvasion. Oncotarget. 2016;7:64182-64190. DOI: 10.18632/oncotarget.11639

[107] Singletary SE, Allred C, Ashley P, Bassett LW, Berry D, Bland KI, et al. Revision of the American joint committee on cancer staging system for breast cancer. Journal of Clinical Oncology: Official Journal of the American Society of Clinical Oncology. 2002;20:3628-3636. DOI: 10.1200/JCO.2002.02.026

[108] Bianchi S, Vezzosi V. Microinvasive carcinoma of the breast. Pathology Oncology Research. 2008;14:105-111. DOI: 10.1007/s12253-008-9054-8

[109] Baxter NN, Virnig BA, Durham SB, Tuttle TM. Trends in the treatment of ductal carcinoma in situ of the breast. Journal of the National Cancer Institute. 2004;96:443-448

[110] Adamovich TL, Simmons RM. Ductal carcinoma in situ with microinvasion. American Journal of Surgery. 2003;186:112-116

[111] Prasad ML, Osborne MP, Giri DD, Hoda SA. Microinvasive carcinoma (T1mic) of the breast: Clinicopathologic profile of 21 cases. The American Journal of Surgical Pathology. 2000;24:422-428

[112] Rosner D, Lane WW, Penetrante R. Ductal carcinoma in situ with microinvasion. A curable entity using surgery alone without need for adjuvant therapy. Cancer. 1991;67:1498-1503

[113] Wong JH, Kopald KH, Morton DL. The impact of microinvasion on axillary node metastases and survival in patients with intraductal breast cancer. Archives of Surgery (Chicago, IL: 1960). 1990;125:1298-1301; discussion 1301-2

[114] Solin LJ, Fowble BL, Yeh IT, Kowalyshyn MJ, Schultz DJ, Weiss MC, et al. Microinvasive ductal carcinoma of the breast treated with breast-conserving surgery and definitive irradiation. International Journal of Radiation Oncology, Biology, Physics. 1992;23:961-968

[115] Padmore RF, Fowble B, Hoffman J, Rosser C, Hanlon A, Patchefsky AS. Microinvasive breast carcinoma: Clinicopathologic analysis of a single institution experience. Cancer. 2000;88:1403-1409

[116] Gojon H, Fawunmi D, Valachis A. Sentinel lymph node biopsy in patients with microinvasive breast cancer: A systematic review and meta-analysis. European Journal of Surgical Oncology: The Journal of the European Society of Surgical Oncology and the British Association of Surgical Oncology. 2014;40:5-11. DOI: 10.1016/j.ejso.2013.10.020

[117] Lyman GH, Giuliano AE, Somerfield MR, Benson AB, Bodurka DC, Burstein HJ, et al. American Society of Clinical Oncology guideline recommendations for sentinel lymph node biopsy in early-stage breast cancer. Journal of Clinical Oncology: Official Journal of the American Society of Clinical Oncology. 2005;23:7703-7720. DOI: 10.1200/JCO.2005.08.001

[118] Dominguez FJ, Golshan M, Black DM, Hughes KS, Gadd MA, Christian R, et al. Sentinel node biopsy is important in mastectomy for ductal carcinoma in situ. Annals of Surgical Oncology. 2008;**15**:268-273. DOI: 10.1245/s10434-007-9610-6

[119] Murphy CD, Jones JL, Javid SH, Michaelson JS, Nolan ME, Lipsitz SR, et al. Do sentinel node micrometastases predict recurrence risk in ductal carcinoma in situ and ductal carcinoma in situ with microinvasion? American Journal of Surgery. 2008;**196**:566-568. DOI: 10.1016/j.amjsurg.2008.06.011

[120] Kinne DW, Petrek JA, Osborne MP, Fracchia AA, DePalo AA, Rosen PP. Breast carcinoma in situ. Archives of surgery (Chicago, IL: 1960). 1989;**124**:33-36

[121] Silverstein MJ, Recht A, Lagios MD, editors. Ductal Carcinoma In Situ of the Breast. Philadelphia, PA, USA: Lippincott Williams & Wilkins; 2002

[122] Parikh RR, Haffty BG, Lannin D, Moran MS. Ductal carcinoma in situ with microinvasion: Prognostic implications, long-term outcomes, and role of axillary evaluation. International Journal of Radiation Oncology, Biology, Physics. 2012;**82**:7-13. DOI: 10.1016/j.ijrobp.2010.08.027

[123] Runowicz CD, Leach CR, Henry NL, Henry KS, Mackey HT, Cowens-Alvarado RL, et al. American Cancer Society/American Society of Clinical Oncology breast cancer survivorship care guideline. Journal of Clinical Oncology: Official Journal of the American Society of Clinical Oncology. 2016;**34**:611-635. DOI: 10.1200/JCO.2015.64.3809

[124] Bertozzi S, Londero AP, Giacomuzzi F, Angione V, Carbone A, Petri R, et al. Applicability of two different validated models to predict axillary non-sentinel lymph node status by sentinel node biopsy in a single Italian center. Breast cancer (Tokyo, Japan). 2015;**22**:350-355. DOI: 10.1007/s12282-013-0485-z

[125] Bernardi S, Bertozzi S, Londero AP, Angione V, Petri R, Giacomuzzi F. Prevalence and risk factors of intraoperative identification failure of sentinel lymph nodes in patients affected by breast cancer. Nuclear Medicine Communications. 2013;**34**:664-673. DOI: 10.1097/MNM.0b013e328361cd84

[126] Bernardi S, Bertozzi S, Londero AP, Giacomuzzi F, Angione V, Dri C, et al. Nine years of experience with the sentinel lymph node biopsy in a single Italian center: A retrospective analysis of 1050 cases. World Journal of Surgery. 2012;**36**:714-722. DOI: 10.1007/s00268-011-1420-0

[127] Cedolini C, Bertozzi S, Seriau L, Londero AP, Concina S, Cattin F, et al. Eight-year experience with the intraoperative frozen section examination of sentinel lymph node biopsy for breast cancer in a North-Italian University Center. International Journal of Clinical and Experimental Pathology. 2014;**7**:364-371

[128] Mansel RE, Fallowfield L, Kissin M, Goyal A, Newcombe RG, Dixon JM, et al. Randomized multicenter trial of sentinel node biopsy versus standard axillary treatment in operable breast cancer: The ALMANAC trial. Journal of the National Cancer Institute. 2006;**98**:599-609. DOI: 10.1093/jnci/djj158

[129] Veronesi U, Paganelli G, Viale G, Luini A, Zurrida S, Galimberti V, et al. A randomized comparison of sentinel-node biopsy with routine axillary dissection in breast cancer. The New England Journal of Medicine. 2003;**349**:546-553. DOI: 10.1056/NEJMoa012782

[130] Veronesi U, Viale G, Paganelli G, Zurrida S, Luini A, Galimberti V, et al. Sentinel lymph node biopsy in breast cancer: Ten-year results of a randomized controlled study. Annals of Surgery. 2010;**251**:595-600. DOI: 10.1097/SLA.0b013e3181c0e92a

[131] Krag DN, Anderson SJ, Julian TB, Brown AM, Harlow SP, Costantino JP, et al. Sentinel-lymph-node resection compared with conventional axillary-lymph-node dissection in clinically node-negative patients with breast cancer: Overall survival findings from the NSABP B-32 randomised phase 3 trial. The Lancet Oncology. 2010;**11**:927-933. DOI: 10.1016/S1470-2045(10)70207-2

[132] Giuliano AE, Kirgan DM, Guenther JM, Morton DL. Lymphatic mapping and sentinel lymphadenectomy for breast cancer. Annals of Surgery. 1994;**220**:391-8; discussion 398-401

[133] Giuliano AE, Jones RC, Brennan M, Statman R. Sentinel lymphadenectomy in breast cancer. Journal of Clinical Oncology: Official Journal of the American Society of Clinical Oncology. 1997;**15**:2345-2350. DOI: 10.1200/JCO.1997.15.6.2345

[134] Solin LJ, Fourquet A, Vicini FA, Haffty B, Taylor M, McCormick B, et al. Mammographically detected ductal carcinoma in situ of the breast treated with breast-conserving surgery and definitive breast irradiation: Long-term outcome and prognostic significance of patient age and margin status. International Journal of Radiation Oncology, Biology, Physics. 2001;**50**:991-1002

[135] Kerlikowske K, Molinaro A, Cha I, Ljung BM, Ernster VL, Stewart K, et al. Characteristics associated with recurrence among women with ductal carcinoma in situ treated by lumpectomy. Journal of the National Cancer Institute. 2003;**95**:1692-1702

[136] Dunne C, Burke JP, Morrow M, Kell MR. Effect of margin status on local recurrence after breast conservation and radiation therapy for ductal carcinoma in situ. Journal of Clinical Oncology: Official Journal of the American Society of Clinical Oncology. 2009;**27**:1615-1620. DOI: 10.1200/JCO.2008.17.5182

[137] MacDonald HR, Silverstein MJ, Mabry H, Moorthy B, Ye W, Epstein MS, et al. Local control in ductal carcinoma in situ treated by excision alone: Incremental benefit of larger margins. American Journal of Surgery. 2005;**190**:521-525. DOI: 10.1016/j.amjsurg.2005.06.005

[138] Jhingran A, Kim JS, Buchholz TA, Katz A, Strom EA, Hunt KK, et al. Age as a predictor of outcome for women with DCIS treated with breast-conserving surgery and radiation: The University of Texas M. D. Anderson Cancer Center experience. International Journal of Radiation Oncology, Biology, Physics. 2002;**54**:804-809

[139] Vicini FA, Recht A. Age at diagnosis and outcome for women with ductal carcinoma-in-situ of the breast: A critical review of the literature. Journal of Clinical Oncology:

Official Journal of the American Society of Clinical Oncology. 2002;**20**:2736-2744. DOI: 10.1200/JCO.2002.07.137

[140] Rodrigues NA, Dillon D, Carter D, Parisot N, Haffty BG. Differences in the pathologic and molecular features of intraductal breast carcinoma between younger and older women. Cancer. 2003;**97**:1393-1403. DOI: 10.1002/cncr.11204

[141] Goldstein NS, Vicini FA, Kestin LL, Thomas M. Differences in the pathologic features of ductal carcinoma in situ of the breast based on patient age. Cancer. 2000;**88**:2553-2560

[142] Carlson GW, Page A, Johnson E, Nicholson K, Styblo TM, Wood WC. Local recurrence of ductal carcinoma in situ after skin-sparing mastectomy. Journal of the American College of Surgeons. 2007;**204**:1074-1078; discussion 1078-80. DOI: 10.1016/j.jamcollsurg.2007.01.063

[143] Provenzano E, Hopper JL, Giles GG, Marr G, Venter DJ, Armes JE. Biological markers that predict clinical recurrence in ductal carcinoma in situ of the breast. European Journal of Cancer (Oxford, England: 1990). 2003;**39**:622-630

[144] Silverstein MJ, Lagios MD, Craig PH, Waisman JR, Lewinsky BS, Colburn WJ, et al. A prognostic index for ductal carcinoma in situ of the breast. Cancer. 1996;**77**:2267-2274. DOI: 10.1002/(SICI)1097-0142(19960601)77:11<2267::AID-CNCR13>3.0.CO;2-V

[145] Silverstein MJ. The University of Southern California/van Nuys prognostic index for ductal carcinoma in situ of the breast. American Journal of Surgery. 2003;**186**:337-343

[146] Fisher ER, Dignam J, Tan-Chiu E, Costantino J, Fisher B, Paik S, et al. Pathologic findings from the National Surgical Adjuvant Breast Project (NSABP) eight-year update of protocol B-17: Intraductal carcinoma. Cancer. 1999;**86**:429-438

7

Applications of Aptamers in Cancer Therapy

Ajda Coker-Gurkan, Pinar Obakan-Yerlikaya and
Elif-Damla Arisan

Abstract

Aptamers are small and specific oligonucleotides [RNA or single-strand DNA (ssDNA)] with a high binding affinity against target protein. *In vitro* selection process of aptamer by selective evolution of ligands by exponential enrichment (SELEX) has been invented in 1990 by Larry Gold and Jack Szostak. SELEX is a random amplification of target protein with combined oligonucleotide libraries and selection of synthesized aptamer by magnetic beads, affinity chromatography, and capillary electrophoresis-based methods. According to their low molecular weight, non-immunogenic feature *in vivo*, low production cost, high thermal stability, increase in production potential, and ample of modification capacities, aptamers are becoming essential medical tools for diagnosis and treatment of diseases such as macular degeneration, hemophilia, heart disease, and various cancer types. The therapeutic potential of aptamers, with high binding affinity against carcinogenesis-associated growth factors, receptors, or proteins frequently overexpressed in specific cancers such as prostate, breast, colon, lung, leukemia, hepatocellular, and cervical carcinoma. The strategies for aptamer-based drugs in cancer therapy design/modify aptamers against cancer biomarkers, accelerate immunotherapy targeting immune system, and increase the drug delivery in cancer cells. In conclusion, aptamers are promising candidate drugs due to their antiproliferative effect on cancer cells and the drug delivery systems during cancer chemotherapy.

Keywords: aptamer, SELEX, cancer, therapy

1. Introduction

Aptamer is derived from one Latin and one Greek word combinations: "aptus," which means "fit," and "meros" meaning "particle" [1]. As a DNA or RNA oligonucleotide, aptamer has low molecular weight (5–40 kDa) and three-dimensional (3D) structure with a high binding affinity against target protein. Synthesis of aptamers by selective evolution of ligands by exponential enrichment (SELEX) has been invented in 1990 by Larry Gold and Jack Szostak and the other laboratories concomitantly [2]. SELEX is a consecutive processes starting with binding of target with random sequence of oligonucleotide library, washing and elution of unbound oligonucleotides, amplification of 3D structure oligonucleotides against the target epitope *via* polymerase chain reaction (PCR), selection of aptamers with high binding affinity and specificity, and finally modifications of novel aptamers to increase stability and function [3]. Through SELEX, an aptamer against various targets can be synthesized such as amino acids, peptides, protein, phospholipids, carbohydrates, nucleic acids, antibiotics, metal ions, and whole cell (bacteria, viruses). Although aptamers are similar to antibodies due to their binding affinity to target molecule, they have a number of advantages such as small and low complexity with low immunogenic activity, high stability, high affinity and specificity for their targets, and easy to synthesize and modify *in vitro* [4].

1.1. SELEX method

The determination of oligonucleotides from a random ssDNA/RNA sequence pool is accomplished through *in vitro* selection referred as SELEX. SELEX method is composed of following various steps: (i) design and synthesis of oligonucleotide library (DNA or RNA), (ii) hybridization of target with oligonucleotide library, (iii) elimination of aptamers unbounded to target, (iv) selection of aptamers that are highly specific against target (4–20 rounds), (v) amplification of selected aptamers by PCR (ssDNA library) or RT-PCR (RNA library) in order to increase aptamer efficacy, (vi) cloning of selected and amplified aptamers in vector (TOPO cloning vector), (vii) sequence determination of cloned aptamers, and (viii) discriminate and identify the novel aptamer from aptamer database tools [5].

Oligonucleotide libraries are the major nucleic acid-based tool to generate aptamer *via* using SELEX method. Classical SELEX libraries are generally 10^{14}–10^{16} molecules with 20–80 nucleotides long and usually amount of 10^{-8}–10^{-10} M. They are arranged in order of sequences with three parts: 5′ sense primer sequence, random nucleotide, and 3′ antisense primer sequence parts, respectively. 5′- sense or 3′-antisense sequence part of the oligonucleotide libraries are 18–22 base long, and the random sequence between 5′ and 3′ sequences ranges from 20 to 40 nucleotides (**Figure 1**) [6].

Besides classical libraries, different featured libraries can be used for SELEX method such as structurally modified, based on a known sequence, free of fixed sequences or genomic sequences. In structurally modified libraries, between two fixed sequences, a random region constructed to form a secondary structure (G-quartets, hairpin, vs) in order to select more stable aptamer against target molecule [7]. A library used for SELEX is constructed with 4–6 nucleotide-fixed regions in both sides called a free of fixed sequence oligonucleotide library (tailored SELEX) [8].

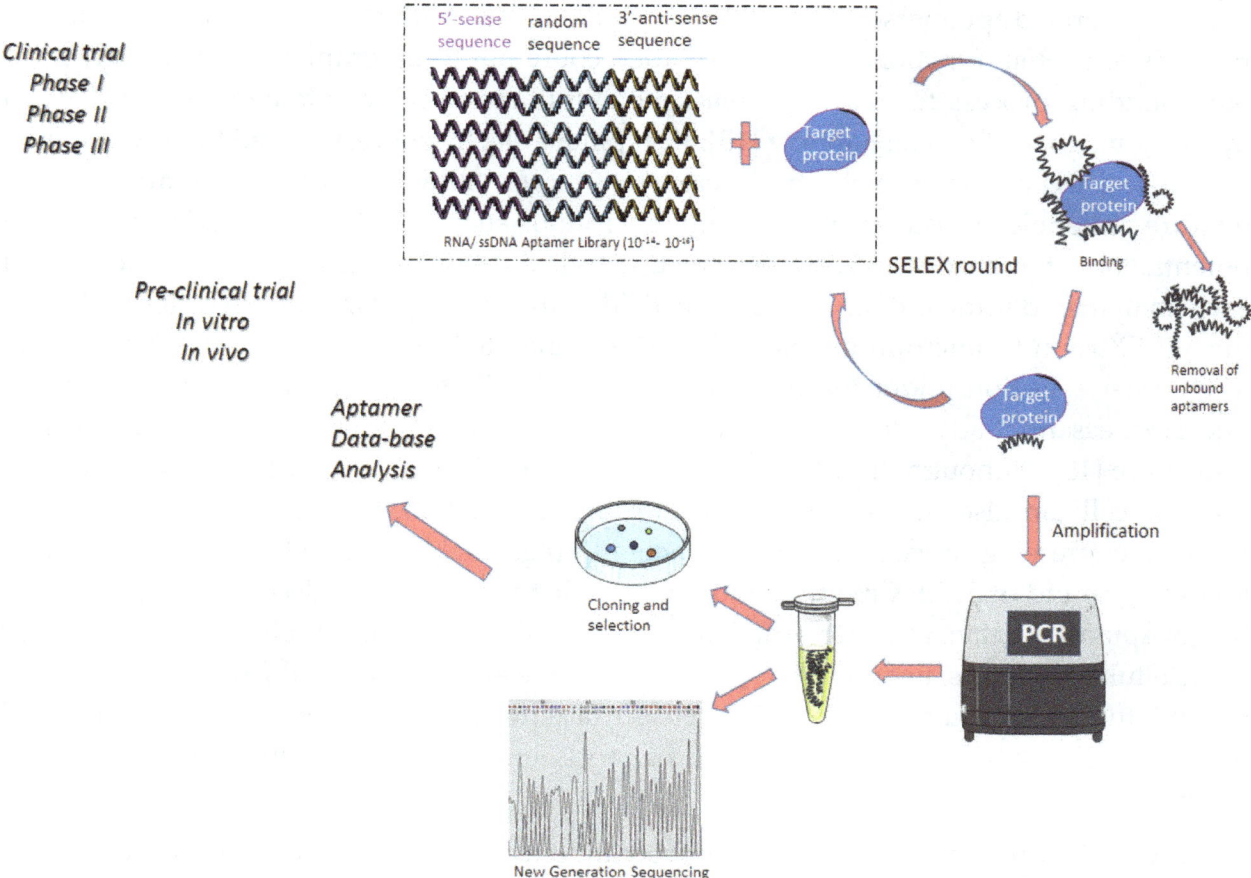

Figure 1. Schematic representation of SELEX method.

In addition, to investigate for sequences such as transcription factors, translation regulators, and splicing sequences, genomic sequence-based libraries are used for genomic SELEX. In genomic SELEX, the oligonucleotide libraries are composed of 50–500 nucleotides long with fixed sequences on each region [9]. In order to protect aptamers from nucleases, chemical modifications such as L-form of nucleotides (L-ribose or L-deoxyribose); 5-iodo-, 4-thiouridine, 5-bromo oligonucleotides; or 5' fluorescein isothiocyanate (FITC) dye and/or 3'- biotin labeling can be performed [10].

Since SELEX method is composed of generation of aptamer against target molecule by using a rich random nucleotide sequence of oligonucleotide libraries, there are modifications on SELEX method according to research aim such as nitrocellulose membrane filtration-based SELEX, affinity chromatography and magnetic bead-based SELEX, capillary electrophoresis-based SELEX, microfluidic-based SELEX, cell SELEX, and others [electromobility shift assay (EMSA), surface plasmon resonance (SPR)]. In nitrocellulose membrane filtration-based SELEX, following at least 12 SELEX selection rounds, aptamers are separated *via* the nitrocellulose membrane [11]. The strategy of affinity chromatography-based SELEX method is depending on the selection of aptamers generated against target protein that is tagged with glutathione-S-transferase (GST) or His-tag and immobilized on beads such as agarose [12]. By using affinity column containing target-immobilized beads to select the

SELEX-generated aptamers, however, the disadvantages of this technique because of untagged proteins or protein functional group unbeaded could not be accomplished. However, without bounding process for target protein, successful and specific aptamers can be selected by using magnetic bead technology [13]. In capillary electrophoresis-based SELEX, aptamer can be selected by electromobility difference of target, library, and target-library complex mixture under electroosmotic flow within few rounds such as 2–4. Theoretically, separation potential of aptamers depends on the speed, sample dilution, resolution, and ionic charge of each analyte under the influence of electric field within the capillary [14]. In order to decline the SELEX rounds, microfluidic-based SELEX is generated to increase the effective capacity of aptamer selection under the influence of microfluidic system principle on microchips. The most essential advantage of this method is rapid and automatically aptamer selection procedure [15]. Although SELEX is generally used for selection of aptamer against proteins, a whole cell can also be used as a target for SELEX method. In cell SELEX, extracellular proteins expressing on cell surface are generally regarded as a target for cell SELEX and, following round of SELEX method with whole cell and the oligonucleotide library, generation of aptamers against surface proteins on target cells. As the target cell expressing various extracellular receptors, ligands, etc. on cell surface, the aptamer selected from cell SELEX can be a mixture of aptamers targeting different surface proteins. However, aptamers generated by cell SELEX can be used for cell-specific diagnosis and therapy, targeting cell drug delivery (**Figure 2**) [16].

The investigation of potential chemotherapeutic effect of selected aptamers generated by SELEX is identified for their novelty in various bioinformatics tools given below [17]:

http://www.cas.org/SCIFINDER/scicover2.html

https://www.hsls.pitt.edu/obrc/index.php?page=URL1096043955

http://connection.ebscohost.com/c/articles/45243053/aptamer-database

By these different and multifunctional SELEX methods, a number of aptamers can be generated and selected. Subsequently, these aptamers can be used for aptamer-based sensors, new drugs, and drug delivery systems. Until now, various aptamers against target proteins are generated and investigated for preclinical studies, and some are under clinical trials such as Phases I and II (**Table 1**) [18]. Macugen (EYE001), FDA-approved modified RNA aptamer, phase II/III completed for the treatment of age-related macular degeneration (AMD). This RNA aptamer is referred as Pegaptanib (Pfizer, NY, USA), and it targets vascular endothelial growth factor (VEGF) [19]. Zimura (ARC1905) is an anti-C5 aptamer that targets essential inflammatory mediator, complement component. Phase I study of zimura and monoclonal antibody fragment for angiogenesis factor VEGF combination treatment was completed in AMD patients [20]. Another RNA aptamer against factor IXa is REG1 that acts as an anticoagulation system, and phase I and phase II trials are successfully accomplished to prevent thrombotic and ischemic complications [21]. Fovista is referred to as E10030, an aptamer against platelet-derived growth factor (PDGF). The phase I and phase II studies of fovista in neovascular AMD have been accomplished. In addition, fovista with anti-VEGF therapy combined treatment is tried in

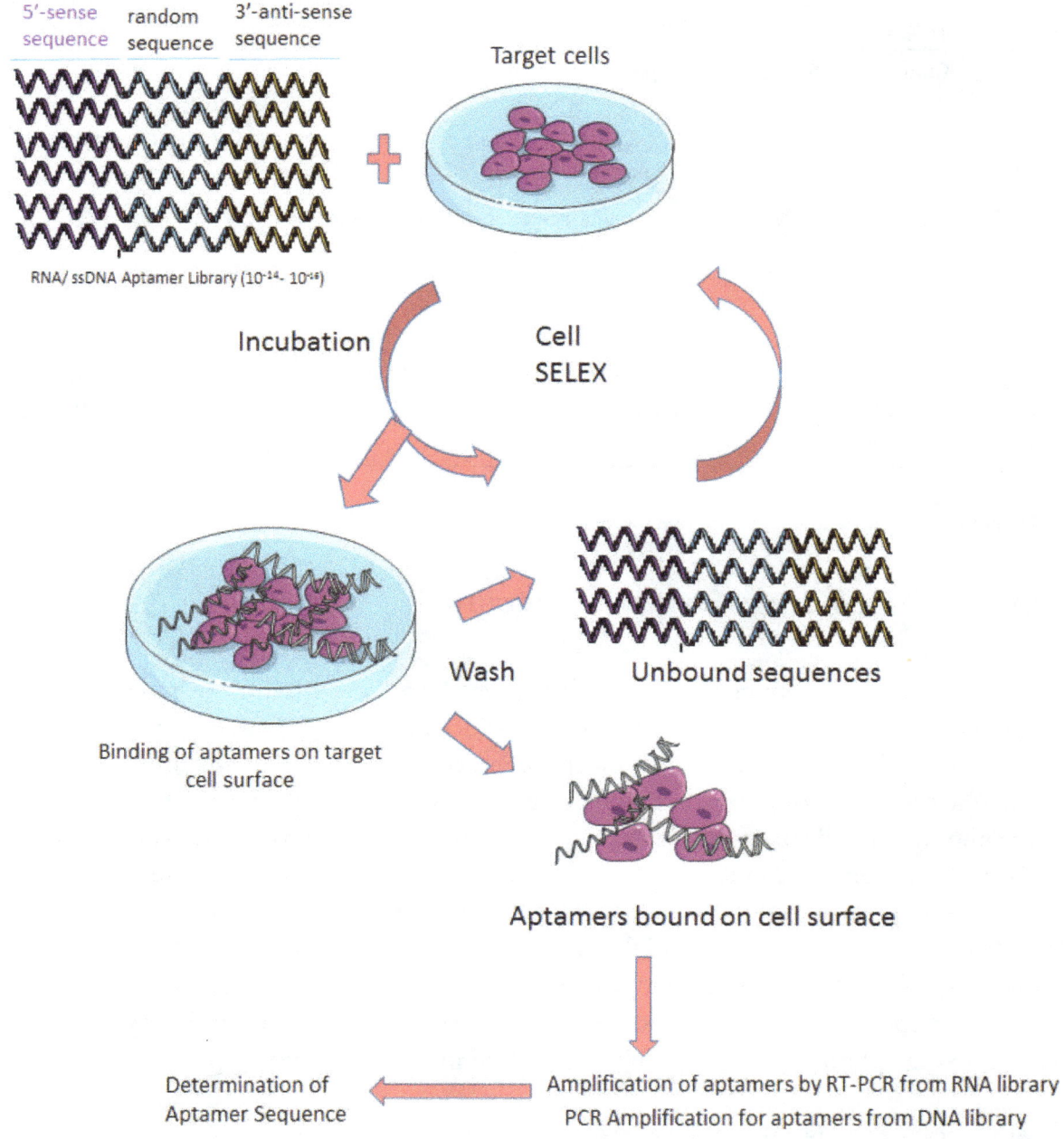

5′-sense   random   3′-anti-sense
sequence   sequence   sequence

RNA/ ssDNA Aptamer Library (10^{-14}- 10^{-16})

Target cells

Incubation

Cell
SELEX

Binding of aptamers on target
cell surface

Wash

Unbound sequences

Aptamers bound on cell surface

Determination of
Aptamer Sequence

Amplification of aptamers by RT-PCR from RNA library
PCR Amplification for aptamers from DNA library

Figure 2. Steps of cell SELEX.

recruited participants [22]. AS1411 is a 26-nucleotide-long guanine-rich oligodeoxynucleotide aptamer that targets nucleolin-1, a phosphoprotein expression on various cancer cell surfaces. Phase II trials of AS1411 in treatment of myeloid leukemia and metastatic renal cell carcinoma have been accomplished. In addition, the treatment potential of AS1411 is inclined by combination of aptamer with chemotherapeutic drugs such as doxorubicin [23]. The AR19499 is a DNA aptamer with high binding affinity against tissue factors Xa and VIIa and leads to tissue factor pathway inhibition. Thus, AR19499 DNA aptamer is used in hemophilia which is a blood clotting deficiency due to improper clotting factor activity [24].

Aptamer	Target	Disease	Trial number	Phase	References
Zimura	Complement 5 (C5)	Idiopathic polypoidal choroidal vasculopathy	NCT02397954	II	[20]
EYE001	VEGF	Neovascular age-related macular degeneration	NCT00021736	II/III	[19]
E10030	PDGF	Neovascular age-related macular degeneration	NCT00569140	I	[22]
REG1	Coagulation factor IXa	Coronary and heart disease	NCT00113997	I	[21]
AS1411	Nucleolin	Acute myeloid leukemia	NCT01034410	II	[23]
AR19499	Tissue factor pathway inhibitor (TFPI)	Hemophilia	NCT01191372	I	[24]

Table 1. Aptamers in the treatment of different diseases.

2. Aptamer-based drugs for cancer therapy

Drugs for the cancer treatment are generally focused on the inhibition of molecular signaling pathways, cell cycle inhibition, and induction of apoptosis. Chemotherapy is one of the major categories for the treatment of cancer; however, its success remains limited due to the ineffective accessibility of drugs to tumor cells. Furthermore, high doses of drugs are used to overcome this handicap causing intolerable toxicity and multidrug resistance. Drug resistance is the major obstacle in cancer therapy; thus the development of new technologies and agents needs to be investigated to overcome drug resistance and prevention of cancer invasion, or metastasis [25]. Because of their high binding affinity and specificity, aptamers become an essential target for cancer drug development. Aptamer-based drug design depends on targeting the cancer-specific biomarker proteins and increases the immunomodulatory functions by aptamers, using aptamers as a drug delivery system in cancer treatment [26].

2.1. Cell-specific targets for aptamer-based therapeutic strategies

New strategies for cancer treatment have been developed on the microarray analysis of cancer tissue samples compared to normal tissue's expression profiles. According to microarray analysis, the significant upregulation of specific genes compared to normal tissue samples is shown with their biomarker potential. Therefore, the development of stable and selective inhibitors for these targets has been analyzed for cancer therapy [27]. One of the essential potential inhibitor for these target molecules are aptamers that are more sensitive and specific to their target *via* high affinity. Thus, aptamer-based drugs are designed and synthesized by SELEX method to investigate first for their binding affinity and potential chemotherapeutic potential in specific cancer types.

2.1.1. Pegaptanib

One of the essential molecules for induction of angiogenesis and to increase vascular permeability is vascular endothelial growth factor (VEGF). The isoforms of VEGF are 206, 189,

165, 145, or 121 amino acids long; one of these isoform VEGF165 overexpression in ovarian cancer cells has been demonstrated. In xenograft mice models, inclined levels of VEGF165 triggered ovarian cancer metastasis, and macrophage infiltration is also determined [28]. The successful designed aptamers against VEGF also put forward a clinical potential in the treatment of metastatic tumors [29]. 0.75–1.4 nm Pegaptanib, RNA aptamer against VEGF-165, inhibited VEGF-associated tumor vascularity, VEGF signaling via blocking phosphorylation of VEGFR2 receptor and phospholipase Cγ, and calcium mobilization [30]. Similar to Pegaptanib, SL(2)-B/RNV66, DNA aptamer is used to inhibit VEGF-mediated tumor neovascularization in hepatic and breast cancer cells [31].

2.1.2. A9g RNA aptamer

Prostate-specific membrane antigen (PSMA), as a prostate cancer marker when overexpressed, is a type II membrane-associated metallopeptidase. Many other solid tumors exhibited PSMA expression in their vasculature. Elevated expression of PSMA on the surface of prostate cancer cell membrane leads scientific focus on PSMA antigen to synthesize aptamer against it. A9g PSMA aptamer is used to target PSMA, which is poorly expressed in normal cells, and it is a transmembrane glycosylated protein (100 kDa), which exerts NAALADase/glutamate carboxypeptidase II activity on surface of the cells [32]. According to previous reports, block PSMA activity was obtained following A9g aptamer, a 2'-F modified RNA treatment. This modification increased the aptamer stability in serum. Although two different modifications were done during the experiments as 2' F and 2' O-Me adducts, 2' O-Methylation did not increase stability. Treating animals with A9g by systemic administration prevented metastatic potential of prostate cells. The therapeutic efficiency of aptamer was high because only 10% mice models showed bone metastasis. When authors checked the safety of aptamer, animals did not exert any change for their weight, blood chemistry, or behavior within 4 weeks [33].

2.1.3. HPV16 E6 (F5) aptamer

Human papillomaviruses (HPVs) are DNA tumor viruses that infect epithelial cells, and they are known widely as causality factors of cervical, head, and neck cancers. Although there are more than 100 different types of HPV strains identified, one of the most common malignancy-associated HPV stain (HPV 16) causes the transformation of viral oncoprotein E6 and E7 in the cervical cells, which leads to inhibition of key tumor suppressors [34]. Postsynaptic density protein (PDZ) domain is discovered as *Drosophila* disk large tumor suppressor and is found in E6 targeting proteins (e.g., Magi, Dlg), which maintains interaction *via* short C-terminal PDZ-domain-binding motif (ETQV). The designed and selected RNA aptamer (F2) against HPV16 E6 was tested in cervical carcinoma cells, which express HPV16 E6 and E7 leading to induction of apoptosis through inhibiting interaction between E6 and the PDZ1 domains from Magi-1 in p53-independent manner [35].

2.1.4. ErbB targeting aptamers

The EGFR/ErbB family of receptor tyrosine kinases (RTK) comprises four members—EGFR (also known as HER1 or ErbB1), ErbB2 (Neu, HER2), ErbB3 (HER3), and ErbB4

(HER4)—containing an extracellular ligand binding region, a single membrane-spanning region, and an intracellular tyrosine kinase-containing domain [36]. Amplification and over-expression of ErbB2 have been also reported in numerous cancers, including breast, ovarian, stomach, bladder, salivary, and lung cancers. One of the promising RNA aptamers is developed against ErbB2, which overexpressed in majority of breast cancer cells. The designed RNA aptamer showed high affinity and specificity against extracellular domain of ErbB2 protein [37]. EGFR is a critical target, and FDA-approved two monoclonal antibodies (cetuximab, panitumumab) and three tyrosine kinase inhibitors (erlotinib, gefitinib, and lapatinib) are effective in the treatment of lung cancer patients [38]. However, the presence of increasing refractory cases is the major obstacle in the treatment of lung cancer. Thereby, more potent or synergizing therapeutically options gain researcher's interest in cancer field. One of suggested therapeutic tools is CL4, a nuclease-resistant RNA aptamer. It is able to bind at high affinity to EGFR (ErbB1, Her1) on the surface of different cancer cells and to block EGFR downstream signaling *via* dimerization of receptors. The apoptotic effect of CL4 was shown in *in vitro* and *in vivo* experimental models. One of the other promising EGFR targeting RNA aptamers is E0727/CL428/KD11 30/TuTu2231, which blocks EGFR phosphorylation and EGFR-mediated PI3K/AKT and MAPK signaling, which led to increased apoptotic ratio in glioblastoma [39] and breast [40] and squamous cell carcinoma [41].

2.1.5. A30 aptamer

One of the members of receptor tyrosine kinase family member type I is human epidermal growth factor receptor-3 (HER3), and upregulation of HER3 expression has been demonstrated in various cancer types. Although the expression of HER3 is not high when compared to HER2 in cancer tissue samples and/or cancer cell lines, increase HER3 levels are evaluated to accelerate the drug resistance. RNA aptamers are selected for the extracellular domain of HER3 (82 kDa domain) by SELEX. One of the RNA aptamers with high binding affinity against HER3ECD is A30 aptamer, which has an inhibitive effect on heregulin-mediated HER2 phosphorylation and MAPK signaling in MCF-7 breast cancer cells [42].

2.1.6. OPN aptamer

Osteopontin (OPN) is a secreted phosphoprotein that induced tumorigenesis, local growth, and metastasis in a variety of cancers. It is a potential therapeutic target for the regulation of cancer metastasis. OPN is also referred to as cell attachment protein and cytokine that signals through two cell adhesion molecules: $\alpha v \beta 3$-integrin and CD44 [43]. The selected RNA aptamer against OPN was effective to block cell migration and invasion in metastatic MDA-MB-231 breast cancer cells. The similar findings were confirmed *in vivo* through xenograft model of MDA-MB-231 cell-mediated tumor formation. OPN-R3 with 2'-O-methyl-substituted nucleotides, 5'-cholesterol modification, and 3'-inverted deoxy thymidine modifications were effective to decrease tumor volume. Therefore it was suggested that small RNA aptamers have potential in the treatment of cancers [44].

2.1.7. NAS-24 aptamer

Vimentin, one of the essential intermediate filamentous protein, play a role during cell adhesions play a role during cell adhesion, migration, and apoptotic cellular processes. Overexpression of vimentin in various cancer cells such as prostate cancer, malignant melanoma, lung cancer, breast cancer, and gastrointestinal tumor is demonstrated [45]. Increased vimentin expression is shown to be linked with cancer invasion and low prognosis potential. NAS-24, an 80-nucleotide-long DNA aptamer, targeting vimentin molecule has been investigated for its apoptotic potential in mouse ascites' adenocarcinoma cells *in vivo* [46]. In order to increase the delivery of NAS-24, additional arabinogalactan (AG) and NAS-24 aptamer complex has been investigated in mice models with exposure of 1.6 µg/kg for 5 days, and treatment significantly triggered twofold apoptotic cell death compared to control mice group [47].

2.1.8. YJ-1 aptamer

According to cancer tissue microarray analysis, ample of tumor antigen is demonstrated in cancer progression, metastasis, and invasion. Overexpression of one of essential antigens, carcinoembryonic antigen (CEA), is associated with cell adhesion, cancer cell migration to the liver, and induction of hepatic metastasis of colon cancer cells. Aptamer against CEA is YJ1 aptamer, which is investigated for potential anticancer agent in colon cancer cells in mice models and revealed inhibition of metastasis of colon cancer to hepatocellular localization. However utilization of CEA aptamers is more potent to monitor disease progression [48].

2.1.9. A-P50 aptamer

A-P50 is a 31-nucleotide RNA aptamer against NF-κB molecule with a high binding affinity against DNA-binding domain of NF-κB p50. As a transcription factor, NF-κB activates various cytokine expressions and takes role in blocking the effect of radiotherapy and chemotherapy in cancer cells. Since NF-κB is a major key molecule in carcinogenesis or cancer drug resistance, potential therapeutic effect of aptamer against NF-κB has been investigated in hepatocellular carcinoma [49]. A-P50 aptamer targeting NF-κB p50 activation inhibition overcomes the doxorubicin-dependent drug resistance in lung cancer *in vitro* and *in vivo* mice models. Therapeutic effect of A-P50 aptamer is increased by Dox combined drug delivery, and this drug delivery system induced apoptotic cell death in A549 and H1299 in non-small cell lung cancer [50].

2.1.10. AP273 AFP aptamer

Hepatic cell proliferation, growth, and differentiation leading to development of hepatocellular carcinoma are associated with alpha fetoprotein (AFP). Active AFP signaling triggered oncogenic mRNA production, which results in investigation of the potential anti-carcinogenic effect of aptamer against AFP [51]. AP273, a DNA aptamer selected by capillary SELEX method, inhibited invasion and migration of HepG2 and SMMC7721 hepatocellular carcinoma cells. Microfluidic chips with magnetic bead bound AFP aptamer are constructed to determine and measure the circulating cancer cells as a diagnosis [52].

As we discussed above, there are a number of DNA or RNA aptamers with increased stability and function which are promising drug candidates in future cancer therapy models. When we checked the patents displaying this potential, aptamers are the important subjects for intellectual property rights. One of pancreatic ductal carcinoma treatment options with aptamers was shown with different functions, as synergistic drug with current therapeutic modalities for pancreatic cancer, single agent, and labeling of cancer cells. The selectivity of designed and selected aptamers for targeted cells, not normal epithelial cells, is one of the most important successful parts of aptamer therapy. Studies on severe combined immunodeficiency (SCID) mice models increased the potential therapeutic advantage of proposed aptamers for the next-term clinical trials. In the treatment of prostate cancer, one of the other promising DNA aptamers is DML-7, which binds to DU145 prostate cancer cells with high affinity in temperature-dependent manner. It is well established that the selectivity of DML-7 against metastatic cell lines was high due to the lack of interaction affinity to LNCaP or 22Rv1 prostate cancer cells [53].

2.2. Immunomodulatory aptamers in the treatment of different solid tumors

Tumor immunity is one of the important subjects in the current cancer therapy understanding. The approval of the immunomodulatory monoclonal antibodies in the treatment of different cancer types highlighted the role of effector T cells in antitumor immunity [54]. The activation of T cells *via* antigen-presenting cells (APCs) is proceeded due to T-cell receptor-triggered antigen-specific signals or co-stimulatory (COS) molecules (such as 4-1BB, CD28, and OX40). Although a number of attempts were done with antibody-based molecules to alter these interactions for COS molecules, the immunogenic properties of antibody-based options are found with limited effectiveness [55]. The designed and selected aptamer against 4-1BB (a COS receptor that is responsible for the activation and expansion of CD8+ T cells) was the first agonistic immunomodulatory aptamer. It is an artificial ligand with high similarity to anti-CTLA that initiates COS signals to boost T-cell survival. The aptamers against tumor necrosis factor receptor family members, OX40 and CD28, potentiated T-cell-mediated tumor immunity in mice models [56]. OX40 RNA aptamer could exert therapeutic potential in melanoma patients. Antagonist effect of Del 60 aptamer (against CTL4) on T-cell proliferation has been demonstrated *in vitro* studies. This RNA aptamer was found effective in *in vivo* tumor growth in melanoma and bladder tumors. In addition, programmed death-1 (PD-1) and PDL1 axis against DNA aptamer (MP7) was reported to inhibit PD-L1-induced apoptosis of tumor-specific T cells and IL-2 secretion [57]. Due to Treg activation following PD-1/PDL1 axis, MP7 aptamer may mediate the Tregs in antitumor immunity [58]. In order to deregulate the immunological functions of tumor microenvironment, inhibition of IL-10 and IL-4Rα-STAT6 signaling with RNA aptamers 5A1 and CL-42 was found effective to decrease tumor growth of colorectal and breast cancer cells. Similar to these achievements, DNA-based aptamers against IL-6 and VR11 prevented IL-6 or TNF-α receptor activation in myeloma cases [59]. In addition, the angiogenesis and invasion inhibition potential of aptamer binding IL-4Rα are demonstrated in myeloid-derived suppressor cells, and also IL4Rα aptamer induced the migration of T lymphocytes in tumor microenvironment in order to decline the cancer volume and size [60]. According to Spiegelmer technology, 2'-Fluoro- or 2'-amino pyrimidines or 2'-O-methyl nucleotides modified L-RNA aptamer generated that are resistant against nucleases. One of the Spiegelmer (L-RNA aptamer, Noxxon Pharma, Germany) forms of L-RNA aptamer is Nox-E36, which is normally used to inhibit monocyte chemoattractant protein-1 (MCP-1) (CCL2). It is suggested to treat glioblastoma multiform patients, which display high MCP-1 expression profile [61]. Potential inhibition effect of Nox-E36 DNA aptamer on MCP-1 molecule revealed the use of Nox-E36 as an immunomodulatory cancer therapy agent in different cancer types. Similar to Nox-E36, Nox-A12 is an anti-chemokine suggested in the treatment of different malignancies. 45-mer L-RNA and PEG-derived formula of Nox-A12 is effective on stromal cell-derived factor-1α (SDF-1α). SDF-1α attracts and activates immune and nonimmune cells that bind to chemokine receptors CXCR4 and CXCR7. The immunological vulnerability potential of cancer cells increased the experimental success of L-RNA aptamers in hematological and solid tumors [62].

2.3. Targeted drug delivery in cancer therapy *via* aptamers

Recently, new targeted drug delivery approaches have been explored such as nanosystems and bio-conjugates leading to successful therapy. Targeted drug delivery systems enable drug accumulation within a target zone and usually catalyze the interaction between a drug and its receptor via four key steps: retain, evade, target, and release. The system selection depends on the specific site of the body. New strategies include the use of aptamers with their high affinity and specificity for targets, easy synthesis, modification, and tissue penetration. In addition, they are even integrated with a number of nanomaterials including gold nanoparticles, carbon nanotubes, DNA micelles, and hydrogels. Such specific approaches are expected to enhance the effect of chemotherapeutics with greater selectivity. In this section of the chapter, a number of aptamers used as effective drug delivery systems were discussed. Aptamer-based drugs for cancer therapy were listed in **Table 2**.

2.3.1. Prostate-specific membrane antigen

Two specific nuclease-stabilized aptamers, xPSM-A9 and xPSM-A10, able to inhibit the enzymatic activity of PSMA, were designed by Lupold et al. in LNCaP cells [63]. The study was the first of its kind that RNA aptamers were evaluated for prostate cancer. The truncated version of xPSM-A10 was highly selective to PSMA, showing strong affinity to LNCaP cells (PSMA+), but not PC3 cells (PSMA-) [64]. The high specificity of the aptamer was further used for silencing RNA (siRNA) delivery to cells. siRNA-aptamer complex knockdown was comparable to the positive control where siRNA-liposomal transfection reagent protocol was used [65, 66]. The study showed the decreasing cell proliferation and apoptosis ratios as a consequence of silencing polo-like kinase (PLK1) and B-cell lymphoma 2 (Bcl-2) genes *via* PSMA aptamer-siRNA complexes in LNCaP cells [67]. In addition, authors also delivered the siRNA-aptamer complex to the LNCaP cell-bearing mice, obtained tumor size and volume reduction, whereas no effect was observed in PC3 (PSMA-) cells. More importantly, siRNA-aptamer delivery overcame the cytotoxicity and immune response problem *in vitro* and *in vivo* experiments associated with the liposomal agent-mediated delivery. Anti-PSMA aptamer-conjugated siRNA strategy was also evaluated for other targets such as eukaryotic elongation factor 2 (EEF2) [68]. Due to the success of anti-PSMA aptamer-siRNA delivery system,

Aptamer name	Aptamer target	Function	Cancer	References
A30	HER3	Inhibition of HER2 and MAPK signaling	HER-3 overexpressing lung cancer, breast cancer, gastric cancer, pancreatic cancer	[42]
A9-g	PSMA	Suppress the enzymatic activity of PSMA	In vivo and in vitro blockage of prostate cancer metastasis	[32, 33]
AFP-apt	Alpha fetoprotein	Suppression of AFP-mediated cancer progression pathways	In vitro hepatocellular carcinoma growth and proliferation inhibition	[51, 52]
A-P50	NF-KB	NF-κB phosphorylation inhibition	Overcoming resistance profile of lung cancer against doxorubicin in vitro and in vivo	[49, 50]
AS1411	Nucleolin	Nucleolin-dependent NF-KB or Bcl2 signaling	Acute myelocytic leukemia, lung cancer, renal cancer, breast cancer, pancreatic cancer	[23, 84–90]
E0727/CL428/KD1130/TuTu2231	Epidermal growth factor receptor (EGFR)	EGFR-mediated PI3K/Akt and MAPK signaling inhibition	Squamous cell carcinoma, breast cancer, glioblastoma multiform, lung cancer	[36–41]
NAS-24	Vimentin	Inhibit cell growth and proliferation	Apoptotic cell death induction in adenocarcinoma in vitro and in vivo	[45–47]
NOX-A12	CXCL12	Suppress the migration and angiogenesis triggered by CXCL12	Multiple myeloma, chronic lymphocytic leukemia, glioblastoma multiform (with radiotherapy)	[62]
NOX-E-36	CXCL12	CXCL12-induced cell migration and angiogenesis inhibition	Incline in vivo drug sensitivity in hematological cancer cells, chronic lymphocytic leukemia, and multiple myeloma and in vivo radiotherapy success in glioblastoma multiform	[62]
OPN-R3	Osteopontin (OPN)	Inhibition of OPN binding to OPN receptor	In vivo and in vitro blocking of breast cancer cell migration and invasion	[43, 44]
Pegaptanib	VEGF-165	Inhibition of angiogenesis via suppressing the VEGF	Solid cancer extends angiogenic potential therapy	[28–31]
YJ-1	Carcinoembryonic antigen (CEA)	Blocking the cross-talk between CEA and ribonucleoprotein M4	Colorectal cancer invasion-metastasis inhibition in vitro and in vivo colorectal cancer	[48]

Table 2. List of aptamer-based drugs for cancer therapy.

researches have also investigated its potential for drug delivery. The first drug used for this purpose was gelonin which is a ribosomal toxin and protein synthesis inhibitor [69]. Studies with gelonin suggested that the effective doses are highly toxic due to its low membrane permeability. Chu et al. exposed LNCaP cells to anti-PSMA aptamer conjugated with gelonin in order to induce cell death [69].

Aptamer direct conjugation with drugs has a major limitation since drug concentration has a direct proportion with aptamer size and binding capacity. To enhance the efficacy of the drug delivery using aptamers, recent approaches focused on the conjugation of aptamers with functional polymers or nanoparticles. Dhar et al. used anti-PSMA aptamer conjugated with poly D, L-lactic-co-glycolic acid (PLGA), and polyethylene glycol (PEG) nanoparticles to deliver cisplatin to LNCaP prostate cancer cells [70]. The success of the entry of the aptamer-nanoparticle-drug complex to the cells was confirmed by fluorescence microscopy through green fluorescent-labeled encapsulation of the nanoparticles. Finally, authors were able to diminish the effective dose of free cisplatin which has a dose-limiting toxicity and acquired resistance problems, with the increase of the drug bioavailability. The same approach was also tested for docetaxel on mice with LNCaP tumor cell [70]. Results were promising in terms of tumor size/volume and survival. xPSM-A10-doxorubicin complex was used for drug delivery studies. The results from these studies increased the efficiency of doxorubicin in LNCaP prostate cancer cells. The aptamer-doxorubicin complex was further conjugated to a fluorescent quantum dot (QD) to provide high targeting potential. The same study revealed that PMSA-mediated endocytosis caused the release of doxorubicin [71]. However, aptamer-QD-doxorubicin complex was as toxic as free doxorubicin. Other anti-PSMA aptamers are the polyethylenimine (PEI)- or polyethylene glycol (PEG)-conjugated ones which were co-delivered with small hairpin RNA (shRNA) against $Bcl-x_L$, the anti-apoptotic gene. These combinations were also succeeded to selectively and potently kill LNCaP cells *in vitro* [72]. Therefore, all these studies demonstrated that aptamer-conjugated nanoparticles with chemotherapeutic drugs can be a powerful approach for targeted drug delivery with minimal side effects.

2.3.2. Tenascin-C

Tenascin-C (TN-C) as an extracellular matrix (ECM) protein having role in tissue remodeling is expressed during embryonic development, tissue repair, and pathological conditions such as chronic inflammation and cancer. It is highly expressed in tumor stroma in glioma and breast cancer [73]. TN-C affects several signaling molecules, Dickkopf-1 (DKK1) and Wnt, e.g., involved in survival, proliferation, invasion, angiogenesis, and metastasis [74]. Researches have designed a single-stranded DNA aptamer *via* SELEX technology to target TN-C in U251 glioblastoma cells and modified them with a metal chelator MAG2 for an ideal binding affinity [75]. While they injected the final radiolabeled MAG2 aptamer to mouse bearing glioblastoma and breast cancer xenografts, resulting positron emission tomography (PET) imaging studies showed that the aptamer was localized in tumors. Recently, it was shown that the modified TN-C aptamer was uptaken by TN-C-positive U87MG glioblastoma and H460 lung cancer cells compared to Sc aptamer, the negative control [76]. In addition, the same study also showed that the aptamer has a fast clearance from the blood stream and kidneys. Further evaluations were obtained in terms of engineering a multimodal nanoparticle-based Simultaneously Multiple

Aptamers and RGD Targeting (SMART) probe that targets TN-C, integrin $\alpha v\beta 3$, and nucleolin at the same time. The SMART probe had a better affinity and specificity to several tumors like glioma, prostate cancer, cervical cancer, and lung cancer cells [77]. The next generation of TN-C aptamer was GBI-10 and shown that it can bind several TN-C peptides *in vitro* [75, 78]. The most important part of the fact that GBI-10 can target several binding sites of TN-C is the ability to address multiple splice variants at the same time. GBI-10 aptamer was also suggested for the diagnosis of tumor during MRI when subjected to gadolinium; a contrast agent helps to determine tumor localization, in a liposome capsule [79]. Therefore, TN-C aptamers due to target specificity, small size, and rapid tissue penetration has potential clinical advantages and is still tested for targeted drug delivery to the ECM of tumors.

2.3.3. Nucleolin

Nucleolin is an abundant nucleolar protein found in eukaryotic organisms including yeast, plants, and mammals. It has several structural domains which help the interaction of nucleolin with various proteins and RNAs, playing role in rDNA transcription and maturation, ribosome biogenesis, and nucleocytoplasmic transport. Although it was first described in 1973 by Orrick et al., its genomic and proteomic organization was clarified by the end of the 1990s [80]. It was elucidated that nucleolin is not only a nucleus resident protein but also is expressed at the cell surface of dividing cells, especially in tumor cells and angiogenic blood vessels in correlation with cell proliferation [81, 82]. The membrane-associated nucleolin has been shown to function as a growth factor receptor [83]. Human gastric cell lines express cell surface nucleolin which functions as receptors for TNF-α-inducing protein (Tipα) of *Helicobacter pylori*. Tipα upon nucleolin binding induced tumor progression *via* the activation of TNFα and NF-κB in human gastric adenocarcinoma cell lines MKN-1 [83]. Nucleolin silencing, by siRNA, resulted in the reduction of cell proliferation and migration. Therefore, studies put forward the cell surface nucleolin as a potential target for anticancer therapies.

AS1411, the first designed anti-nucleolin aptamer, is a 26-nucleotide-long guanosine-rich DNA sequence having antiproliferative activity [84]. It forms a G-quartet-containing structure which is resistant to nuclease degradation and remarkably stable in serum. AS1411 treatment caused the inhibition of NF-κB signaling, DNA replication, cell cycle arrest, and apoptotic induction. In addition, it was shown that AS1411 can bind Bcl-2 mRNA resulting its destabilization and consequent downregulation in breast cancer cells [85]. *In vivo* preclinical studies demonstrated the antitumor effect of AS1411 in mice bearing tumor xenografts with breast and lung cancer cells [86]. AS1411 was also tested in Phase II clinical trials on five patients with renal carcinoma and leukemia. The response against the aptamer was very promising in one renal cell carcinoma patient with 84% tumor size reduction and 2-year tumor-free progression. The patient whole exome sequencing revealed that AS1411 caused missense mutation in mammalian target of rapamycin (mTOR) and fibroblast growth factor receptor 2 (FGFR2) genes [23].

Besides the direct anticancer strategy using aptamers acting on nucleolin, cargo delivery into cancer cells was tested due to the fact that nucleolin shuttles between the cell surface, cytoplasm, and nucleus in dividing cells. Before aptamer strategy, F3, a 34-amino acid peptide able to recognize nucleolin on the cell surface of angiogenic cells, has been used to target cancer cells [81]. Radio-labeled F3 peptide was used to deliver α-particle resulting tumor volume reduction in mouse xenograft models [87]. Aptamers are potentially better over peptides due to their high serum stability and immune tolerance. Therefore, AS1411 has been used for imaging and drug delivery systems in conjunction with nanoparticles. AS1411-human serum albumin (HSA) nanoparticles was used as drug carrier, and the uptake of the complex is increased compared to only-aptamer condition in MCF-7 breast cancer cells, but not in MCF-10A normal breast epithelial cells. This simple complex by modified HSA nanoparticles has been used for paclitaxel delivery and suggested as a way to overcome the limitations of paclitaxel toxicity [88]. A similar strategy was followed in gastric cancer. Behrooz et al. designed a single-stranded AS1411 together with polyamidoamine (PAMAM)-polyethylene glycol (PEG) complex. PAMAM-PEG-AS1411 complex dramatically increased the uptake of 5-FU by MKN45 gastric cancer cells without toxic effects [89]. PEG conjugated to AS1411 complex was also used to deliver Bcl-x$_L$-specific shRNA and doxorubicin in AGS gastric adenocarcinoma which inhibited the cell growth and enhanced tumoricidal effect of doxorubicin [89]. AS1411 aptamer was conjugated to multimodal nanoparticles also (MFR-AS1411). MFR-AS1411-injected mouse bearing C6 rat glioma cell line was observed for the nanoparticle uptake. Authors suggested that aptamer-nanoparticle complex is a candidate for cancer diagnosis with MR imaging [90]. All these findings concluded that AS1411 is a particularly promising agent for targeted delivery approaches.

2.3.4. Mucin-1

Mucin-1 is a glycoprotein modified by O-glycosylation expressed on epithelial cell surfaces. Its expression is increased tenfold in malignancies such as breast, lung, and colon cancer [91]. Altschuler et al. showed that glycosylated MUC-1 is subjected to clathrin-coated endocytosis as well [92]. Since MUC-1 is a membrane protein and overexpressed in cancer cells with relatively low expression in normal tissue, it is an attractive tumor marker for targeted therapy. Therefore, MUC-1 aptamer, MA3, was developed to selectively deliver anticancer agents to cancer cells such as doxorubicin *in vitro*. Eighty six base DNA aptamer MA3 was applied to MUC1-positive A549 lung cancer and MUC1-negative HepG2 hepatocellular carcinoma cells [93]. The study showed that MA3-doxorubicin complex selectively delivered doxorubicin to MUC1-positive cells with minimal cross reactivity to albumin. Unlike free doxorubicin which enters cells by passive diffusion, aptamer-doxorubicin chooses receptor-mediated endocytosis in A549 cells [94]. In addition, three more anti-MUC-1 DNA aptamers were selected by Ferreira et al. that can selectively bind breast and pancreatic cancer cells [95]. The efficacy of the aptamer was also tested on ovarian cancer cells in a quantum dot-MUC-1-doxorubicin (QD-MUC-1-Dox) combination. *In vivo* imaging studies revealed that QD-MUC-1-Dox conjugate in a lower concentration was highly cytotoxic than free doxorubicin even in multidrug-resistant ovarian cancer cells [96]. MUC-1 aptamer was also conjugated to other nanoparticle structures such as mesoporous silica nanoparticles (MSNs). Confocal microscopy studies showed that MDA-MB-231 breast cancer cells that overexpress MUC-1 and MDA-MB-231 tumor-bearing Balb/c mice showed increased MSN-MUC-1 aptamer, but not the same scenario for non-tumorigenic MCF-10A breast epithelial cells. The complex was also used for a successful delivery of doxorubicin to MCF-7 cells [97]. Another MUC-1-targeted aptamer L3 was combined with doxorubicin and exhibited selective toxicity to MCF-7 breast cancer cells. Most importantly, L3 aptamer was able to evade macrophages [98]. All these results indicated that anti-MUC-1 aptamers have potential for targeted drug delivery, diagnosis, and staging of cancer.

2.3.5. Protein tyrosine kinase 7

Protein tyrosine kinase 7 (PTK7) is one of the members of receptor tyrosine kinase family, also known as colon carcinoma-4 (CCK-4). PTK7 is highly expressed not only in colon but in various human malignancies inducing cell proliferation and metastasis. The first DNA aptamer targeting PTK7 was developed in 2006 by Shangguan et al. as the consequence of a cell SELEX protocol used in cancer biomarker search for acute lymphoblastic leukemia [99]. Forty-one-nucleotide-long aptamer called sgc8c was found selectively bound to PTK7. Subsequent studies are performed by other research groups with sgc8c internalized into PTK7 overexpressing cells [100, 101]. Sgc8c was conjugated with viral capsid protein MS2 linked to AlexaFluor488 in Jurkat T leukemia cells, and its efficient binding was determined by confocal microscopy [102]. Liposomal nanoparticles were also used for PTK7 aptamer delivery into CEM-CCRF cells with low molecular weight dextran as a simulation of drug delivery [103]. Next, researchers have conjugated sgc8 to various chemotherapeutics such as anthracycline for drug delivery experiments. Huang et al. were able to design the aptamer suitable for internalization and transportation to endosome in order to drug release in CCRF-CEM cancer cells [100]. Other anthracyclines were also combined with sgc8 such as daunoru-bicin which was highly effective to kill PTK7-expressing cancer cells but not PTK7 negative cells [104, 105]. More recently Sgc8 was labeled with a radiochemical, F-18 (^{18}F-fluorobenzyl azide). Sgc8-F18 showed high affinity to PTK7 expressing HCT 116 colon cancer and U87MG glioblastoma cell lines. The aptamer was rapidly cleared from the blood through kidneys. The study suggested that this complex may be suitable for aptamer targeting and drug delivery tracking in cancer cells [106]. Consequently, PTK7 targeting aptamers were suggested an effective strategy for the specific uptake of chemotherapeutic drugs and minimize their toxic effects on normal cells.

2.3.6. Epidermal growth factor receptor

Epidermal growth factor receptor (EGFR) is a transmembrane receptor tyrosine kinase which belongs to the ErbB family of receptor tyrosine kinases. EGFR is also considered as the pro-totype for receptor-mediated endocytosis. Upon binding with growth factors of EGF fam-ily, EGFR dimerization and autophosphorylation occur. Overexpression or mutant receptor expression lead a mitogen signals in various cancer types [107]. The inhibition of EGFR by monoclonal antibodies or small molecules such as cetuximab or erlotinib, respectively, has been shown as an effective strategy in the combat against cancer; however, it is not the case for all tumor types. The ability of ligand binding and endocytosis makes EGFR an ideal target for aptamer-mediated drug delivery. First experiments performed by Li et al. evaluated the EGFR aptamer conjugation with gold nanoparticles targeting human epithelial carcinoma cells line, A431 [108]. EGFR-overexpressing A431 cells were able to internalize the aptamer, however MDA-MB-453 cells with low level of EGFR expression. Li et al. also suggested the aptamer has high *in vivo* stability [109]. Although the strategy is promising, currently there is only limited information for EGFR aptamer-mediated targeting.

In conclusion, a number of SELEX method-based aptamers have clinical potential to treat different malignancies as single agents or combination with another classical chemotherapeutics. In addition, the novel drug delivery methods enhanced the target-specific therapeutic potential of aptamers. Although early versions of aptamers exerted stability problems, chemical modifications increased their physiological availability. However, limited number of clinical trials for the treatment of malignancies with specific aptamers is an obstacle for near-future clinical modalities based on aptamers. Due to high specificity with increased stability, aptamers are more potent than monoclonal antibody-based drugs with low cost in cancer therapy.

Author details

Ajda Coker-Gurkan*, Pinar Obakan-Yerlikaya and Elif-Damla Arisan

*Address all correspondence to: a.coker@iku.edu.tr

Science and Leters Faculty, Department of Molecular Biology and Genetics, Istanbul Kultur University, Istanbul, Turkey

References

[1] Tuerk C, Gold L. Systematic evolution of ligands by exponential enrichment – Rna ligands to bacteriophage-T4 DNA-polymerase. Science. 1990;**249**(4968):505-510

[2] Ellington AD, Szostak JW. *In vitro* selection of Rna molecules that bind specific ligands. Nature. 1990;**346**(6287):818-822

[3] Stoltenburg R, Reinemann C, Strehlitz B. SELEX-A (r)evolutionary method to generate high-affinity nucleic acid ligands. Biomolecular Engineering. 2007;**24**(4):381-403

[4] Jayasena SD. Aptamers: An emerging class of molecules that rival antibodies in diagnostics. Clinical Chemistry. 1999;**45**(9):1628-1650

[5] Musheev MU, Krylov SN. Selection of aptamers by systematic evolution of ligands by exponential enrichment: Addressing the polymerase chain reaction issue. Analytica Chimica Acta. 2006;**564**(1):91-96

[6] Conrad RC et al. *In vitro* selection of nucleic acid aptamers that bind proteins. Combinatorial Chemistry. 1996;**267**:336-367

[7] Hamm J. Characterisation of antibody-binding RNAs selected from structurally constrained libraries. Nucleic Acids Research. 1996;**24**(12):2220-2227

[8]   Vater A, Klussmann S. Toward third-generation aptamers: Spiegelmers and their thera-peutic prospects. Current Opinion in Drug Discovery & Development. 2003;**6**(2):253-261

[9]   Gold L et al. SELEX and the evolution of genomes. Current Opinion in Genetics & Development. 1997;**7**(6):848-851

[10] Golden MC et al. Diagnostic potential of PhotoSELEX-evolved ssDNA aptamers. Journal of Biotechnology. 2000;**81**(2-3):167-178

[11] Gopinath SCB. Methods developed for SELEX. Analytical and Bioanalytical Chemistry. 2007;**387**(1):171-182

[12] Wang C et al. Strategies for combination of Aptamer and targeted drug delivery. Journal of Nanoscience and Nanotechnology. 2014;**14**(1):501-512

[13] Joyce GF. In-vitro evolution of nucleic-acids. Current Opinion in Structural Biology. 1994;**4**(3):331-336

[14] Wang JH et al. Novel application of fluorescence coupled capillary electrophoresis to resolve the interaction between the G-quadruplex aptamer and thrombin. Journal of Separation Science. 2017;**40**(15):3161-3167

[15] Cho M et al. Quantitative selection of DNA aptamers through microfluidic selection and high-throughput sequencing. Proceedings of the National Academy of Sciences of the United States of America. 2010;**107**(35):15373-15378

[16] Kunii T et al. Selection of DNA aptamers recognizing small cell lung cancer using living cell-SELEX. Analyst. 2011;**136**(7):1310-1312

[17] Lee JF et al. Aptamer database. Nucleic Acids Research. 2004;**32**:D95-D100

[18] Keefe AD, Pai S, Ellington A. Aptamers as therapeutics. Nature Reviews Drug Discovery. 2010;**9**(7):537-550

[19] Kourlas H, Schiller DS. Pegaptanib sodium for the treatment of neovascular age-related macular degeneration: A review. Clinical Therapeutics. 2006;**28**(1):36-44

[20] Biesecker G et al. Derivation of RNA aptamer inhibitors of human complement C5. Immunopharmacology. 1999;**42**(1-3):219-230

[21] Rusconi CP et al. RNA aptamers as reversible antagonists of coagulation factor IXa. Nature. 2002;**419**(6902):90-94

[22] Rohloff JC et al. Nucleic acid ligands with protein-like side chains: Modified aptamers and their use as diagnostic and therapeutic agents. Molecular Therapy-Nucleic Acids. 2014;**3**:1-13

[23] Rosenberg JE et al. A phase II trial of AS1411 (a novel nucleolin-targeted DNA aptamer) in metastatic renal cell carcinoma. Investigational New Drugs. 2014;**32**(1):178-187

[24] Waters EK et al. Aptamer ARC19499 mediates a procoagulant hemostatic effect by inhib-iting tissue factor pathway inhibitor. Blood. 2011;**117**(20):5514-5522

[25] Gottesman MM. Mechanisms of cancer drug resistance. Annual Review of Medicine. 2002;**53**:615-627

[26] Phillips JA et al. Applications of aptamers in cancer cell biology. Analytica Chimica Acta. 2008;**621**(2):101-108

[27] Sreekumar A et al. Profiling of cancer cells using protein microarrays: Discovery of novel radiation-regulated proteins. Cancer Research. 2001;**61**(20):7585-7593

[28] Duyndam MCA et al. Vascular endothelial growth factor-165 overexpression stimulates angiogenesis and induces cyst formation and macrophage infiltration in human ovarian cancer xenografts. American Journal of Pathology. 2002;**160**(2):537-548

[29] Sia D et al. VEGF signaling in cancer treatment. Current Pharmaceutical Design. 2014;**20**(17):2834-2842

[30] Niu G, Chen X. Vascular endothelial growth factor as an anti-angiogenic target for cancer therapy. Current Drug Targets. 2010;**11**(8):1000-1017

[31] Nagpal M, Nagpal K, Nagpal PN. A comparative debate on the various anti-vascular endothelial growth factor drugs: Pegaptanib sodium (Macugen), ranibizumab (Lucentis) and bevacizumab (Avastin). Indian Journal of Ophthalmology. 2007;**55**(6):437-439

[32] Chang SS. Monoclonal antibodies and prostate-specific membrane antigen. Current Opinion in Investigational Drugs. 2004;**5**(6):611-615

[33] de Franciscis V. A theranostic "SMART" aptamer for targeted therapy of prostate cancer. Molecular Therapy. 2014;**22**(11):1886-1888

[34] Furumoto H, Irahara M. Human papilloma virus (HPV) and cervical cancer. The Journal of Medical Investigation. 2002;**49**(3-4):124-133

[35] Belyaeva TA et al. An RNA Aptamer targets the PDZ-binding motif of the HPV16 E6 Oncoprotein. Cancers (Basel). 2014;**6**(3):1553-1569

[36] Masuda H et al. Role of epidermal growth factor receptor in breast cancer. Breast Cancer Research and Treatment. 2012;**136**(2):331-345

[37] Kim MY, Jeong S. *In vitro* selection of RNA aptamer and specific targeting of ErbB2 in breast cancer cells. Nucleic Acid Therapeutics. 2011;**21**(3):173-178

[38] Thomas A, Rajan A, Giaccone G. Tyrosine kinase inhibitors in lung cancer. Hematology/ Oncology Clinics of North America. 2012;**26**(3):589-605 viii

[39] Camorani S et al. Aptamer targeting EGFRvIII mutant hampers its constitutive autophosphorylation and affects migration, invasion and proliferation of glioblastoma cells. Oncotarget. 2015;**6**(35):37570-37587

[40] Buerger C et al. Sequence-specific peptide aptamers, interacting with the intracellular domain of the epidermal growth factor receptor, interfere with Stat3 activation and inhibit the growth of tumor cells. The Journal of Biological Chemistry. 2003;**278**(39):37610-37621

[41] Li N et al. Inhibition of cell proliferation by an anti-EGFR aptamer. PLoS One. 2011; **6**(6):e20299

[42] Chen CH et al. Inhibition of heregulin signaling by an aptamer that preferentially binds to the oligomeric form of human epidermal growth factor receptor-3. Proceedings of the National Academy of Sciences of the United States of America. 2003;**100**(16):9226-9231

[43] Furger KA et al. The functional and clinical roles of osteopontin in cancer and metastasis. Current Molecular Medicine. 2001;**1**(5):621-632

[44] Mi Z et al. RNA aptamer blockade of osteopontin inhibits growth and metastasis of MDA-MB231 breast cancer cells. Molecular Therapy. 2009;**17**(1):153-161

[45] Rho JH, Roehrl MH, Wang JY. Glycoproteomic analysis of human lung adenocarcinomas using glycoarrays and tandem mass spectrometry: Differential expression and glycosylation patterns of vimentin and fetuin A isoforms. The Protein Journal. 2009;**28**(3-4):148-160

[46] Lehr CM, Gabor F. Lectins and glycoconjugates in drug delivery and targeting. Advanced Drug Delivery Reviews. 2004;**56**(4):419-420

[47] Zamay TN et al. DNA-aptamer targeting vimentin for tumor therapy *in vivo*. Nucleic Acid Therapeutics. 2014;**24**(2):160-170

[48] Lee YJ et al. An RNA aptamer that binds carcinoembryonic antigen inhibits hepatic metastasis of colon cancer cells in mice. Gastroenterology. 2012;**143**(1):155-165 e8

[49] Wurster SE, Maher 3rd LJ. Selection and characterization of anti-NF-kappaB p65 RNA aptamers. RNA Journal. 2008;**14**(6):1037-1047

[50] Mi J et al. RNA aptamer-targeted inhibition of NF-kappa B suppresses non-small cell lung cancer resistance to doxorubicin. Molecular Therapy. 2008;**16**(1):66-73

[51] Lee YJ, Lee SW. Regression of hepatocarcinoma cells using RNA aptamer specific to alpha-fetoprotein. Biochemical and Biophysical Research Communications. 2012;**417**(1):521-527

[52] Dong L et al. Screening and identifying a novel ssDNA Aptamer against alpha-fetoprotein using CE-SELEX. Scientific Reports. 2015;**5**:15552

[53] Duan M et al. Selection and characterization of DNA aptamer for metastatic prostate cancer recognition and tissue imaging. Oncotarget. 2016;**7**(24):36436-36446

[54] Kim HJ, Cantor H. The path to reactivation of antitumor immunity and checkpoint immunotherapy. Cancer Immunology Research. 2014;**2**(10):926-936

[55] Peggs KS, Quezada SA, Allison JP. Cancer immunotherapy: Co-stimulatory agonists and co-inhibitory antagonists. Clinical and Experimental Immunology. 2009;**157**(1):9-19

[56] Soldevilla MM, Villanueva H, Pastor F. Aptamers: A feasible technology in cancer immunotherapy. Journal of Immunology Research. 2016;**2016**:1083738

Applications of Aptamers in Cancer Therapy

[57] Zhou G et al. Aptamers: A promising chemical antibody for cancer therapy. Oncotarget. 2016;**7**(12):13446-13463

[58] Santulli-Marotto S et al. Multivalent RNA aptamers that inhibit CTLA-4 and enhance tumor immunity. Cancer Research. 2003;**63**(21):7483-7489

[59] Berezhnoy A et al. Isolation and optimization of murine IL-10 receptor blocking oligonucleotide aptamers using high-throughput sequencing. Molecular Therapy. 2012;**20**(6):1242-1250

[60] Roth F et al. Aptamer-mediated blockade of IL4Ralpha triggers apoptosis of MDSCs and limits tumor progression. Cancer Research. 2012;**72**(6):1373-1383

[61] Vater A, Klussmann S. Turning mirror-image oligonucleotides into drugs: The evolution of Spiegelmer((R)) therapeutics. Drug Discovery Today. 2015;**20**(1):147-155

[62] de Nigris F et al. CXCR4 inhibitors: Tumor vasculature and therapeutic challenges. Recent Patents on Anti-Cancer Drug Discovery. 2012;**7**(3):251-264

[63] Lupold SE et al. Identification and characterization of nuclease-stabilized RNA molecules that bind human prostate cancer cells via the prostate-specific membrane antigen. Cancer Research. 2002;**62**(14):4029-4033

[64] McNamara 2nd JO et al. Cell type-specific delivery of siRNAs with aptamer-siRNA chimeras. Nature Biotechnology. 2006;**24**(8):1005-1015

[65] Li X, Zhao Q, Qiu L. Smart ligand: Aptamer-mediated targeted delivery of chemotherapeutic drugs and siRNA for cancer therapy. Journal of Controlled Release. 2013;**171**(2):152-162

[66] Chu TC et al. Aptamer mediated siRNA delivery. Nucleic Acids Research. 2006;**34**(10):e73

[67] Dassie JP et al. Systemic administration of optimized aptamer-siRNA chimeras promotes regression of PSMA-expressing tumors. Nature Biotechnology. 2009;**27**(9):839-849

[68] Wullner U et al. Cell-specific induction of apoptosis by rationally designed bivalent aptamer-siRNA transcripts silencing eukaryotic elongation factor 2. Current Cancer Drug Targets. 2008;**8**(7):554-565

[69] Chu TC et al. Aptamer: Toxin conjugates that specifically target prostate tumor cells. Cancer Research. 2006;**66**(12):5989-5992

[70] Dhar S et al. Targeted delivery of cisplatin to prostate cancer cells by aptamer functionalized Pt(IV) prodrug-PLGA-PEG nanoparticles. Proceedings of the National Academy of Sciences of the United States of America. 2008;**105**(45):17356-17361

[71] Bagalkot V et al. Quantum dot-aptamer conjugates for synchronous cancer imaging, therapy, and sensing of drug delivery based on bi-fluorescence resonance energy transfer. Nano Letters. 2007;**7**(10):3065-3070

[72] Kim E et al. Prostate cancer cell death produced by the co-delivery of Bcl-xL shRNA and doxorubicin using an aptamer-conjugated polyplex. Biomaterials. 2010;**31**(16):4592-4599

[73] Jahkola T et al. Expression of tenascin-C in intraductal carcinoma of human breast: Relationship to invasion. European Journal of Cancer. 1998;**34**(11):1687-1692

[74] Saupe F et al. Tenascin-C downregulates wnt inhibitor dickkopf-1, promoting tumorigenesis in a neuroendocrine tumor model. Cell Reports. 2013;**5**(2):482-492

[75] Daniels DA et al. A tenascin-C aptamer identified by tumor cell SELEX: Systematic evolution of ligands by exponential enrichment. Proceedings of the National Academy of Sciences of the United States of America. 2003;**100**(26):15416-15421

[76] Jacobson O et al. PET imaging of tenascin-C with a radiolabeled single-stranded DNA aptamer. Journal of Nuclear Medicine. 2015;**56**(4):616-621

[77] Ko HY et al. A multimodal nanoparticle-based cancer imaging probe simultaneously targeting nucleolin, integrin alphavbeta3 and tenascin-C proteins. Biomaterials. 2011;**32**(4):1130-1138

[78] Li K et al. Chemical modification improves the stability of the DNA aptamer GBI-10 and its affinity towards tenascin-C. Organic & Biomolecular Chemistry. 2017;**15**(5):1174-1182

[79] Gu MJ et al. *In vitro* study of novel gadolinium-loaded liposomes guided by GBI-10 aptamer for promising tumor targeting and tumor diagnosis by magnetic resonance imaging. International Journal of Nanomedicine. 2015;**10**:5187-5204

[80] Orrick LR, Olson MO, Busch H. Comparison of nucleolar proteins of normal rat liver and Novikoff hepatoma ascites cells by two-dimensional polyacrylamide gel electrophoresis. Proceedings of the National Academy of Sciences of the United States of America. 1973;**70**(5):1316-1320

[81] Christian S et al. Nucleolin expressed at the cell surface is a marker of endothelial cells in angiogenic blood vessels. The Journal of Cell Biology. 2003;**163**(4):871-878

[82] Westmark CJ, Malter JS. Up-regulation of nucleolin mRNA and protein in peripheral blood mononuclear cells by extracellular-regulated kinase. The Journal of Biological Chemistry. 2001;**276**(2):1119-1126

[83] Fujiki H, Watanabe T, Suganuma M. Cell-surface nucleolin acts as a central mediator for carcinogenic, anti-carcinogenic, and disease-related ligands. Journal of Cancer Research and Clinical Oncology. 2014;**140**(5):689-699

[84] Bates PJ et al. Discovery and development of the G-rich oligonucleotide AS1411 AS a novel treatment for cancer. Experimental and Molecular Pathology. 2009;**86**(3):151-164

[85] Soundararajan S et al. The nucleolin targeting aptamer AS1411 destabilizes Bcl-2 messenger RNA in human breast cancer cells. Cancer Research. 2008;**68**(7):2358-2365

[86] Ireson CR, Kelland LR. Discovery and development of anticancer aptamers. Molecular Cancer Therapeutics. 2006;**5**(12):2957-2962

[87] Drecoll E et al. Treatment of peritoneal carcinomatosis by targeted delivery of the radiolabeled tumor homing peptide bi-DTPA-[F3]2 into the nucleus of tumor cells. PLoS One. 2009;**4**(5):e5715

[88] Wu J et al. Nucleolin targeting AS1411 modified protein nanoparticle for antitumor drugs delivery. Molecular Pharmaceutics. 2013;**10**(10):3555-3563

[89] Taghavi S et al. Polyethylenimine-functionalized carbon nanotubes tagged with AS1411 aptamer for combination gene and drug delivery into human gastric cancer cells. International Journal of Pharmaceutics. 2017;**516**(1-2):301-312

[90] Hwang DW et al. A nucleolin-targeted multimodal nanoparticle imaging probe for tracking cancer cells using an aptamer. Journal of Nuclear Medicine. 2010;**51**(1):98-105

[91] Taylor-Papadimitriou J et al. MUC1 and the immunobiology of cancer. Journal of Mammary Gland Biology and Neoplasia. 2002;**7**(2):209-221

[92] Altschuler Y et al. Clathrin-mediated endocytosis of MUC1 is modulated by its glycosylation state. Molecular Biology of the Cell. 2000;**11**(3):819-831

[93] Hu Y et al. Novel MUC1 aptamer selectively delivers cytotoxic agent to cancer cells *in vitro*. PLoS One. 2012;**7**(2):e31970

[94] Lee Y et al. Synthesis, characterization, antitumor activity of pluronic mimicking copolymer micelles conjugated with doxorubicin via acid-cleavable linkage. Bioconjugate Chemistry. 2008;**19**(2):525-531

[95] Ferreira CS et al. Phototoxic aptamers selectively enter and kill epithelial cancer cells. Nucleic Acids Research. 2009;**37**(3):866-876

[96] Savla R et al. Tumor targeted quantum dot-mucin 1 aptamer-doxorubicin conjugate for imaging and treatment of cancer. Journal of Controlled Release. 2011;**153**(1):16-22

[97] Pascual L et al. MUC1 aptamer-capped mesoporous silica nanoparticles for controlled drug delivery and radio-imaging applications. Nanomedicine. 2017;**13**(8):2495-2505

[98] Tan L et al. Designer tridentate mucin 1 aptamer for targeted drug delivery. Journal of Pharmaceutical Sciences. 2012;**101**(5):1672-1677

[99] Shangguan D et al. Aptamers evolved from live cells as effective molecular probes for cancer study. Proceedings of the National Academy of Sciences of the United States of America. 2006;**103**(32):11838-11843

[100] Huang YF et al. Molecular assembly of an aptamer-drug conjugate for targeted drug delivery to tumor cells. Chembiochem. 2009;**10**(5):862-868

[101] Xiao Z et al. Cell-specific internalization study of an aptamer from whole cell selection. Chemistry. 2008;**14**(6):1769-1775

[102] Tong GJ et al. Viral capsid DNA aptamer conjugates as multivalent cell-targeting vehicles. Journal of the American Chemical Society. 2009;**131**(31):11174-11178

[103] Kang H et al. A liposome-based nanostructure for aptamer directed delivery. Chem Commun (Camb). 2010;**46**(2):249-251

[104] Danesh NM et al. Targeted and controlled release delivery of daunorubicin to T-cell acute lymphoblastic leukemia by aptamer-modified gold nanoparticles. International Journal of Pharmaceutics. 2015;**489**(1-2):311-317

[105] Taghdisi SM et al. Targeted delivery of daunorubicin to T-cell acute lymphoblastic leukemia by aptamer. Journal of Drug Targeting. 2010;**18**(4):277-281

[106] Jacobson O et al. 18F-Labeled single-stranded DNA Aptamer for PET imaging of protein tyrosine Kinase-7 expression. Journal of Nuclear Medicine. 2015;**56**(11):1780-1785

[107] Normanno N et al. Epidermal growth factor receptor (EGFR) signaling in cancer. Gene. 2006;**366**(1):2-16

[108] Li N et al. Directed evolution of gold nanoparticle delivery to cells. Chemical Communications (Camb). 2010;**46**(3):392-394

[109] Master AM, Sen Gupta A. EGF receptor-targeted nanocarriers for enhanced cancer treatment. Nanomedicine (London, England). 2012;**7**(12):1895-1906

8

Physical Therapy in Patients with Cancer

Shinichiro Morishita and Atsuhiro Tsubaki

Abstract

Physical therapists often treat cancer patients. Cancer treatment includes chemotherapy, radiotherapy, and surgery, which are being continuously developed and thus increase survival of patients with each cancer diagnosis. More specifically, 5-year survival rates increase with each cancer diagnosis. Cancer patients have many problems including muscle weakness, pulmonary dysfunction, fatigue, and pain. In the end, patients with cancer tend to have a decline in activities of daily living (ADL) and quality of life (QOL). Additionally, cancer patients often have progressive disease, depression, and anxiety. Physical therapy often helps patients regain strength and physical function and improve their QOL and independence of daily living that they may have lost due to cancer or its treatment. Physical therapy has an important role in increasing physical function of cancer patients, cancer survivors, and children with cancer. In the future, physical therapy may be progressively needed for management of cancer patients.

Keywords: physical therapy, cancer, cancer survivor, ADL, QOL

1. Introduction

Cancer and its treatments are associated with a wide range of distressing physical and psychological symptoms that can affect patients for many years following treatment [1]. Many cancer patients also have physical dysfunction and experience deficits in muscle strength, flexibility, and endurance as a result of chemotherapy, radiation therapy, and surgery [2]. Physical therapy is a comprehensive, multidisciplinary approach to the evaluation and treatment of patients diagnosed with various forms of cancer. Physical therapy can improve functional problems such as weakness, soft tissue tightness, joint stiffness, fatigue, and swelling or edema [3, 4]. Physical therapy allows experts to find the best ways for cancer patients to stay active. Physical therapy-led exercise is clinically effective and can help cancer patients improve their quality of life (QOL) [5]. Physical therapy includes stretching, strengthening, and aerobic exercises for the inpatients, outpatients, and cancer survivors. It often helps patients regain strength, physical functioning, quality of life, and independence in activities of daily living (ADL) that they may have lost due to cancer or its treatment. Physical therapists are available in multiple treatment settings, including preoperative, postoperative, acute care, nursing home, and inpatient and outpatient rehabilitation. Physical therapists also work in conjunction with the rehabilitation team to design components of a survivorship care plan in order to optimize overall functional outcomes (**Figure 1**) [6]. Cancer has four stages, and cancer patients have differences in disease and disabilities during each stage (**Table 1**). Physical therapists often use four cancer rehabilitation stages and identify the stage before physical therapy for cancer patients (**Table 2**) [7]. There are different approaches for therapy of cancer patients during each stage.

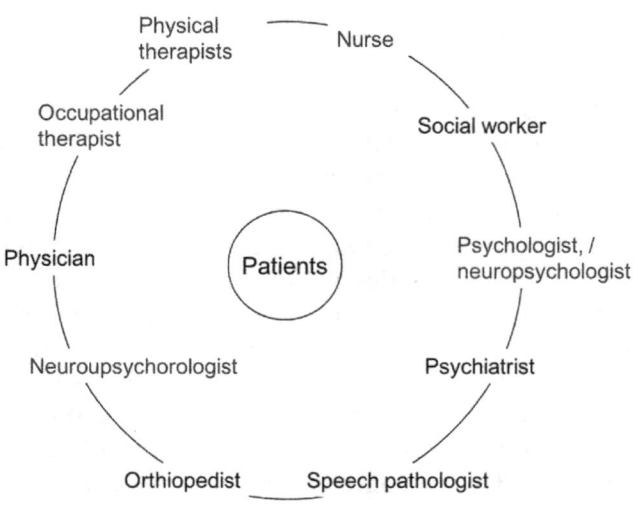

Figure 1. Rehabilitation team for cancer patients.

Stage	Characteristics
Stage 1	Cancer is relatively small and contained within the organ it originated from. This stage describes cancer in situ, which means "in place." Stage 1 cancers have not spread to nearby tissues. This stage of cancer is often highly curable, usually by removing the entire tumor with surgery
Stage 2	Cancer has not started to spread into surrounding tissue but the tumor is larger than in Stage 1. Sometimes, Stage 2 means that cancer cells have spread into lymph nodes close to the tumor. At this stage, cancer or tumor is relatively small and has not grown deeply into the nearby tissues. It also has not spread to the lymph nodes or other parts of the body. It is often called an early-stage cancer
Stage 3	Cancer is larger. It may have started to spread into surrounding tissues, and cancer cells may be present in the lymph nodes of the area. This stage indicates larger cancers or tumors
Stage 4	Cancer has spread from where it started to another organs or parts of the body. This is also called a secondary, advanced, or metastatic cancer

Table 1. Cancer stage.

Stage
(1) Preventive
Intervention focused on improving the patient's level of function prior to the onset of the effects of the cancer and its treatment, patient education, and psychological support
(2) Restorative rehabilitation
Intervention focused on returning the patient to a previous level of function and addressing impairments from cancer and its treatment
(3) Supportive rehabilitation
Intervention is meant to assist the cancer patient to function at the highest level within the context of his or her impairments, activity limitations, and participation restrictions
(4) Palliative rehabilitation
Intervention focused on minimizing complications such as pressure ulcers, contractures, and muscle deconditioning ensuring adequate pain control and emotional support for the family

Table 2. Four cancer rehabilitation stages.

This chapter introduces overview, treatment, common dysfunctions, physical therapy assessment, physical therapy, key points in diagnosis, and palliative care of following cancer types: breast cancer, gynecologic cancers, brain tumor, head and neck cancer, lung cancer, esophagus cancer, bone cancer, and blood cancer. This chapter also shows the important role of physical therapy in cancer patients.

2. General concept of physical therapy

Physical therapists must undergo assessment based on the International Classification of Functioning, Disability and Health (ICF) model before, during, and after physical therapy for each cancer patient (**Figure 2**). ICF enables physical therapist to provide cancer patients with therapy. Cancer patients have many problems caused by cancer treatment or cancer itself. Physical therapy assessment should include manual muscle testing (MMT), range of motion (ROM), balance test, endurance test, and ADL test. Performance status (PS; **Table 3**) [8], Palliative Performance Scale (PPS; **Table 4**) [9], Barthel index (BI) [10], functional independence measure (FIM) [11, 12], and QOL are also used as assessment tools for cancer patients. Physical therapists should be aware that cancer patients are exposed to various risks such as infectious diseases due to immunosuppressive effects of the treatment. Thus, physical therapists must manage risks that are related to cancer and its treatment (**Table 5**) [13]. Additionally, physical therapists must recognize that cancer is a progressive disease. In general, cancer patients have a gradual decline in their physical function. Once a goal is set, physical therapists must be aware of cancer progression and patients' prognosis [14]. Physical therapists also must know a variety of other problems that occur in cancer patients. Cancer patients might not only have physical function problems but may also develop depression and anxiety in the future [15]. Cancer patients might feel the fear of cancer recurrence or death. Physical therapy may be effective in reducing fatigue, increasing muscle strength and exercise capacity, and improving QOL in various cancer patients.

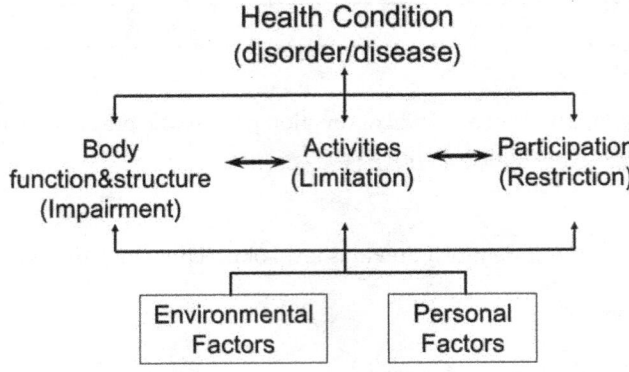

Figure 2. International Classification of Functioning, Disability, and Health.

Grade	ECOG performance status
0	Fully active, able to carry on all pre-disease performance without restriction
1	Restricted in physically strenuous activity but ambulatory and able to carry out work of a light or sedentary nature, e.g., light house work, office work
2	Ambulatory and capable of all self-care but unable to carry out any work activities. Up and about more than 50% of waking hours
3	Capable of only limited self-care, confined to bed or chair more than 50% of waking hours
4	Completely disabled. Cannot carry on any self-care. Totally confined to bed or chair
5	Dead

Table 3. Performance status (PS).

PPS level	Ambulation	Activity and evidence of disease	Self-care	Intake	Conscious level
100	Full	Normal activity and work no evidence of disease	Full	Normal	Full
90	Full	Normal activity and work Some evidence of disease	Full	Normal	Full
80	Full	Normal activity with effort Some evidence of disease	Full	Normal or reduced	Full
70	Reduced	Unable normal job/ work Significant disease	Full	Normal or reduced	Full
60	Reduced	Unable hobby/house work Significant disease	Occasional assistance necessary	Normal or reduced	Full or confusion

PPS level	Ambulation	Activity and evidence of disease	Self-care	Intake	Conscious level
50	Mainly sit/lie	Unable to do any work Extensive disease	Considerable assistance required	Normal or reduced	Full or confusion
40	Mainly in bed	Unable to do most activity Extensive disease	Mainly assistance	Normal or reduced	Full or drowsy ± confusion
30	Totally bed bound	Unable to do any activity Extensive disease	Total care	Normal or reduced	Full or drowsy ± confusion
20	Totally bed bound	Unable to do any activity Extensive disease	Total care	Minimal to sips	Full or drowsy ± confusion
10	Totally bed bound	Unable to do any activity Extensive disease	Total care	Mouth care only	Drowsy or coma ± confusion
0	Death				

[1]PPS scores are determined by reading horizontally at each level to find a "best fit" for the patient who is then assigned as the PPS% score.

[2]Begin at the left column, read downward until the appropriate ambulation level is reached, and then read across to the next column and downward again until the activity/evidence of disease is located. These steps are repeated until all five columns are covered before assigning the actual PPS for that patient. In this way, "leftward" columns (columns to the left of any specific column) are "stronger" determinants and generally take precedence over others.

[3]PPS scores are in 10% increments only. Sometimes, there are several columns easily placed at one level but one or two which seem better at a higher or lower level. One then needs to make a "best fit" decision. Choosing a "halfwit" value of PPS 45%, for example, is not correct. The combination of clinical judgment and "leftward precedence" is used to determine whether 40% or 50% is the more accurate score for that patient.

Table 4. Palliative Performance Scale (PPSv2).

1. Hematologic profile: hemoglobin <7.5 g, platelets <20,000, white blood cell count <3000

2. Metastatic bone disease

3. Compression of a hollow viscous (bowel, bladder, or ureter) vessel or spinal cord

4. Fluid accumulation in the pleura, pericardium, abdomen, or retroperitoneum associated with persistent pain, dyspnea, or problems with mobility

5. CNS depression or coma or increased intracranial pressure

6. Hypokalemia/hyperkalemia, hyponatremia, or hypocalcemia/hypercalcemia

7. Orthostatic hypotension

8. Heart rate in excess 110 beat/min or ventricular arrhythmia

9. Fever greater than 101°F

Table 5. Precaution rehabilitation for cancer patients.

3. Physical therapy in cancer patients

3.1. Breast cancer

3.1.1. Overview

Breast cancer is the most common invasive cancer in women worldwide [16]. Breast cancer alone accounts for 25% of all cancer cases and 15% of all cancer deaths among women [17]. Breast cancer starts when cells in the breast begin to grow out of control. These cells usually form a tumor that can be often seen on an X-ray or felt as a lump. Breast cancer can develop following changes in genetic material leading to cellular changes that causes cells to start multiplying in an uncontrolled fashion, forming lumps or nodules.

3.1.2. Treatment

In general, breast cancer patients have few treatment options such as surgery (breast-conserving surgery and mastectomy), radiation therapy, chemotherapy, and hormone therapy [18, 19]. In some cases, lymph nodes located close to the affected breast need to be surgically removed.

3.1.3. Common dysfunctions in breast cancer

Muscle weakness around the shoulder joint, decline of ADL using upper extremities, dizziness, loss of appetite, shortness of breath, depression are present in a substantial majority of patients during or after their initial treatment (surgery, radiation, and/or chemotherapy) [20, 21]. Physical therapists must pay attention to the occurrence of musculoskeletal disorders and lymph vascular disorders following breast surgery. Musculoskeletal disorders include postsurgical pain, rotator cuff disease, and adhesive capsulitis [22]. Lymph vascular disorders are common after removal of lymph nodes [23]. As a result, breast cancer patients have limited range of motion, muscle weakness, pain, and ADL decline such as difficulties while brushing hair or taking off the jacket. In some cases of breast cancer, cellulitis occurs that can become a potentially serious bacterial skin infection [21, 24].

3.1.4. Physical therapy assessment

Physical therapy assessment of cancer patients includes the ICF, examination of shoulder ROM, MMT, pain levels, fatigue, upper limb volume, an upper limb disability questionnaire, and QOL evaluation. Additionally, in the cases of breast cancer patients, physical therapists assess exercise tolerance.

3.1.5. Physical therapy

Many previous studies showed that physical therapy has effectiveness in breast cancer patients [25, 26]. In general, combined physical therapy is effective to treat postoperative lymphedema, pain, and impaired ROM after treatment for breast cancer [26]. Physical therapy for breast cancer patients includes lymphatic drainage massage, vantage, manual stretching, myofascial therapy, relaxation massage, stretching, strengthening, resisted exercise, proprioceptive neuromuscular facilitation (PNF) exercises, isometric exercises, aerobic exercises, transcutaneous electrical nerve stimulation (TENS), heat and cold, patient education, and behavioral training. Breast cancer patients also receive ADL training such as bathing, showering (washing the body), and dressing.

3.1.6. Key points

Physical therapists should improve mobility of upper extremities with a reduction of their volume. This should be followed by an attempt to recover upper limb function in ADL.

3.2. Gynecologic cancers

3.2.1. Overview

Gynecologic cancers accounted for 19% of the 5.1 million estimated new cancer cases and 13 million 5-year prevalent cancer cases among women in the world in 2002 [27]. Gynecologic cancer is described as the uncontrolled growth and spread of abnormal cells originating in the female reproductive organs. They are found in different places within a woman's pelvis, which is the area below the stomach and in between the hip bones. Five main types of gynecologic cancers are present: cervical, ovarian, uterine, vaginal, and vulvar.

3.2.2. Treatment

In general, gynecologic cancers can be cured with aggressive treatment involving surgery, chemotherapy, and/or radiation. Treatment goal in recurrent and metastatic cancer is to decrease progression of the disease [28, 29].

3.2.3. Common dysfunctions in gynecologic cancer

Weakness of pelvic floor muscles, decline in ADL, dizziness, loss of appetite, shortness of breath, depression are the symptoms present in a substantial majority of patients during or after their initial treatment (surgery, radiation, and/or chemotherapy) [30]. Lower extremity weakness often occurs in gynecologic cancer patients; thus, locomotion disability is common [31]. Physical therapists must pay attention to occurrence of musculoskeletal and lymph vascular disorders at the lower extremities following gynecologic surgery [32]. Lymphovascular disorders cause problems after removal of lymph nodes [33]. As a result, patients experience limited ROM, muscle weakness, pain, and decline in ADL.

3.2.4. Physical therapy assessment

First, physical therapists should assess pelvic floor muscle strength as gynecologic cancers have urinary incontinence after the treatment [34, 35]. Second, physical therapists should assess ICF category: lower extremities such as hip, knee, and ankle ROM; MMT; assessment of pain levels; fatigue; upper limb volume; locomotion ability such as gait speed; balance function; QOL; ADL; and sexual function [36]. Additionally, physical therapists should assess exercise tolerance.

3.2.5. Physical therapy

A few previous reports showed that physical therapy has a positive effect on gynecologic cancer patients [37]. Physical therapists should perform pelvic floor physical therapy as a tool to aid in addressing pelvic floor symptoms [37]. In general, physical therapy for gynecologic cancer patients includes locomotion ability exercises such as standing and walking, lymphatic drainage massage, vantage, manual stretching, myofascial therapy, relaxation massage, stretching, strengthening, resisted exercise, PNF, aerobic exercise, TENS, patient education, and behavioral training.

3.2.6. Key points

Physical therapists should improve muscle strength of lower extremities and reduce their volume as soon as possible. This should be followed by acquiring locomotion.

3.3. Brain tumor

3.3.1. Overview

The worldwide cancer incidence of a malignant brain tumor is 3.4 per 100,000 for men and 3.0 per 100,000 for women [38]. Brain tumor is the most common neurological complication related to cancer [39]. Brain tumors can originate from the patient's brain (primary brain tumors) or from other parts of the patient's body (secondary or metastatic brain tumors) [40, 41]. Brain tumors can destroy brain cells, increase inflammation, and elevate brain pressure. Brain tumors may cause a wide range of neurological dysfunctions, including disorders of the nervous system.

3.3.2. Treatment

In general, treatment options include surgery, radiation therapy, chemotherapy, targeted biological agents, or a combination of these [42]. Surgical resection is commonly the first recommended treatment in order to rapidly reduce brain pressure.

3.3.3. Common dysfunctions in brain tumor

Brain tumor patients commonly experience weakness, sensory loss, and abnormal muscle tone. These include spasticity, visuospatial deficits, hemi-neglect or bilateral visual deficits, ataxia, cognitive deficits (thought processes, memory changes, apraxia, etc.), speech difficulties, dysphagia, bowel and bladder dysfunction, psychological problems, and fatigue. As a result, ADL decline and lower QOL are common in brain tumor patients [43, 44].

3.3.4. Physical therapy assessment

Physical therapists often assess ICF category, Glasgow Coma Scale, Mini-Mental State Examination, Fugl-Meyer, Motor Assessment Scale, Motricity Index, Berg Balance Assessment, Beck Depression Inventory (BDI), and Hospital Anxiety and Depression Scale (HADS). They examine pain levels and locomotion ability such as gait speed, QOL, and sexual function. Additionally, physical therapists should assess exercise tolerance in brain tumor patients [45, 46].

3.3.5. Physical therapy

To date, no previous study has reported positive effects of physical therapy in adult brain tumor patients. However, a few reports showed that physical therapy may be effective in pediatric brain tumor patients [47]. In general, physical therapy performed in brain tumor patients is also performed in stroke patients [48]. It includes neurofacilitation techniques such as Bobath, PNF, Brunnstrom, motor relearning, functional electrical stimulation (FES), biofeedback, balance retraining, gait reeducation, and use of supportive equipment. Physical therapists must be aware of the progress of paralysis in brain tumor patients as a result of increasing tumor size. Physical therapists should know how to improve convalescence of the brain. Additionally, cognitive dysfunction, apraxia, and aphasia should be assessed [49].

3.3.6. Key points

Physical therapists should aim to treat paralysis and improve ADL as soon as possible. Attention should be paid to progressive paralysis in brain tumor patients.

3.4. Head and neck cancer

3.4.1. Overview

Overall, the annual incidence of head and neck cancer worldwide is more than 550,000 cases with around 300,000 deaths [50]. Men are affected significantly more than women [51]. Head and neck cancer includes cancers of the mouth, nose, sinuses, salivary glands, throat, and lymph nodes in the neck. Most originate from the moist tissues that line the mouth, nose, and throat. Head and neck cancers can also originate within the salivary glands. Salivary glands contain many different types of cells that can become cancerous leading to many different types of salivary gland cancers.

3.4.2. Treatment

Treatment options include surgery, radiation therapy, chemotherapy, and targeted therapy [52]. Surgery or radiation therapy alone or a combination of these treatments may be part of a patient's treatment plan [53]. Tracheostomy is performed when there are concerns about breathing due to airway obstruction associated with a throat cancer or treatment side effects [54]. Nutritional status of patients declines following tracheostomy. As patients are not able to eat, they usually receive intravenous feeding.

3.4.3. Common dysfunctions in head and neck tumor

Aspiration pneumonia after concurrent chemoradiation therapy and surgery is seen in head and neck cancer patients [55]. Most patients have dysphagia and are at increased risk of having aspiration and subsequent pneumonia [56]. Additionally, physical therapists must be aware of the decline in nutritional status after surgery or chemoradiation in these patients [57]. Paralysis of accessory nerve that causes trapezius muscle dysfunction is often seen following neck dissection [58]. This dysfunction leads to shoulder syndrome with adhesive capsulitis. Muscle weakness, decline of ADL, dizziness, loss of appetite, shortness of breath, depression are observed in a substantial majority of patients during or after their initial treatment (surgery, radiation, and/or chemotherapy) [59]. Upper and lower extremities tend to be weaker following long-term bedridden and sedentary treatment.

3.4.4. Physical therapy assessment

General pulmonary function tests are performed: spirometry; breathing pattern and cough; breath sounds including wheezing, coarse crackles, fine crackles, and rhonchi; and posture deformities in the chest or the spine; dysphagia evaluation; and ADL. Additionally, physical therapists should perform exercise tolerance test in gynecologic cancer patients. Furthermore, physical therapists should assess shoulder function including strength, mobility, and pain after surgery or chemoradiotherapy. Physical therapists often assess ICF category and lower and upper joint ROM; perform MMT; and evaluate pain levels, fatigue, and locomotion ability such as gait speed, balance function, and QOL.

3.4.5. Physical therapy

Physical therapy of the arms is performed to improve locomotion and pulmonary dysfunction. Some previous reports showed that physical therapy has effectiveness in head and neck cancer patients [60, 61]. When patients have paralysis of the accessory nerve, physical therapists perform exercises for the trapezius muscle to reduce its dysfunction [62]. Additionally, physical therapy of head and neck cancer patients includes locomotion ability exercises such as standing and walking, massage, manual stretching, myofascial therapy, relaxation massage, stretching, strengthening, resisted exercise, PNF, aerobic exercise, TENS, patient education, and behavioral training [63, 64]. However, if patients are fasting and have aspiration, they may have lower nutritional status requiring physical function recovery to be delayed.

3.4.6. Key points

Physical therapists must recognize that head and neck cancer patients tend to experience decline of the pulmonary function and paralysis of accessory nerve following the neck surgery. Physical therapists should recover pulmonary and shoulder function and improve ADL in such patients.

3.5. Lung cancer

3.5.1. Overview

Lung cancer is the most frequently diagnosed cancer worldwide with about 1.35 million new cases diagnosed each year [65]. Lung cancer starts with uncontrollable growth of abnormal cells in the lung. These cells can invade nearby tissues and form tumors. Lung cancer can start anywhere in the lungs and affect any part of the respiratory system. Cancer cells can spread, or metastasize, to the lymph nodes and other parts of the body. There are two main types of lung cancer: small-cell lung cancer (SCLC) and non-small-cell lung cancer (NSCLC). Small-cell lung cancers usually grow quicker and are more likely to spread to other body parts. Non-small-cell lung cancer accounts for about 85% of all lung cancer cases, whereas small-cell lung cancer accounts for about 15% of all lung cancer cases [50, 66].

3.5.2. Treatments

Lung cancer treatment depends on its type. Small-cell lung cancer is mostly treated with chemotherapy [67]. Non-small-cell lung cancer can be treated with surgery, chemotherapy, radiotherapy, or a combination of these depending on the stage at which the cancer is diagnosed [68, 69].

3.5.3. Common dysfunctions in lung cancer

When lung cancer treatment involves chemotherapy only, patients experience a decrease in physical function including decreased muscle strength and flexibility, which is also observed before the treatment. However, if lung cancer patients receive surgery, they encounter more problems than without the surgery. These problems include pulmonary dysfunction and decline of locomotion and ADL. Additionally, lung cancer patients experience pain of a surgical wound following thoracotomy and costectomy. Muscle weakness, decline of ADL, dizziness, loss of appetite, shortness of breath, and depression occur in a substantial majority of patients during or after their initial treatment (surgery, radiation, and/or chemotherapy). Upper and lower extremity and trunk muscle strength decreases following long-term bedridden and sedentary treatment.

3.5.4. Physical therapy assessment

General pulmonary function tests include spirometry; breathing pattern and cough; breath sounds like wheezing, coarse crackles, fine crackles, and rhonchi; postural deformities in the chest or the spine; and dysphagia evaluation on ADL [70, 71]. Additionally, physical therapists should assess exercise tolerance and shoulder function including its strength, mobility, and pain following surgery or chemoradiotherapy in patients with lung cancer. Physical therapists often assess ICF category and lower and upper joint ROM; perform MMT; and assess pain levels, fatigue, and locomotion ability such as gait speed, balance function, and QOL.

3.5.5. Physical therapy

Physical therapy of the arms is done in order to improve locomotion and pulmonary dysfunction after the treatment [72]. Some previous studies reported that preoperative physical therapy has effectiveness in lung cancer patients [73, 74]. Intensive physical therapy appears to increase oxygen saturation, reduce hospital stay, and change ventilation/perfusion distribution in lung cancer patients [73]. Following surgery with resection, physical therapists promote mobilization starting at the intensive care unit (ICU) because lung cancer patients tend to be sedentary leading to progressive decline in their physical function. Physical therapy for lung cancer patients includes massage, manual stretching, myofascial therapy, relaxation massage, stretching, strengthening, resisted exercise, PNF, aerobic exercise, TENS, patient education, and behavioral training.

3.5.6. Key points

Physical therapists should prevent development of further weakness after the treatment. Following surgery, physical therapists must make lung cancer patients perform pulmonary and mobilization exercises as soon as possible.

3.6. Esophageal cancer

3.6.1. Overview

Esophageal carcinoma affects more than 450,000 people worldwide, and the incidence is rapidly increasing [75]. Esophageal cancer is a disease in which malignant (cancer) cells form in the tissues of the esophagus. The most common types of esophageal cancer are squamous cell carcinoma and adenocarcinoma. Smoking and heavy alcohol use increase the risk of esophageal squamous cell carcinoma [76]. Esophageal cancer is often diagnosed at an advanced stage because there are no early signs or symptoms. A cancerous tumor is malignant, meaning it can grow and spread to other parts of the body. Esophageal cancer can also spread into the lungs, liver, stomach, and other parts of the body.

3.6.2. Treatment

Chemotherapy, radiotherapy, and surgery are often used as treatments for esophageal cancers [77]. Chemotherapy by itself rarely is effective. It is often combined with radiation therapy. Chemoradiation is often used before the surgery aiming to remove the cancer and some of the normal surrounding tissues. In some cases it might be combined with other treatments, such as chemotherapy and/or radiation therapy [78].

3.6.3. Common dysfunctions in esophageal cancer

If esophageal cancer patients receive chemotherapy or radiotherapy alone, they tend to have decreased physical function including loss of muscle strength and flexibility which is also observed before treatment. However, if surgery is performed, patients have more problems than without surgery, including pulmonary dysfunction and decline of locomotion and ADL. Following surgery, patients have to stay in ICU for few days. During this period, patients may develop a decline in pulmonary function and as a result, they may be intubated for a long time. Additionally, fasting is common for a few weeks until patients can eat food without aspiration. Muscle weakness, decline of ADL, dizziness, loss of appetite, shortness of breath, depression are observed in a substantial majority of patients during or after their initial treatment (surgery, radiation, and/or chemotherapy). Upper and lower extremity and trunk muscle strength decreases following long-term bedridden and sedentary treatment.

3.6.4. Physical therapy assessment

General pulmonary function tests should be performed in cancer patients. This includes spirometry; breathing pattern and cough; breath sounds like wheezing, coarse crackles, fine crackles, and rhonchi; and postural deformities in the chest or the spine. Evaluation of dysphagia on ADL should be also often assessed. Additionally, physical therapists should assess exercise tolerance in esophageal cancer patients and shoulder function including strength, mobility, and pain after surgery or chemoradiotherapy in patients with esophageal cancers. Physical therapists often assess ICF category and lower and upper joint ROM; perform MMT; and assess pain levels, fatigue, and locomotion ability such as gait speed, balance function, and QOL [79].

3.6.5. Physical therapy

To date, there are no previous studies reporting that physical therapy is effective in esophageal cancer patients. In general, physical therapy has few aims in these patients. First, performance of pulmonary exercises including positioning and breathing exercises promotes weaning of the ventilator and extubating. Second, improvement of locomotion promotes mobilization in patient's bedside [80]. Third, physical therapy aims to improve muscle strength and exercise tolerance during hospitalization. Physical therapy often includes massage, manual stretching, myofascial therapy, relaxation massage, stretching, strengthening, resisted exercise, PNF, aerobic exercise, TENS, patient education, and behavioral training.

3.6.6. Key points

Physical therapists should aim to prevent further weakness after the treatment. Following surgery, physical therapists must make patients perform pulmonary exercise and mobilization as soon as possible.

3.7. Bone cancer

3.7.1. Overview

The age-adjusted incidence rate of primary malignant bone tumors in the United States is 0.9 per 100,000 persons per year, accounting for approximately 0.2% of all malignancies [81]. Bone cancer is a rare form of cancer that can affect any bone in the body. Bone cancer is a cancer that arises from the cells that make up the bones. When cancer is detected in the bone, it most often has started somewhere else (e.g., in another organ) and then spread to the bones. This is known as cancer that has metastasized to the bone and is named after the site where the original cancer began. Bone cancer can vary widely from person to person depending on its location and size. The most common type of malignant bone tumor is osteosarcoma, which most often develops in the bones of the arms, legs, and pelvis. Other types of bone cancer include the following: chondrosarcoma, Ewing's tumor, chordoma, fibrosarcoma, giant cell tumor, and malignant fibrous histiocytoma [82].

3.7.2. Treatment

Treatment includes surgery, chemotherapy, and radiation therapy [83, 84]. Amputation may be necessary if limb-sparing surgery is not possible or had no positive outcomes [85].

3.7.3. Common dysfunctions in bone cancer

Chemotherapy or radiotherapy alone results in and improvement of physical function including muscle strength and flexibility. However, if bone cancer patients received surgery, they could develop some problems. Patients may have pain and weakness of the affected limb and may have restricted weight bearing and movement of limbs or the spine. In addition, when amputation of the arm, leg, hand, or foot is performed, patients become more physically disabled. Bone cancer patients with spine tumor, paraplegia, or quadriplegia have declined motor and sensory function in addition to bladder and bowel dysfunction [86].

3.7.4. Physical therapy assessment

Physical therapists should often assesses ICF category; pain levels; affected bone tumor; ROM; MMT; fatigue; ADL; and locomotion ability such as gait speed, balance function, and QOL. Physical therapists should be aware of motion and weight-bearing restrictions that occur after the surgery. In case of amputation, physical therapists should assess phantom limb pain, muscle strength, and mobility of the affected limb. Patients with spine tumor have paralysis; hence, physical therapists should use the American Spinal Injury Association (ASIA) scores for evaluation of sensory function, strength, mobility, and pain after the surgery or chemoradiotherapy.

3.7.5. Physical therapy

To date, there are no previous studies reporting that physical therapy is effective in bone cancer patients. In general, physical therapists must pay attention to fragile bones. Bone tumors make bones easy to fracture with vigorous movements. Physical therapy differs depending on the treatment of bone cancer. When bone cancer patients receive chemotherapy and radiotherapy only, muscle strengthening and endurance exercises are performed. However, when patients receive surgery, physical therapists must pay attention to contraindicative exercises. When patients receive amputation, limb prosthetics should be considered by the physiotherapist together with a prosthetist and an orthotist. In bone cancer patients with paraplegia such as bone tumor in the spinal cord, physical therapy is carried out in accordance with physical therapy of spinal cord injury. Otherwise, physical therapy often includes stretching, strengthening, resisted exercise, PNF, aerobic exercise, patient education, and behavioral training.

3.7.6. Key points

Physical therapists must know the location and progression of bone tumor as it is an important factor allowing improvement of physical function after treatment.

3.8. Blood cancer including hematopoietic stem cell transplantation (HSCT)

3.8.1. Overview

The number of new cases of leukemia is 4.5–9.1 per 100,000 men and 3.6–6.0 per 100,000 women per year [50]. Blood cancer affects the blood and lymph systems. Bone marrow has a function of producing blood cells such as red blood cells, white blood cells, and platelets. Bone marrow is a flexible soft tissue found in the hollow interior of the bones. Blood cancer may begin in blood-forming tissue (e.g., bone marrow) or in the cells of the immune system. There are different types of hematological cancers including leukemia, non-Hodgkin lymphoma, Hodgkin lymphoma, and multiple myeloma. Leukemia is a cancer that originates in the white blood cells and affects people of all ages [87].

3.8.2. Treatment

In general, blood cancer treatment includes chemotherapy, corticosteroids, radiation, and HSCT.

3.8.3. Common dysfunctions in blood cancer

First, blood cancer patients that have received chemotherapy experience a decrease in physical function including muscle strength and endurance capacity. Second, if complete remission is not achieved after chemotherapy, HSCT has to be chosen. In this case, patients experience even more decreased muscle strength and endurance capacity as they have to stay in a hospital for a few weeks [88, 89]. Hospitalized patients often have graft-versus-host disease (GVHD). GVHD normally affects the skin, liver, and gastrointestinal system resulting in further dysfunctions. Furthermore, following HSCT treatment, patients must stay in the isolation room to prevent infection; hence, a decrease in physical activity during these days will occur [90].

3.8.4. Physical therapy assessment

Physical therapists should assess muscle strength, body composition, mobility, and endurance capacity in blood cancer patients. Physical therapists often assess ICF category, lower and upper joint ROM, balance function, MMT, fatigue, and locomotion ability such as gait speed, balance function, and QOL [91–94].

3.8.5. Physical therapy

Physical therapy focused on the arms is performed in order to improve locomotion and muscle strength after treatment. Some previous reports showed that physical therapy is effective in pediatric leukemia patients [95, 96]. Additionally, some previous reports showed that physical therapy is effective in patients with HSCT [90, 97]. Following HSCT, physical therapists must wear a mask, plastic grove, and apron during physical therapy. The most common physical therapy of blood cancer includes massage, manual stretching, myofascial therapy, relaxation massage, stretching, strengthening, resisted exercise, PNF, aerobic exercise, balance training, TENS, patient education, and behavioral training.

3.8.6. Key points

Physical therapists should aim to increase muscle strength and exercise capacity in blood cancer patients. Additionally, physical therapists must be aware that patients may have myelosuppression as a result of chemotherapy. Physical therapy should be performed in such a way that it prevents infection in these patients.

3.9. Palliative care in cancer

Palliative care helps people cope with the symptoms of cancer and cancer treatment [98]. Palliative care aims to improve the quality of life of patients who have serious or life-threatening diseases [99]. The goal of palliative care is to prevent or treat the symptoms and side effects of the disease and its treatment in addition to related psychological, social, and spiritual problems [100]. However, the main goal is not to cure patients [101]. When many different treatments have been tried and showed no control over cancer, it could be the time to weigh the benefits and risks of continuing trying new treatments. Palliative care provides patients of any age or disease stage with relief from symptoms, pain, and stress and should be provided along curative treatment. Palliative care focuses on helping people get relief from symptoms caused by serious illness (e.g., nausea, pain, fatigue, or shortness of breath) [102].

3.9.1. Treatment

Palliative treatment is designed to relieve symptoms and often includes medication, nutritional support, relaxation techniques, spiritual support, emotional support, and other therapies [103, 104]. Palliative treatment improves patient's quality of life. It can be used at any stage of an illness and also if there are troubling symptoms such as pain or sickness. Palliative treatment can also mean using medicines to reduce or control side effects of cancer treatments.

3.9.2. Common dysfunctions in palliative care in cancer patients

Cancer patients have many problems making palliative care a good additional treatment option. Patients have many symptoms including pain, fatigue, loss of appetite, nausea, vomiting, shortness of breath, insomnia, thirst, dry mouth, bad taste, and difficulty swallowing. Gradually, patients may become bedridden and sedentary. Patients usually have a bigger decrease in muscle strength, pulmonary function, ADL, and locomotion after they received palliative care. In some cases, cancer patients have lymphedema. Unfortunately, patients may die in a few weeks or months.

3.9.3. Physical therapy assessment

Physical therapists should often assess ICF category, pain levels, ROM, MMT, fatigue, ADL, and QOL. Additionally, physical therapists should perform pulmonary function tests including spirometry; breathing pattern; cough; breath sounds such as wheezing, coarse crackles, fine crackles, and rhonchi; and postural deformities in the chest or the spine and evaluate dysphagia on ADL. If cancer patients become bedridden for a long time, physical therapists should assess pressure ulcers at the sacrum and coccyx.

3.9.4. Physical therapy

A few previous reports showed that physical therapy may be effective in cancer patients who receive palliative care [105, 106]. In general, physical therapy helps to maintain mobility and improves body movements [7, 107]. Physical therapists improve locomotion ability by exercises that include standing and walking, massage, manual stretching, strengthening, resisted exercises, aerobic exercises, patient education, and behavioral training. If patients have severe pain related to cancer, physical therapy includes myofascial therapy, relaxation massage, TENS, heat and cold, and positioning. If patients are bedridden or sedentary for a long time, physical therapists should relieve pressure to prevent pressure ulcers on bones such as the sacrum and coccyx.

3.9.5. Key points

Physical therapists must be aware that cancer patients experience more fatigue and pain while improving their locomotion. When cancer patients cannot receive progressive physical therapy, physical therapists should use myofascial therapy, relaxation massage, TENS, heat and cold, and positioning to relieve pain.

4. Summary and conclusion

Cancer patients have some physical impairment. Physical therapy is helpful and contributes to patients' recovery. Cancer patients are exposed to some risk factors during physical therapy. Therefore, physical therapists must pay attention and manage those risk factors. Cancer survivors increase 5 years of survival in various cancer diseases. Physical therapy may have an important role to improve physical function, ADL, and QOL of cancer patients and cancer survivors.

Author details

Shinichiro Morishita* and Atsuhiro Tsubaki

*Address all correspondence to: ptmorishin@yahoo.co.jp

Institute for Human Movement, Medical Sciences, Niigata University of Health and Welfare, Niigata, Japan

References

[1] de Haes JC, van Knippenberg FC, Neijt JP: Measuring psychological and physical distress in cancer patients: structure and application of the Rotterdam Symptom Checklist. Br J Cancer 1990, 62(6):1034–1038.

[2] Fialka-Moser V, Crevenna R, Korpan M, Quittan M: Cancer rehabilitation: particularly with aspects on physical impairments. J Rehabil Med 2003, 35(4):153–162.

[3] Fernández-Lao C, Cantarero-Villanueva I, Fernández-de-Las-Peñas C, del Moral-Ávila R, Castro-Sánchez AM, Arroyo-Morales M: Effectiveness of a multidimensional physical therapy program on pain, pressure hypersensitivity, and trigger points in breast cancer survivors: a randomized controlled clinical trial. Clin J Pain 2012, 28(2):113–121.

[4] Carmeli E, Bartoletti R: Retrospective trial of complete decongestive physical therapy for lower extremity secondary lymphedema in melanoma patients. Support Care Cancer 2011, 19(1):141–147.

[5] Swenson KK, Nissen MJ, Knippenberg K, Sistermans A, Spilde P, Bell EM, Nissen J, Chen C, Tsai ML: Cancer rehabilitation: outcome evaluation of a strengthening and conditioning program. Cancer Nurs 2014, 37(3):162–169.

[6] Kirschner KL, Eickmeyer S, Gamble G, Spill GR, Silver JK: When teams fumble: cancer rehabilitation and the problem of the "handoff". PM R 2013, 5(7):622–628.

[7] Silver JK, Raj VS, Fu JB, Wisotzky EM, Smith SR, Kirch RA: Cancer rehabilitation and palliative care: critical components in the delivery of high-quality oncology services. Support Care Cancer 2015, 23(12):3633–3643.

[8] Oken MM, Creech RH, Tormey DC, Horton J, Davis TE, McFadden ET, Carbone PP: Toxicity and response criteria of the Eastern Cooperative Oncology Group. Am J Clin Oncol 1982, 5(6):649–655.

[9] Lau F, Maida V, Downing M, Lesperance M, Karlson N, Kuziemsky C: Use of the palliative performance scale (PPS) for end-of-life prognostication in a palliative medicine consultation service. J Pain Symptom Manage 2009, 37(6):965–972.

[10] Collin C, Wade DT, Davies S, Horne V: The Barthel ADL index: a reliability study. Int Disabil Stud 1988, 10(2):61–63.

[11] Hamilton BB, Laughlin JA, Fiedler RC, Granger CV: Interrater reliability of the 7-level functional independence measure (FIM). Scand J Rehabil Med 1994, 26(3):115–119.

[12] Linacre JM, Heinemann AW, Wright BD, Granger CV, Hamilton BB: The structure and stability of the functional Independence measure. Arch Phys Med Rehabil 1994, 75(2):127–132.

[13] Vargo MM, Gerber LH: Rehabilitation for patients with cancer diagnosis. In: Physical medicine and rehabilitation: principles and practice. edn. Edited by Delisa JA, Gans BM, Walsh NE. Philadelphia: Lippincott Williams & Wilkins; 2005: 1771–1794.

[14] Gerber LH, Stout NL, Schmitz KH, Stricker CT: Integrating a prospective surveillance model for rehabilitation into breast cancer survivorship care. Cancer 2012, 118(8 Suppl):2201–2206.

[15] Buffart LM, van Uffelen JG, Riphagen II, Brug J, van Mechelen W, Brown WJ, Chinapaw MJ: Physical and psychosocial benefits of yoga in cancer patients and survivors, a systematic review and meta-analysis of randomized controlled trials. BMC Cancer 2012, 12:559.

[16] Parkin DM, Bray F, Ferlay J, Pisani P: Global cancer statistics, 2002. CA Cancer J Clin 2005, 55(2):74–108.

[17] Torre LA, Bray F, Siegel RL, Ferlay J, Lortet-Tieulent J, Jemal A: Global cancer statistics, 2012. CA Cancer J Clin 2015, 65(2):87–108.

[18] Yadav BS, Sharma SC, Singh R, Singh G: Patterns of relapse in locally advanced breast cancer treated with neoadjuvant chemotherapy followed by surgery and radiotherapy. J Cancer Res Ther 2007, 3(2):75–80.

[19] Mannino M, Yarnold JR: Local relapse rates are falling after breast conserving surgery and systemic therapy for early breast cancer: can radiotherapy ever be safely withheld? Radiother Oncol 2009, 90(1):14–22.

[20] Rietman JS, Dijkstra PU, Hoekstra HJ, Eisma WH, Szabo BG, Groothoff JW, Geertzen JH: Late morbidity after treatment of breast cancer in relation to daily activities and quality of life: a systematic review. Eur J Surg Oncol 2003, 29(3):229–238.

[21] Chan DN, Lui LY, So WK: Effectiveness of exercise programmes on shoulder mobility and lymphoedema after axillary lymph node dissection for breast cancer: systematic review. J Adv Nurs 2010, 66(9):1902–1914.

[22] Stubblefield MD, Custodio CM: Upper-extremity pain disorders in breast cancer. Arch Phys Med Rehabil 2006, 87(3 Suppl 1):S96–S99; quiz S100–101.

[23] Armer J, Fu MR, Wainstock JM, Zagar E, Jacobs LK: Lymphedema following breast cancer treatment, including sentinel lymph node biopsy. Lymphology 2004, 37(2):73–91.

[24] Stuiver MM, ten Tusscher MR, Agasi-Idenburg CS, Lucas C, Aaronson NK, Bossuyt PM: Conservative interventions for preventing clinically detectable upper-limb lymphoedema

in patients who are at risk of developing lymphoedema after breast cancer therapy. Cochrane Database Syst Rev 2015(2):CD009765.

[25] Cho Y, Do J, Jung S, Kwon O, Jeon JY: Effects of a physical therapy program combined with manual lymphatic drainage on shoulder function, quality of life, lymphedema incidence, and pain in breast cancer patients with axillary web syndrome following axillary dissection. Support Care Cancer 2016, 24(5):2047–2057.

[26] De Groef A, Van Kampen M, Dieltjens E, Christiaens MR, Neven P, Geraerts I, Devoogdt N: Effectiveness of postoperative physical therapy for upper-limb impairments after breast cancer treatment: a systematic review. Arch Phys Med Rehabil 2015, 96(6):1140–1153.

[27] Sankaranarayanan R, Ferlay J: Worldwide burden of gynaecological cancer: the size of the problem. Best Pract Res Clin Obstet Gynaecol 2006, 20(2):207–225.

[28] Bhoola S, Hoskins WJ: Diagnosis and management of epithelial ovarian cancer. Obstet Gynecol 2006, 107(6):1399–1410.

[29] Fader AN, Rose PG: Role of surgery in ovarian carcinoma. J Clin Oncol 2007, 25(20): 2873–2883.

[30] Gonzalez BD, Manne SL, Stapleton J, Myers-Virtue S, Ozga M, Kissane D, Heckman C, Morgan M: Quality of life trajectories after diagnosis of gynecologic cancer: a theoretically based approach. Support Care Cancer 2017, 25(2):589–598.

[31] Abu-Rustum NR, Rajbhandari D, Glusman S, Massad LS: Acute lower extremity paralysis following radiation therapy for cervical cancer. Gynecol Oncol 1999, 75(1):152–154.

[32] Deura I, Shimada M, Hirashita K, Sugimura M, Sato S, Oishi T, Itamochi H, Harada T, Kigawa J: Incidence and risk factors for lower limb lymphedema after gynecologic cancer surgery with initiation of periodic complex decongestive physiotherapy. Int J Clin Oncol 2015, 20(3):556–560.

[33] Lagoo AS, Robboy SJ: Lymphoma of the female genital tract: current status. Int J Gynecol Pathol 2006, 25(1):1–21.

[34] Yang EJ, Lim JY, Rah UW, Kim YB: Effect of a pelvic floor muscle training program on gynecologic cancer survivors with pelvic floor dysfunction: a randomized controlled trial. Gynecol Oncol 2012, 125(3):705–711.

[35] Rutledge TL, Rogers R, Lee SJ, Muller CY: A pilot randomized control trial to evaluate pelvic floor muscle training for urinary incontinence among gynecologic cancer survivors. Gynecol Oncol 2014, 132(1):154–158.

[36] Thorsen L, Nystad W, Stigum H, Hjermstad M, Oldervoll L, Martinsen EW, Hornslien K, Strømme SB, Dahl AA, Fosså SD: Cardiorespiratory fitness in relation to self-reported physical function in cancer patients after chemotherapy. J Sports Med Phys Fitness 2006, 46(1):122–127.

[37] Huffman LB, Hartenbach EM, Carter J, Rash JK, Kushner DM: Maintaining sexual health throughout gynecologic cancer survivorship: A comprehensive review and clinical guide. Gynecol Oncol 2016, 140(2):359–368.

[38] Ferlay J, Soerjomataram I, Dikshit R, Eser S, Mathers C, Rebelo M, Parkin DM, Forman D, Bray F: Cancer incidence and mortality worldwide: sources, methods and major patterns in GLOBOCAN 2012. Int J Cancer 2015, 136(5):E359–E386.

[39] Williams BJ, Suki D, Fox BD, Pelloski CE, Maldaun MV, Sawaya RE, Lang FF, Rao G: Stereotactic radiosurgery for metastatic brain tumors: a comprehensive review of complications. J Neurosurg 2009, 111(3):439–448.

[40] Sontheimer H: Ion channels and amino acid transporters support the growth and invasion of primary brain tumors. Mol Neurobiol 2004, 29(1):61–71.

[41] Yamamoto M, Ueno Y, Hayashi S, Fukushima T: The role of proteolysis in tumor invasiveness in glioblastoma and metastatic brain tumors. Anticancer Res 2002, 22(6C):4265–4268.

[42] Bouffet E, Tabori U, Huang A, Bartels U: Possibilities of new therapeutic strategies in brain tumors. Cancer Treat Rev 2010, 36(4):335–341.

[43] Schiff D, Lee EQ, Nayak L, Norden AD, Reardon DA, Wen PY: Medical management of brain tumors and the sequelae of treatment. Neuro Oncol 2015, 17(4):488–504.

[44] Correa DD: Cognitive functions in brain tumor patients. Hematol Oncol Clin North Am 2006, 20(6):1363–1376.

[45] Giordana MT, Clara E: Functional rehabilitation and brain tumour patients. A review of outcome. Neurol Sci 2006, 27(4):240–244.

[46] Vargo M: Brain tumor rehabilitation. Am J Phys Med Rehabil 2011, 90(5 Suppl 1):S50–S62.

[47] Panossian A: Facial paralysis reconstruction in children and adolescents with central nervous system tumors. J Pediatr Rehabil Med 2014, 7(4):295–305.

[48] Van Peppen RP, Kwakkel G, Wood-Dauphinee S, Hendriks HJ, Van der Wees PJ, Dekker J: The impact of physical therapy on functional outcomes after stroke: what's the evidence? Clin Rehabil 2004, 18(8):833–862.

[49] Day J, Gillespie DC, Rooney AG, Bulbeck HJ, Zienius K, Boele F, Grant R: Neurocognitive deficits and neurocognitive rehabilitation in adult brain tumors. Curr Treat Options Neurol 2016, 18(5):22.

[50] Jemal A, Bray F, Center MM, Ferlay J, Ward E, Forman D: Global cancer statistics. CA Cancer J Clin 2011, 61(2):69–90.

[51] Gupta B, Johnson NW, Kumar N: Global epidemiology of head and neck cancers: a continuing challenge. Oncology 2016, 91(1):13–23.

[52] Merlano M, Mattiot VP: Future chemotherapy and radiotherapy options in head and neck cancer. Expert Rev Anticancer Ther 2006, 6(3):395–403.

[53] Nelke KH, Pawlak W, Gerber H, Leszczyszyn J: Head and neck cancer patients' quality of life. Adv Clin Exp Med 2014, 23(6):1019–1027.

[54] Siddiqui AS, Dogar SA, Lal S, Akhtar S, Khan FA: Airway management and postoperative length of hospital stay in patients undergoing head and neck cancer surgery. J Anaesthesiol Clin Pharmacol 2016, 32(1):49–53.

[55] Nguyen NP, Smith HJ, Dutta S, Alfieri A, North D, Nguyen PD, Lee H, Martinez T, Lemanski C, Ludin A et al.: Aspiration occurrence during chemoradiation for head and neck cancer. Anticancer Res 2007, 27(3B):1669–1672.

[56] Eisbruch A, Schwartz M, Rasch C, Vineberg K, Damen E, Van As CJ, Marsh R, Pameijer FA, Balm AJ: Dysphagia and aspiration after chemoradiotherapy for head-and-neck cancer: which anatomic structures are affected and can they be spared by IMRT? Int J Radiat Oncol Biol Phys 2004, 60(5):1425–1439.

[57] Prevost V, Joubert C, Heutte N, Babin E: Assessment of nutritional status and quality of life in patients treated for head and neck cancer. Eur Ann Otorhinolaryngol Head Neck Dis 2014, 131(2):113–120.

[58] McGarvey AC, Chiarelli PE, Osmotherly PG, Hoffman GR: Physiotherapy for accessory nerve shoulder dysfunction following neck dissection surgery: a literature review. Head Neck 2011, 33(2):274–280.

[59] van Wilgen CP, Dijkstra PU, van der Laan BF, Plukker JT, Roodenburg JL: Shoulder and neck morbidity in quality of life after surgery for head and neck cancer. Head Neck 2004, 26(10):839–844.

[60] Murphy BA, Deng J: Advances in supportive care for late effects of head and neck cancer. J Clin Oncol 2015, 33(29):3314–3321.

[61] Tacani PM, Franceschini JP, Tacani RE, Machado AF, Montezello D, Góes JC, Marx A: Retrospective study of the physical therapy modalities applied in head and neck lymphedema treatment. Head Neck 2016, 38(2):301–308.

[62] McGarvey AC, Osmotherly PG, Hoffman GR, Chiarelli PE: Scapular muscle exercises following neck dissection surgery for head and neck cancer: a comparative electromyographic study. Phys Ther 2013, 93(6):786–797.

[63] Guru K, Manoor UK, Supe SS: A comprehensive review of head and neck cancer rehabilitation: physical therapy perspectives. Indian J Palliat Care 2012, 18(2):87–97.

[64] Espitalier F, Testelin S, Blanchard D, Binczak M, Bollet M, Calmels P, Couturaud C, Dreyer C, Navez M, Perrichon C et al.: Management of somatic pain induced by treatment of head and neck cancer: postoperative pain. Guidelines of the French oto-rhino-laryngology—head and neck surgery Society (SFORL). Eur Ann Otorhinolaryngol Head Neck Dis 2014, 131(4):249–252.

[65] Dela Cruz CS, Tanoue LT, Matthay RA: Lung cancer: epidemiology, etiology, and prevention. Clin Chest Med 2011, 32(4):605–644.

[66] Herbst RS, Heymach JV, Lippman SM: Lung cancer. N Engl J Med 2008, 359(13):1367–1380.

[67] Noonan KL, Ho C, Laskin J, Murray N: The influence of the evolution of first-line chemotherapy on steadily improving survival in advanced non-small-cell lung cancer clinical trials. J Thorac Oncol 2015, 10(11):1523–1531.

[68] Xu YP, Li B, Xu XL, Mao WM: Is there a survival benefit in patients with stage IIIA (N2) non-small cell lung cancer receiving neoadjuvant chemotherapy and/or radiotherapy prior to surgical resection: a systematic review and meta-analysis. Medicine (Baltimore) 2015, 94(23):e879.

[69] Vandenbroucke E, De Ryck F, Surmont V, van Meerbeeck JP: What is the role for surgery in patients with stage III non-small cell lung cancer? Curr Opin Pulm Med 2009, 15(4):295–302.

[70] Rivas-Perez H, Nana-Sinkam P: Integrating pulmonary rehabilitation into the multidisciplinary management of lung cancer: a review. Respir Med 2015, 109(4):437–442.

[71] Nazarian J: Cardiopulmonary rehabilitation after treatment for lung cancer. Curr Treat Options Oncol 2004, 5(1):75–82.

[72] Nici L: The role of pulmonary rehabilitation in the lung cancer patient. Semin Respir Crit Care Med 2009, 30(6):670–674.

[73] Pehlivan E, Turna A, Gurses A, Gurses HN: The effects of preoperative short-term intense physical therapy in lung cancer patients: a randomized controlled trial. Ann Thorac Cardiovasc Surg 2011, 17(5):461–468.

[74] Morano MT, Araújo AS, Nascimento FB, da Silva GF, Mesquita R, Pinto JS, de Moraes Filho MO, Pereira ED: Preoperative pulmonary rehabilitation versus chest physical therapy in patients undergoing lung cancer resection: a pilot randomized controlled trial. Arch Phys Med Rehabil 2013, 94(1):53–58.

[75] Pennathur A, Gibson MK, Jobe BA, Luketich JD: Oesophageal carcinoma. Lancet 2013, 381(9864):400–412.

[76] Peng Q, Chen H, Huo JR: Alcohol consumption and corresponding factors: A novel perspective on the risk factors of esophageal cancer. Oncol Lett 2016, 11(5):3231–3239.

[77] Carcaterrra M, Osti MF, De Sanctis V, Caruso C, Berardi F, Enrici RM: Adjuvant radiotherapy and radiochemotherapy in the management of esophageal cancer: a review of the literature. Rays 2005, 30(4):319–322.

[78] Siersema PD, van Hillegersberg R: Treatment of locally advanced esophageal cancer with surgery and chemoradiation. Curr Opin Gastroenterol 2008, 24(4):535–540.

[79] Gimigliano R, Bertella M, Gimigliano F, Iolascon G: Rehabilitation in esophageal cancer. Rays 2005, 30(4):295–298.

[80] Aceto P, Congedo E, Cardone A, Zappia L, De Cosmo G: Postoperative management of elective esophagectomy for cancer. Rays 2005, 30(4):289–294.

[81] Franchi A: Epidemiology and classification of bone tumors. Clin Cases Miner Bone Metab 2012, 9(2):92–95.

[82] Bertoni F, Bacchini P: Classification of bone tumors. Eur J Radiol 1998, 27 Suppl 1:S74–S76.

[83] O'Toole GC, Boland P: Metastatic bone cancer pain: etiology and treatment options. Curr Pain Headache Rep 2006, 10(4):288–292.

[84] Anderson P, Salazar-Abshire M: Improving outcomes in difficult bone cancers using multimodality therapy, including radiation: physician and nursing perspectives. Curr Oncol Rep 2006, 8(6):415–422.

[85] Bekkering WP, Vliet Vlieland TP, Fiocco M, Koopman HM, Schoones JW, Nelissen RG, Taminiau AH: Quality of life, functional ability and physical activity after different surgical interventions for bone cancer of the leg: a systematic review. Surg Oncol 2012, 21(2):e39–e47.

[86] Baines MJ: Spinal cord compression—a personal and palliative care perspective. Clin Oncol (R Coll Radiol) 2002, 14(2):135–138.

[87] Dores GM, Devesa SS, Curtis RE, Linet MS, Morton LM: Acute leukemia incidence and patient survival among children and adults in the United States, 2001–2007. Blood 2012, 119(1):34–43.

[88] Morishita S, Kaida K, Yamauchi S, Wakasugi T, Ikegame K, Kodama N, Ogawa H, Domen K: Early-phase differences in health-related quality of life, psychological status, and physical function between human leucocyte antigen-haploidentical and other allogeneic haematopoietic stem cell transplantation recipients. Eur J Oncol Nurs 2015, 19(5):443–450.

[89] Morishita S, Kaida K, Yamauchi S, Sota K, Ishii S, Ikegame K, Kodama N, Ogawa H, Domen K: Relationship between corticosteroid dose and declines in physical function among allogeneic hematopoietic stem cell transplantation patients. Support Care Cancer 2013, 21(8):2161–2169.

[90] Morishita S, Kaida K, Setogawa K, Kajihara K, Ishii S, Ikegame K, Kodama N, Ogawa H, Domen K: Safety and feasibility of physical therapy in cytopenic patients during allogeneic haematopoietic stem cell transplantation. Eur J Cancer Care (Engl) 2013, 22(3):289–299.

[91] Morishita S, Kaida K, Aoki O, Yamauchi S, Wakasugi T, Ikegame K, Ogawa H, Domen K: Balance function in patients who had undergone allogeneic hematopoietic stem cell transplantation. Gait Posture 2015, 42(3):406–408.

[92] Morishita S, Kaida K, Yamauchi S, Wakasugi T, Yoshihara S, Taniguchi K, Ishii S, Ikegame K, Kodama N, Ogawa H et al.: Gender differences in health-related quality of life, physical function and psychological status among patients in the early phase following allogeneic haematopoietic stem cell transplantation. Psychooncology 2013, 22(5):1159–1166.

[93] Morishita S, Kaida K, Ikegame K, Yoshihara S, Taniguchi K, Okada M, Kodama N, Ogawa H, Domen K: Impaired physiological function and health-related QOL in patients before hematopoietic stem-cell transplantation. Support Care Cancer 2012, 20(4):821–829.

[94] Morishita S, Kaida K, Tanaka T, Itani Y, Ikegame K, Okada M, Ishii S, Kodama N, Ogawa H, Domen K: Prevalence of sarcopenia and relevance of body composition, physiological function, fatigue, and health-related quality of life in patients before allogeneic hematopoietic stem cell transplantation. Support Care Cancer 2012, 20(12):3161–3168.

[95] Vercher P, Hung YJ, Ko M: The effectiveness of incorporating a play-based intervention to improve functional mobility for a child with relapsed acute lymphoblastic leukaemia: a case report. Physiother Res Int 2016, 21(4):264–270.

[96] Esbenshade AJ, Friedman DL, Smith WA, Jeha S, Pui CH, Robison LL, Ness KK: Feasibility and initial effectiveness of home exercise during maintenance therapy for childhood acute lymphoblastic leukemia. Pediatr Phys Ther 2014, 26(3):301–307.

[97] van Haren IE, Timmerman H, Potting CM, Blijlevens NM, Staal JB, Nijhuis-van der Sanden MW: Physical exercise for patients undergoing hematopoietic stem cell transplantation: systematic review and meta-analyses of randomized controlled trials. Phys Ther 2013, 93(4):514–528.

[98] Armes J, Crowe M, Colbourne L, Morgan H, Murrells T, Oakley C, Palmer N, Ream E, Young A, Richardson A: Patients' supportive care needs beyond the end of cancer treatment: a prospective, longitudinal survey. J Clin Oncol 2009, 27(36):6172–6179.

[99] Peters L, Sellick K: Quality of life of cancer patients receiving inpatient and home-based palliative care. J Adv Nurs 2006, 53(5):524–533.

[100] Jocham HR, Dassen T, Widdershoven G, Halfens R: Quality of life in palliative care cancer patients: a literature review. J Clin Nurs 2006, 15(9):1188–1195.

[101] Gattellari M, Voigt KJ, Butow PN, Tattersall MH: When the treatment goal is not cure: are cancer patients equipped to make informed decisions? J Clin Oncol 2002, 20(2):503–513.

[102] Dy SM, Harman SM, Braun UK, Howie LJ, Harris PF, Jayes RL: To stent or not to stent: an evidence-based approach to palliative procedures at the end of life. J Pain Symptom Manage 2012, 43(4):795–801.

[103] Mansky PJ, Wallerstedt DB: Complementary medicine in palliative care and cancer symptom management. Cancer J 2006, 12(5):425–431.

[104] True G, Phipps EJ, Braitman LE, Harralson T, Harris D, Tester W: Treatment preferences and advance care planning at end of life: the role of ethnicity and spiritual coping in cancer patients. Ann Behav Med 2005, 30(2):174–179.

[105] Kumar P, Casarett D, Corcoran A, Desai K, Li Q, Chen J, Langer C, Mao JJ: Utilization of supportive and palliative care services among oncology outpatients at one academic cancer center: determinants of use and barriers to access. J Palliat Med 2012, 15(8):923–930.

[106] López-Sendín N, Alburquerque-Sendín F, Cleland JA, Fernández-de-las-Peñas C: Effects of physical therapy on pain and mood in patients with terminal cancer: a pilot randomized clinical trial. J Altern Complement Med 2012, 18(5):480–486.

[107] Olson E, Cristian A: The role of rehabilitation medicine and palliative care in the treatment of patients with end-stage disease. Phys Med Rehabil Clin N Am 2005, 16(1):285–305, xi.

9

Local Treatment Options for Unresectable Liver Metastases in Colorectal Cancer

Mark McGregor, Gonzalo Tapia Rico,
Amanda Townsend and Tim Price

Abstract

Despite the increase in effectiveness of systemic therapy, cure for colorectal cancer with liver metastases (CRLM) is rarely achieved without surgical resection, with less than 20% of patients initially suitable for surgery. Liver-directed therapies are continually being investigated in the hope of improving cure rates in patients with unresectable liver metastases. These modalities include selective internal radiation therapy (SIRT), radiofrequency ablation (RFA), transarterial chemoembolization (TACE) and hepatic artery infusion (HAI) chemotherapy. While there is evidence of activity for all these treatments, they are somewhat lacking in high level randomized, controlled trial evidence (RCT) with appropriate control arms relevant to current standard of care. This review examines the efficacy and safety of these treatments in unresectable CRLM.

Keywords: colorectal cancer, SIRT, RFA, HAI, TACE, liver metastases

1. Introduction

Colorectal cancer is the fourth most common cancer and third leading cause of cancer death worldwide [1]. Approximately 20% of patients have stage 4 disease at diagnosis with 5 year overall survival rate traditionally not exceeding 13% [2, 3] or 20% in more recent clinical trial populations on multi-agent chemotherapy [4]. The venous drainage of the intestinal tract is through the portal system and hence the first site of dissemination is usually the liver. Up to 25% of patients present with synchronous hepatic metastases with a further 50% developing liver metastases during the course of their illness [5]. This is the most common site for metastases in colorectal cancer and the leading cause of death [6].

Surgical resection of liver metastases remains the only potentially curative treatment modality in patients with colorectal liver metastases (CRLM). Resection of liver metastases can result in 3 year survival rates of 76% [7] and an average 5 year overall survival of 40–45% [8, 9]. At the time of diagnosis, fewer than 20% of patients are considered suitable for resection due to tumor size and location, inadequate hepatic reserve or presence of extra-hepatic metastases [5, 10, 11].

Patients with unresectable disease and best supportive care alone have a median overall survival of less than 10 months [10]. This significantly increases with the use of multiagent chemotherapy of fluoropyrimidine and oxaliplatin or irinotecan [12–14]. The additional use of biological agents such as bevacizumab (VEGF inhibitor) or cetuximab and pantimumab (EGFR inhibitors) have further improved response rates and duration of survival. Further discovery of predictive and prognostic biomarkers such as activating RAS mutation and BRAF mutations are also helping to assist in personalizing treatment decisions and improve survival (EGFR inhibitors in RAS wild type). More recently, the location (left versus right) of the primary colorectal tumor has been found to have prognostic and predictive significance with left sided tumors having an improved prognosis versus right side, as well as predicting for improved efficacy of first-line cetuximab [15]. Despite these advances, systemic therapy alone still does not offer a meaningful chance of cure.

The use of systemic therapy including chemotherapy and biological agents (VEGF and EGFR inhibitors) can be used to downstage liver metastases to allow for subsequent resection in a small proportion of patients, with 5 year survival rates of these patients 33% [16–19].

The low rates of resectable liver metastases combined with the limitations of systemic therapy alone has led to multiple trials of a number of different loco-regional therapies to achieve better control of liver metastases and improve long term outcomes for those with unresectable disease. These therapies utilize the predominant hepatic arterial perfusion of liver metastases compared to portal venous supply of non-cancerous liver parenchymal tissue. Locoregional therapies include selective internal radiation therapy (SIRT), radio-frequency ablation (RFA), trans-arterial chemoembolization (TACE) and hepatic artery infusion (HAI) chemotherapy. With multiple treatment options now available for metastatic colorectal cancer, and their potential for sequential use, it is unclear how and when locoregional therapies should be utilized. The magnitude of clinical benefit of these therapies must be weighed against cost, toxicity and inconvenience. This chapter will examine the efficacy and toxicity of some of these therapies, with particular focus on the use of SIRT and concentrating on results from the small number of randomized controlled trials that have been conducted for these treatment modalities.

2. Selective internal radiation therapy

Normal liver parenchyma has an inherently low radiation threshold of approximately 30–40 Gy before developing the clinical syndrome of radiation induced liver dysfunction [20].

This has limited the utility and efficacy of external beam radiation in those with liver metastases.

SIRT involves the embolization of radiolabelled spheres into the hepatic artery, preferentially lodging in vasculature surrounding tumor deposits and delivering high doses of radiation to these specific sites. Yttrium-90 (Y90) is a high energy beta emitting radioisotope which can be incorporated into glass or resin microspheres. The mean and maximum tissue penetration of radiation from Y90 is 2.5 and 11 mm respectively, resulting in delivery of effective doses of radiation (200–300 Gy) to tumor tissue without significant toxicity to surrounding normal liver tissue [21–23].

The commercially available product for use in colorectal cancer with liver metastases is the SIR-Sphere (SIRTex Medical, Sydney, Australia), which is a resin microsphere of 32 μm diameter, embedded with Y90. Given the small mean diameter, absolute contraindications include excessive (>20%) hepatopulmonary shunting or shunting to the gastrointestinal tract due to the risks of radiation pneumonitis and gastrointestinal ulceration. Prior to the use of SIRT, angiography is performed to ensure arterial anatomy is favorable to proceed. Macroaggregated albumin labeled Technetium 99 m is subsequently injected into the hepatic artery to determine the degree of shunting with the option of occlusion of potential enteric channels such as the gastroduodenal artery. Further adverse effects include abdominal pain, liver function abnormalities and fatigue [22, 24, 25]. As well as excessive shunting, other relative contraindications include significant synthetic liver dysfunction, high extrahepatic burden predicting short-term mortality and extensive portal vein thrombosis [26].

2.1. Efficacy

A phase 3 randomized, controlled trial from Gray et al. [27], demonstrating the activity of SIRT in combination with HAI chemotherapy, led to SIR-Spheres obtaining FDA approval in treatment of colorectal cancer live metastases in 2002. In this trial, 74 patients with unresectable liver metastases from colorectal cancer were randomized to HAI chemotherapy using floxuridine alone versus HAI floxuridine with the addition of SIRT. Treatment protocol excluded those with extra-hepatic metastases at time of trial entry; however, 41 patients were found to have extra-hepatic disease post randomization. Patients were treatment naïve, except for 11 patients (15%) who had previously received chemotherapy, with trial treatment either commencing for progressive disease after first-line chemotherapy or post a short course of bridging chemotherapy. For the total study population, the addition of SIRT resulted in a higher response rate (44 versus 18%) and time to progression of disease in the liver (12.0 versus 7.6 months) compared to HAI alone. No statistically significant difference was found in median overall survival (OS) between the two groups (17 months versus 15.9 months, p = 0.18). Five-year OS was 6% in SIRT + HAI group and 0% in HAI alone group. Those receiving HAI alone were 3.1 times more likely to die from progression of liver metastases. Exploratory Cox regression analysis found a survival advantage for SIRT + HAI in those patients who survived at least 15 months, with a possible explanation that those who did not rapidly develop extra-hepatic metastases benefited more from the improved locoregional control of additional

SIRT. Only two patients had liver metastases resected after treatment, one from each group. Significant numbers of patients in both groups received extra off-protocol chemotherapy, adding further limitation to the analysis.

Using individual patient data, analysis was performed on only those patients who had not had any prior chemotherapy (excluding 11 patients). In the 63 first-line therapy patients, response rate was 37 versus 14% (p = 0.051). There was no significant improvement in median progression free survival (PFS) when SIRT was added to HAI (7.3 months versus 5.9 months, HR 0.72, p = 0.21). Median OS also was not significantly different (17.6 months versus 15.9 months, HR 0.62, p = 0.07). In the 22 patients with no extra-hepatic disease, there was also no significant benefit on median progression free or overall survival although 2 year overall survival was 50% with SIRT + HAI versus 21% with HAI alone.

How generalizable these findings are in today's treatment of colorectal cancer is debateable given the more widespread use of systemic rather than regional chemotherapy, particularly in the first-line setting. Since this trial, there have been numerous trials demonstrating activity in various lines of treatment, with and without the use of systemic therapy.

2.1.1. Refractory setting

In the setting of colorectal cancer with liver metastases refractory to systemic chemotherapy, SIRT has shown significant activity in numerous single arm trials. Kennedy et al. treated 208 patients with liver metastases, refractory to oxaliplatin and irinotecan, with unimodality SIRT achieving response rates (RR) of 35% by RECIST, 91% RR by PET scanning and 70% RR by CEA. Response was a predictor of survival with median OS 10.5 months in RECIST responders and only 4.5 months in non-responders [28]. Mulcahy et al. administered SIRT to 72 pretreated patients with liver metastases and minimal extra-hepatic disease with a response rate of 40.3% and median overall survival of 14.5 months, with significant differences in survival in those with and without extra-hepatic disease (7.9 versus 21 months) [29]. A phase 2 trial by Cosimelli et al. used SIRT also in the population with disease refractory to oxaliplatin and irinotecan, with most having at least 4 lines of prior treatment and high volume liver metastases. Response rate was 24 with 2% complete response (CR) and 24% stable disease. Once again, response predicted improvement in overall survival with a median OS of 16 months in responders versus 8 months in non-responders. Two year OS for all participants was 19.6% [30]. Further phase 1 and 2 trials of SIRT alone or with chemotherapy in second line or later settings, achieved response rates of 17–32% with consistent findings of improved survival being associated with radiological and CEA response and lack of extrahepatic disease [31–33].

The only prospective randomized controlled trial of the use of SIRT in chemotherapy refractory CRLM was from Hendlisz et al., who enrolled 44 patients progressing on standard chemotherapy of fluorouracil (5FU), oxaliplatin and irinotecan and randomized them to protracted 5FU infusion alone versus SIRT + protracted 5FU infusion. All patients had no extrahepatic disease at randomization. Response rate was low with no significant difference found between groups (10 versus 0%, p = 0.22) although stabilization rate (PR + stable disease) was significantly higher in the SIRT +5FU group (86 versus 35%, p = 0.001). One patient who gained a response underwent resection of hepatic metastasis. PFS was significantly increased in the SIRT +5FU group compared to 5FU alone, with median PFS of 4.5 versus 2.1 months (HR 0.51, p = 0.03). Median time to progression in liver was similar at 5.5 versus 2.1 months, suggesting systemic control was not a major factor in this population of liver limited disease. Despite the PFS benefit, there was no significant overall survival benefit with the addition of SIRT (median OS 10 months versus 7.3 months, p = 0.80). Potential reasons for this include small study numbers as well as the high number of subsequent treatments in chemotherapy alone arm with 70% (16/23) of patients in chemotherapy alone arm treated with further therapies, and 10 of those 16 treated with radioembolization. This compared to only 39% of the SIRT group receiving further lines of treatment [34].

Although this randomized trial examined only a small number of participants, PFS and OS figures of the experimental arm were similar to some of the single arm trials of SIRT in refractory disease previously described [29, 30, 33], suggesting there is activity in selected patients with CRLM refractory to standard treatments. A meta-analysis of patients with unresectable, chemorefractory CRLM patients, including 20 studies of 979 patients prior to 2012, showed an average response rate of 31% and disease control rate of 71.5% with median time to intrahepatic progression at 9 months. Median overall survival was 12 months [35]. Poorer overall survival was associated with multiple previous lines of chemotherapy, lack of radiological response, extra-hepatic disease and extensive liver disease >25%. There was a very wide range of delivered radioactivity, treatment volume, extrahepatic disease and concurrent use of chemotherapy between included trials, compromising the ability to interpret results to a wider population.

There is still no definitive evidence that the activity described in this refractory group of patients results in an overall survival benefit compared to other available systemic treatments. Although EGFR antagonists were used in a number of patients prior to randomization and post progression, they were not routinely available and RAS testing was not commonplace as part of patient selection for these agents. With EGFR antagonists now used much more frequently in RAS wild-type disease, including as single agents in refractory disease, further randomized, controlled trials assessing the benefit of SIRT in those refractory to all standard treatments, including EGFR inhibitors and bevacizumab, are required to better understand the efficacy, patient selection and sequence of use of SIRT. These potential trials may be inhibited by poor recruitment given the development and study of newer systemic agents such as TAS-102 and regorafenib in the refractory setting [36, 37].

2.1.2. First-line combination with chemotherapy

After Gray et al. showed improved response rate and time to progression in the liver when SIRT was used with HAI chemotherapy as first-line treatment [27], numerous studies have been conducted to assess the benefit of SIRT in combination with systemic chemotherapy in the first-line setting.

A small randomized, controlled phase 2 study by van Hazel et al. compared SIRT in addition to fluorouracil and leucovorin (5FU/LV) with 5FU/LV alone in 21 patients with unresectable liver metastases and no previous treatment [38]. Six of the twenty-one patients had extrahepatic disease present at randomization and the data for these patients were not reported separately. Response rate was significantly increased with the addition of SIRT (73 versus 0%) as well as median time to progression (18.6 months versus 3.6 months, p = 0.004). Median overall survival was also significantly increased with SIRT (29.4 months versus 12.8 months). Similar to Gray's earlier trial in 2001 [27], the application of these results to standard clinical practice is limited by small numbers as well as the superseded nature of the control arm of 5FU/LV alone as a standard chemotherapy regime in first-line metastatic colorectal cancer. For that reason, a planned phase 3 trial of these groups was abandoned with further trials set up to examine the addition of SIRT to combination chemotherapy such as FOLFOX.

A phase 1 trial from Sharma et al. combined SIRT with FOLFOX4 systemic therapy in 20 treatment-naïve patients with unresectable CRLM. Overall response rate was 90% with stable disease in the remaining 10%. Median PFS was 9.3 months and median time to progression in the liver was 12.3 months. Two patients underwent resection of liver metastases at completion of protocol treatment [39].

Larger phase 3 trials have since been carried out adding SIRT to more modern conventional chemotherapy regimes, first in the SIRFLOX trial by van Hazel et al. published in 2016 [40], followed by a combined analysis of SIRFLOX, FOXFIRE and FOXFIRE-Global from Wasan et al. published in 2017 [41].

The SIRFLOX trial enrolled 530 patients with colorectal cancer with unresectable liver metastases who had no prior systemic treatment [40]. Liver only metastases or limited extrahepatic metastases (fewer than 5 lung nodules of ≤1 cm diameter or a single nodule of ≤1.7 cm diameter, and/or lymph node involvement with a single anatomic area of <2 cm diameter) were included. Patients were randomized to receive mFOLFOX6 ± bevacizumab (physician's choice) and SIRT (with cycle 1) or mFOLFOX6 ± bevacizumab alone. The SIRT arm received lower doses of oxaliplatin and no bevacizumab for the first 3 cycles based on toxicity seen in the previous phase 1 trial [39]. Primary end point was progression free survival and secondary endpoints included PFS in liver, response rate at any site, response rate in liver, liver resection rate and overall survival. Both arms had 40% of participants with extrahepatic metastases. There was no difference between the groups in primary endpoint with median PFS 10.7 months in SIRT + chemotherapy versus 10.2 months in chemotherapy alone (p = 0.43). Difference in overall response rate did not reach statistical significance (76.4 versus 68.0%, p = 0.113). Despite lack of overall response or PFS benefit when including all sites of metastases, SIRT did lead to an improvement in response rates in liver (78.7 versus 68.8%, p = 0.042) as well as liver-specific progression free survival (20.5 months versus 12.6 months). This did not lead to a significant difference in liver resection rates (13.7 versus 14.2%). This trial was underpowered to meaningfully assess overall survival and thus was not published in this original paper, with survival data reported and published in the combined analysis of SIRFLOX with FOXFIRE and FOXFIRE-Global. The site of first disease progression appeared to explain the discrepancy between PFS at all sites and PFS in the liver with 77% of the control arm progressing first in the liver compared to 52.4% of SIRT arm, while the SIRT arm had a higher rate of first progression at non-liver sites (27.7 versus 7.9%). Other proposed factors for lack of PFS benefit were the 8% of patients assigned SIRT who did not undergo the procedure, 8% of patients with bilobar liver disease who received SIRT to only one lobe and the large proportion (45%) of patients who had an intact primary tumor.

Prior to publication of the combined analysis, the authors postulated that liver-specific PFS and response could translate into an overall survival benefit in this population of patients. Liver PFS was a new endpoint used in this trial and interpreting across trials was difficult. If the extra-hepatic disease at diagnosis and progression was more indolent in nature, such as is often seen in lung metastases in colorectal cancer [42], then liver PFS may be more important to survival in the liver-dominant metastatic colorectal cancer setting. This hypothesis is also the premise behind increasing rates of hepatic resection in the setting of coexistent low volume lung metastases [43]. A similar hypothesis was used in explaining the improved overall survival of RFA when combined with chemotherapy in metastatic colorectal cancer with metastases confined to liver in the CLOCC study [44]. The authors of that trial postulated the lower incidence of liver metastases as the first site of recurrence (45 versus 76%) contributed to the median overall survival benefit (45.6 months in RFA + chemotherapy versus 40.5 months in chemotherapy alone). However, that population also had an improved overall PFS with the addition of RFA as well as an increased hepatic resection rate of 45 versus 10% with RFA, limiting the ability to directly compare these studies and assign meaningful benefit to liver-specific PFS as an endpoint.

Wasan et al. published a combined analysis of three multicentre, randomized phase 3 trials evaluating the addition of SIRT to standard chemotherapy in the first-line setting for patients with unresectable colorectal liver metastases [41]. Limited extra-hepatic metastases were permitted. 1103 patients were recruited in total across 14 countries. The three individual trials each had very similar designs to allow for this pre-planned combined analysis, randomizing patients to FOLFOX chemotherapy with SIRT or FOLFOX chemotherapy alone. Use of bevacizumab or cetuximab (in RAS wild-type tumors) was permitted and overall survival was the primary endpoint. There was no significant difference in patient characteristics between the two groups with 35.9% of SIRT group and 34.8% of control arm having extra-hepatic metastases; 50.2 versus 55% having primary tumor in situ and 32.3 versus 30.6% having >25% liver involvement of metastatic disease. There was a significant difference in the number of patients receiving bevacizumab with 35.6% receiving bevacizumab in the SIRT group compared to 46.6% in the control arm. Only 0.6 versus 1.7% received cetuximab.

There was no difference in overall survival between those receiving SIRT + chemotherapy versus those receiving chemotherapy alone (median OS 22.6 versus 23.3 months, p = 0.61) with no difference found in the liver-metastasis only subgroup. Median PFS was also not significantly impacted (11.0 versus 10.3 months, p = 0.11). Compared to the SIRFLOX trial, increase in overall response rate reached statistical significance in the SIRT group (72 versus 63%, p = 0.001) with no impact on hepatic resection rate (17 versus 16%). Liver specific progression free survival was increased in the SIRT + FOLFOX group with first progression in the liver occurring in 31 versus 49% in FOLFOX alone (HR 0.51, p < 0.0001). Non-liver progression and death without liver progression occurred in 54% of SIRT + FOLFOX group versus 36% in FOLFOX alone (HR 1.76, p < 0.0001).

There are a number of potential factors to explain the improved response and liver specific PFS not translating to an overall survival or PFS benefit, even in liver only metastatic disease. These include reduced oxaliplatin dose and reduced and delayed bevacizumab usage in SIRT patients, as well as fewer patients from SIRT group receiving subsequent systemic therapy compared to chemotherapy alone group (67.9 versus 74%). Eight percent of patients assigned to SIRT did not receive the treatment while 3% of patients in FOLFOX alone group crossed over to SIRT, and 12% received it as a later line of therapy. Likely to be of more significance is the high proportion of patients developing extra-hepatic progression in the SIRT group and the impact this may have had on liver resection rates, which was equal between groups despite a higher liver response rate with SIRT. The low overall survival rates in both groups compared to other more recent trials likely reflects the relative lack of use of bevacizumab and EGFR inhibitors [4].

An unplanned subgroup analysis did show a significant PFS and OS advantage for SIRT + FOLFOX versus FOLFOX alone in those with right sided primary tumors (overall survival HR 0.67, p = 0.007) [45]. Right sided tumors have recently been shown to be predictive of poorer response and prognosis compared to left sided tumors when systemic chemotherapy is used [15]. The use of SIRT in this population appears to overcome this intrinsic resistance to chemotherapy, although this is hypothesis generating only given the unplanned, post-hoc nature of this subgroup analysis. Further research into this patient group and analysis of various other biological subtypes (RAS and BRAF mutant disease) is required to aid patient selection.

The results of these large phase 3 trials do not currently support the use of SIRT in combination with chemotherapy for liver-only or liver-dominant unresectable metastatic colorectal cancer in the first-line setting.

A summary of the completed RCT's in SIRT is provided in **Table 1**.

2.2. Toxicity and quality of life

SIRT has been demonstrated to be a relatively safe procedure when the appropriate pre-treatment investigations are carried out correctly. Recognized toxicities include post-radioembolization syndrome with transient liver toxicity characterized by elevation of ALP, ALT and bilirubin [46], although the severity of this syndrome in SIRT is milder than the post-embolization syndrome in TACE [47]. Other radioembolization specific complications include gastric ulceration, pancreatitis, portal hypertension from liver fibrosis, radiation induced liver disease and radiation pneumonitis. In meta-analysis in 2009, the rates of all of these complications were <1% with the exception of gastric ulceration which was <5% [46]. There is a lack of reporting of delayed radiation toxicity such as liver dysfunction and gastric ulceration with rates reported in the range of 4–10% in a small number of phase 2 and observational trials [30, 33, 48, 49] and interpreting etiology of liver dysfunction (treatment related versus disease related) is difficult.

There is increased toxicity with the addition of SIRT to systemic chemotherapy compared to chemotherapy alone in the first-line setting. The addition of SIRT to 5FU/LV in the small trial of 21 patients by Van hazel [38] led to increase in grade 3/4 toxicities compared to

Study	Response rate	Liver resection rate	Median progression free survival	Median overall survival
Gray [27] HAI floxuridine + SIRT versus HAI floxuridine 74 patients, 11 with prior systemic treatment	*All patients (n = 74)* 44 versus 17.6% (p = 0.01) *First line (n = 63)* 37 versus 14% (p = 0.051) *Liver only disease (n = 22)* 25 versus 14% (p = 0.60)	*All patients (n = 74)* 2.9 versus 2.8% (1 in each group)	*All patients (n = 74)* 12 versus 7.6 months (p = 0.04) *First line (n = 63)* 7.3 versus 5.9 months (p = 0.21) *Liver only disease (n = 22)* 2.7 versus 4.3 months HR 0.72 (CI 0.27–1.90)	*All patients (n = 74)* 17 versus 15.9 months (p = 0.18) *First line (n = 63)* 17.6 versus 15.6 months (p = 0.07) *Liver only disease (n = 22)* 14.2 versus 15.6 months HR 0.54 (CI 0.20–1.44)
van Hazel [38] FU/LV + SIRT versus FU/LV 21 patients, previously untreated	*All patients (n = 21)* 73 versus 0% (p = 0.001) *Liver only disease (n = 15)* 78 versus 0% (p = 0.007)	*All patients (n = 21)* 0 versus 0%	*All patients (n = 21)* 11.5 versus 4.6 months HR 0.23 (CI 0.08–0.68) *Liver only disease (n = 15)* 19.1 versus 4.9 months HR 0.23 (CI 0.06–0.96)	*All patients (n = 21)* 29.4 versus 11.8 months HR 0.22 (CI 0.07–0.74) *Liver only disease (n = 15)* 31.9 versus 13.8 months HR 0.24 (CI 0.06–0.99)
Hendlisz [34] 5FU infusion + SIRT versus 5FU infusion 44 patients, refractory to chemotherapy, liver only disease	*All patients (n = 44)* 10 versus 0% (p = 0.22)	*All patients (n = 44)* 0 versus 4.7% (1 patient)	*All patients (n = 44)* 4.5 versus 2.1 months (p = 0.03)	*All patients (n = 44)* 10.0 versus 7.3 months (p = 0.80)
van Hazel [40] mFOLFOX6 + SIRT versus mFOLFOX6 530 patients, previously untreated, liver dominant disease	*All patients (n = 530)* 76.4 versus 68.1% (p = 0.113) *Liver specific response* 78.7 versus 68.8% (p = 0.042)	*All patients (n = 530)* 14.2 versus 13.7% (p = 0.86)	*All patients (n = 530)* 10.7 versus 10.2 months HR 0.93; (CI 0.77–1.12) *Liver only disease (n = 318)* Not published HR 0.9 (0.70–1.15)	Not published
Wasan [41] mFOLFOX6 ± bev + SIRT versus mFOLFOX6 ± bev 1103 patients from three trials, previously untreated, liver dominant disease	*All patients (n = 1103)* 72.4 versus 62.8% (p = 0.0012) *Liver specific response* Not available	*All patients (n = 530)* 17 versus 16% (p = 0.67)	*All patients (n = 1103)* 11.0 v 10.3 months HR 0.90; (CI 0.79–1.02) *No extrahepatic disease (n = 713)* Not reported	*All patients (n = 1103)* 22.6 versus 23.3 months HR 1.04; (CI, 0.90–1.19) *No extrahepatic disease (n = 713)* 24.5 versus 24.6 months HR 1.00; (CI 0.85–1.19)

Table 1. Outcomes of randomized trials in SIRT.

chemotherapy alone (13 versus 4 events), including nausea, abdominal pain, radiation hepatitis and hematological abnormalities. In the combination group, there was one death due to neutropenic sepsis, one liver abscess and one episode of radiation induced cirrhosis in a group of only 11 patients. In the much larger and more recent trial population of SIRFLOX, FOXFIRE and FOXFIRE-Global [41], there also was an increase in grade 3/4 adverse effects with the addition of SIRT (74 versus 66.5%) including neutropenia (36.7 versus 24.2%), febrile neutropenia (6.5 versus 2.8%), thrombocytopenia (7.7 versus 1.2%), fatigue (8.5 versus 4.9%) and abdominal pain (6.1 versus 2.3%). Only 0.8% of SIRT patients developed radiation hepatitis. Adverse events leading to treatment discontinuation were higher in the SIRT group in FOXFIRE population (14 versus 8%) with data not fully available for the other two trials. There were eight treatment related deaths in FOLFOX + SIRT group and three treatment related deaths in FOLFOX alone group. Of the eight deaths in the SIRT group, three were due to radiation induced liver disease, two due to complications from surgery, one due to liver failure, one due to radiation pneumonitis and one due to off-target delivery of microspheres. Long-term toxicity data showed two deaths due to hepatic failure after the end of the main safety window. Any potential use of SIRT in the first-line setting where overall survival is often over 2 years, would require close monitoring for long-term toxicity that may not be well described in trials.

Perhaps surprisingly by contrast, there was no significant increase in toxicity in the randomized controlled trial conducted in the chemotherapy refractory setting, albeit with a very small patient population [34]. There was one reported grade 3 event in SIRT + chemotherapy group compared to 6 in chemotherapy alone. Grade 1–2 nausea was more common in the combination group (5 events versus 0). Addition of SIRT to HAI also was not shown to have higher grade 3 or 4 events compared to HAI alone in the trial by Gray et al. [27], with a slight increase in grade 1–2 nausea and diarrhea.

Given the palliative nature of these treatments, quality of life is an important consideration when assessing the utility of SIRT. Despite this, there is a relatively limited amount of data on SIRT's impact on quality of life. The most recent analysis by Wasan et al. [41] incorporated quality of life analysis into their study using a EuroQol-5D three level questionnaire to measure health in five dimensions and summarized as utility score between 0 (death) and 1 (full health). This was done at baseline, 2–3 months, 6 months and 12 months followed by annually. The average unadjusted utility scores were not significantly different between treatment groups at any time except at 2–3 months (0.828 in SIRT + chemotherapy versus 0.846 in chemotherapy alone), although this was by a magnitude that would not be considered clinically meaningful. Lack of analysis during the first six weeks of treatment, the period where SIRT was administered, may have potentially missed a period of time where quality of life suffered due to the invasive nature of the procedure. Van Hazel et al. [38] used a Functional Living Index-Cancer questionnaire which found no change from baseline but did not report the impact of treatment.

In the refractory setting, Cosimelli et al. collected quality of life data, however only 28% of patients completed questionnaires with potentially biased results [30]. Further trials did not report quality of life data [34, 35], an unfortunate omission in a chemotherapy refractory population in whom any measurement of treatment effectiveness should include quality of life.

2.3. Summary

The lack of definite PFS and OS benefit and lack of increased hepatic resection rates, as well as increased toxicity and no improvement on quality of life, suggests there is no strong evidence to recommend SIRT's routine use with chemotherapy in the first-line setting in those with unresectable CRLM. Particular subgroups of patients who may be predisposed to resistance to chemotherapy (right sided tumors, BRAF mutant) need further trials exploring any potential benefits specific to them. SIRT has activity and improves PFS in the chemotherapy refractory setting with tolerable toxicity in small trials, although its impact on quality of life is unknown and has no proven benefit on overall survival. The potential benefit of SIRT needs to be weighed against the invasive nature, costs and risks of toxicity of the procedure, with assessment for treatment based on individual patient factors.

3. Radiofrequency ablation

Over the recent years, RFA has become a widely accepted liver-directed option for the treatment of hepatocellular carcinomas (HCC) and liver metastases, especially from colorectal cancers. Unlike other liver-targeted modalities for unresectable colorectal liver metastases, such as SIRT or TACE, RFA can be used with curative intent [50, 51].

A high-frequency alternating electric current is delivered through metal probes which are conveniently inserted into the target lesion. These needle electrodes can be placed percutaneously using imaging guidance, via laparoscopy or during abdominal laparotomy. When this electrical current is applied, heat is generated (with temperatures ranging from 60–100°C), which causes localized coagulative necrosis and protein denaturation within the tumor along with a margin of healthy tissue [52, 53].

3.1. Efficacy

In current clinical practice, RFA is being used as an alternative to liver resection in patients ineligible for surgery due to comorbidities or poor performance status or for those colorectal cancer patients with unresectable liver metastases. For patients with cirrhosis, poor liver reserve or chemotherapy-associated steatohepatitis or for those with recurrences posthepatectomy with minimal hepatic reserve, RFA may also be beneficial since it minimizes the destruction of the surrounding healthy hepatic tissue [54]. However, all of these theoretical indications are conditioned by the fact that liver metastases have to be limited in number (usually less than 5) and size (generally no more than 5 cm) [55]. Although there are no randomized clinical trials data demonstrating survival equivalence between hepatectomy and RFA for colorectal cancer liver metastases, some retrospective studies have shown that RFA may provide similar outcomes to those of liver surgery when the lesions are completely ablated and clear margins are achieved [56–58]. However there is no consensus on this with other authors suggesting alternate views [59–61]. Therefore prospective trials comparing RFA and liver surgery are necessary to definitively answer this question [62, 63].

Among several cohort studies looking at RFA as primary treatment for liver metastases, the 5-year survival and local tumor recurrence rates reported vary widely, mainly due to variable patient selection, imbalance in the baseline patients' characteristics and different techniques and probes used over time. The 5-year survival reported in the literature ranges from 15–50% after RFA for liver-only metastatic colorectal cancers [55, 63–66]. As mentioned, the local recurrence rates reported also vary widely (2–40%), although there is the suggestion from these studies that the smaller the treated lesion is (<3 cm) and the longer the distance from major vessels, the better the outcome [55, 57, 67].

In order to select the most suitable liver-only metastatic colorectal cancer patients for RFA, as well as systemic chemotherapy, to attempt to achieve long-term disease control, Stang et al. proposed a score based on four clinical variables: response to systemic therapy, ≤3 liver metastases, ≤3 cm in size and low carcinoembryonic antigen (CEA) value [68]. In this retrospective study, patients who fulfilled all four criteria (score 4) had significantly higher probabilities for overall survival and recurrence-free survival at 5 years after RFA (39 and 22%, respectively) compared to those patients who scored ≤3 (0–27 and 0–9%, respectively). As discussed by the authors in the paper, the clinical significance of this proposed score needs to be validated in a prospective manner.

Evrard et al. investigated in a phase II prospective study (EORTC 40004) whether the use of intraoperative RFA in conjunction with hepatic resection could increase the cure rate in colorectal cancer patients with unresectable liver metastases [69]. Fifty-two patients were included in the analysis. The primary endpoint was complete hepatic response at 3 months which was reached in a total of 39 patients. The 5-year overall survival rate was 43%. Karanicolas et al. reached the same conclusion in their study that combining liver resection and ablation may increase the cure for selected patients with bilateral hepatic colorectal metastases [70]. A total of 141 patients were treated with bilateral resection and 95 underwent ablation in this study. Long-term outcome was not significantly different between groups (5-year overall survival rate with ablation was 56% versus resection: 49%; p = 0.16).

Another interesting study was conducted by Ruers et al., which prospectively evaluated long-term outcomes of combining RFA plus chemotherapy versus chemotherapy alone. This study was originally designed as a randomized phase III study to detect a difference in survival between both arms; however, due to slow recruitment, the study was downsized to a randomized phase II trial with 10 year overall survival results reported in 2015 [44, 71]. The *EORTC-NCRI-CCSG-ALM Intergroup 40,004 (CLOCC) study* included 119 patients randomized to either chemotherapy alone (n = 59) or RFA plus chemotherapy (n = 60). At a median follow-up of 9.7 years, the median progression-free survival was 16.8 months for the combined arm compared with 9.9 months for the chemotherapy-only arm (hazard ratio [HR] = 0.57; 95% confidence interval [CI], 0.38–0.85; p = 0.005). The median overall survival was 45.6 months for the combined arm compared with 40.54 months for the chemotherapy arm (HR = 0.58; 95% CI, 0.38–0.88; p = 0.010). These results suggest that combining RFA with chemotherapy for unresectable liver metastases in colorectal cancer patients can considerably change the outcome for some patients, improving overall survival. However, these results require careful interpretation and indeed, have been questioned on the basis of the imbalance of patient characteristics between treatment arms, as well as the fact that some of the ablated patients included in the study underwent further liver resection following RFA.

3.2. Toxicity and quality of life

RFA is a minimally invasive liver-targeted modality with a favorable safety profile with low rate of major complications and deaths (around 1–3 and <1%, respectively) [56, 59, 67]. Information regarding tolerability and quality of life is scarce given the retrospective nature of the vast majority of evidence around RFA for liver-only metastatic colorectal cancers. Solbiati et al., for instance, reported major adverse events incidence in 1.3% of the patients (one bowel perforation and one intrahepatic hematoma) although no deaths occurred [72]. Minor adverse event rate was 10% and fever was the most common complication reported (8 of a total of 156 patients). On the other hand, Ruers included in his study health-related quality of life questionnaires (EORTC QLQ-C30) at baseline and every 6 weeks afterwards. Quality of life after RFA showed only a short decline with recovery to baseline levels within 2 months after RFA [44].

3.3. Summary

RFA is a reasonable option for metastatic colorectal cancer patients with unresectable liver metastases or for those with recurrent disease after hepatectomy with small liver metastases providing that adequate margins are thought to be achievable. Given the lack of randomized controlled trial data, liver resection remains the standard treatment for the local treatment of resectable liver metastases. More prospective clinical trials looking at RFA in different settings (for example, RFA + resection, RFA + adjuvant systemic chemotherapy, etc.) are needed.

4. Trans-arterial chemo-embolization

TACE is a locoregional therapy, which uses hepatic artery catheterization to deliver chemo-therapy locally followed by embolization with vessel occlusion, delivering high doses of che-motherapy to the target lesion. Combinations of doxorubicin, mitomycin-C and cisplatin are most commonly used as the chemotherapeutic agents in what is known as conventional TACE (cTACE) [73]. For a number of years, TACE has been used in the treatment of unresectable hepatocellular carcinoma (HCC) and is now the standard of care for particular subgroups of HCC after showing survival benefit over best supportive care [74, 75].

4.1. Conventional TACE (cTACE)

In the setting of metastatic colorectal cancer with liver metastases, the use of cTACE has been limited by a paucity of standardized data, with evidence limited to heterogenous single arm trials, to the extent that consensus guidelines are unable to provide recommendation for its use [50]. Initial non-randomized, single arm trials in the 1990s using cTACE in first and second line of treatment showed modest response rates of 17–25% [76, 77]. Two more recent trials have examined the effectiveness of cTACE across multiple lines of therapy. Vogl et al. administered repeated cycles of cTACE to 463 patients with unresectable liver metastases not responding to chemotherapy [78]. Response rate was 14.7% with stable disease rate of 48.2% and 12 month survival of 62%. Retrospective analysis of cTACE in patients refractory to 1st–5th line chemotherapy by Albert et al., showed only a 2% response rate and 43% disease stability rate with a 9 month median overall survival from the time of cTACE [79]. The lack of control arms in these trials significantly limits any interpretation of the efficacy of cTACE and its possible role among multiple other locoregional and systemic therapies in colorectal cancer.

Furthermore, toxicity is a significant issue in those undergoing cTACE. Post-embolization syndrome (PES) due to ischaemia induced inflammation occurs in 30–80% of patients with symptoms including abdominal pain, fever, nausea and vomiting and deranged liver function tests [47, 80]. Other complications can include liver abscess, pancreatitis and biliary sclerosis [77, 81].

The lack of evidence showing response or survival rates comparable or superior to current standard treatments, in addition to the toxicity of PES and other complications, leaves cTACE without a clear role in treating colorectal cancer liver metastases.

4.2. Drug-eluting bead TACE (DEB-TACE)

More recent developments have focused on TACE with the use of drug eluting polyvinyl alcohol beads (DEB-TACE), which allow a sustained release of chemotherapy agents, in particular irinotecan, to the vascular supply of the tumor. Embolization with these beads reduces flow in vessels feeding the tumor, hence increasing dwell time and reducing washout of the active drug [82]. Despite a similar toxicity profile to cTACE, DEB-TACE appears to have fewer drug-related adverse events.

Single arm phase 2 trials showed promising results with response rates between 48 and 75% and downstaging of liver metastases to allow surgical resection or ablation in 7–20% [83, 84].

A small phase 3 trial from Fiorentini et al. has been the only randomized, controlled trial to show a survival benefit from TACE in metastatic colorectal cancer [85]. This study enrolled 74 patients with liver limited disease occupying <50% of parenchyma, having progressed on at least 2 lines of therapy. They were randomized to receive two treatments of TACE with drug eluting beads containing irinotecan (DEBIRI) or FOLFIRI systemic chemotherapy for 4 months. No cross-over was allowed. Primary end point of overall survival was found to be significantly increased in the DEBIRI group compared to FOLFIRI group (median OS 22 versus 15 months, p = 0.031). Overall response rates were 69 versus 20%. PFS was also significantly increased in DEBIRI group (7 versus 4 months). Interestingly time to extra-hepatic progression was higher in DEBIRI group (13 versus 9 months) although this did not reach statistical significance, potentially suggesting some activity outside of the liver. Poor prognostic indicators for survival included high percentage of liver involvement, low albumin, high ALP and high LDH. As expected, hematological toxicity and mucositis were higher in the FOLFIRI group, with LFT and bilirubin derangement higher in DEBIRI group and PES occurring in approximately 30% of patients. Quality of life analysis showed significantly higher scores at both 1 and 3 months in those receiving DEBIRI.

Another randomized, controlled phase 2 trial by Martin et al. investigated the use of DEBIRI in combination with chemotherapy in the first-line setting [86]. Seventy patients with liver dominant disease and no prior chemotherapy were randomized to FOLFOX ± bevacizumab + DEBIRI versus FOLFOX ± bevacizumab alone. There were some imbalances in treatment groups with DEBIRI combination arm having a higher proportion of patients ECOG 1–2 and a higher proportion of patients with extra-hepatic disease. Response rate was higher in the DEBIRI combination group compared to chemotherapy alone with 4 month response rate 95 versus 70%. Downstaging of liver metastases to resection occurred in 35% in DEBIRI combination arm versus 16% in chemotherapy alone. Despite the improved response and resection rate in DEBIRI group, it was the chemotherapy alone control arm which showed a trend toward improvement in PFS with median PFS 12 months in DEBIRI arm versus 15 months in control arm (p = 0.18). There was significantly higher serious adverse event rate in the DEBIRI combination group. Overall survival data was not published.

4.3. Summary

Both trials show promising results, particularly in Fiorentini's trial in the refractory setting, given the overall survival advantage occurred without any crossover of groups and with similar rates of post-progression chemotherapy [85]. Quality of life improvement was also an important endpoint. The first-line trial from Martin et al., was unable to show a significant PFS benefit with overall survival data not yet known [86].

This would suggest that the role of DEB TACE is more likely to be in later lines of therapy based on current evidence. Replication of these results in a larger population, with control arms using more active chemotherapy regimens including bevacizumab or EGFR inhibitors, is required to better define the role of DEB-TACE in the sequence of treatments for CRLM. This is already underway with a recent publication of a prospective single arm trial treating patients with DEBIRI and cetuximab concurrently with encouraging median PFS and OS data (9.8 months and 24 months) [87].

5. Hepatic artery infusion chemotherapy

Liver metastases from colorectal cancer generally receive the majority of their blood supply through the hepatic artery, while conversely, the portal vein supplies irrigation to the normal hepatic tissue. Taking advantage of this dual hepatic blood supply, HAI was developed with the aim of delivering high chemotherapy concentrations within hepatic metastases, while minimizing systemic toxicity [88, 89]. HAI can be administered either through a surgically implanted port or via percutaneous catheter connected to a pump. Multiple agents have been tested to be infused via hepatic artery, although Floxuridine (FUDR) is the most widely used drug, thanks to its short half-life and high first-pass metabolism rate which allow the intrametastatic drug concentrations to be increased without significant systemic side effects [88]. On that basis, HAI has been investigated as a treatment for heavily treated metastatic colorectal cancer with liver metastases, as well as in the perioperative liver resection setting [90, 91]. In the following paragraphs, we will review the evidence for HAI in these different categories.

5.1. Unresectable liver metastases

In the literature, three meta-analyses [92–94] have undertaken comparisons of FUDR or 5-FU HAI versus systemic chemotherapy for the treatment of unresectable colorectal liver metastases. Their results have been contradictory. In all three, the response rate has universally reported to be in favor of the loco-regional modality comparing to (currently obsolete) systemic chemotherapy regimens. Moreover, while the two earlier meta-analyses [93, 94] detected a survival advantage for HAI, the more recent one by Mocellin et al. failed to demonstrate statistical survival superiority (15.9 versus 12.4 months, HR = 0.90, p = 0.24) [92]. However, these results should be interpreted with caution due to limitations in the studies' designs, the use of old-fashioned chemotherapy regimens and selection bias.

Since these initial studies of HAI-FUDR/5-FU alone were reported, other treatment strategies combining HAI and modern systemic chemotherapy have been tested in order to improve long-term outcomes for patients with liver metastases in different settings. Along with the improvement in systemic chemotherapy, HAI in combination with systemic chemotherapy agents has been tested with some success in single-arm single institutional trials [95, 96]. In the refractory setting for instance, Fazio et al. recruited 45 heavily treated colorectal cancer patients with liver-only or liver-dominant metastases who were then exposed to HIA with 5-FU, cisplatin and mitomycin C using a temporary subclavian catheter [97]. Of the 44 patients evaluable, 68% showed response to treatment (35% had a partial response and 33% stable disease). However, this strategy was not exempt from serious complications: grades 3–4 neutropenia and thrombocytopenia were reported in 22 and 15% of patients, respectively, and 20% of the patients developed gastro-duodenal ulcers. Also in the pretreated setting, Boige et al. conducted a retrospective study using HAI-oxaliplatin plus systemic 5-FU/ leucovorin (LV) in 44 patients after failure of prior systemic chemotherapy [98]. The authors reported an impressive median overall survival and progression-free survival of 16 and 7 months, respectively. Toxicity included grade 3–4 neutropenia (43%), grade 2–3 neuropathy (43%), and grade 3–4 abdominal pain (14%). Neyns et al. explored the combination of HAI and systemic cetuximab for the treatment of colorectal cancer patients with liver metastases who failed at least one line of treatment [99]. Although theirs' was a very small early study (only eight patients included), it showed that this combination may warrant further investigation.

HAI has also been investigated in patients with *a priori* unresectable liver metastases. One of the first randomized studies comparing HAI plus systemic bolus 5-FU/LV (n = 40) versus HAI alone (n = 36) for patients with non-resectable liver metastases demonstrated an increase in survival in the combined group (20 versus 14 months, p = 0.0033), although no significant increase in response rate was seen [100]. With the introduction of better systemic chemotherapy, such as oxaliplatin- or irinotecan-based regimens associated with HAI, the liver metastases conversion rates seem to improve. There are several examples in the literature of prospective (although small) trials combining HAI and systemic oxaliplatin- or irinotecan-based chemotherapy showing encouraging conversion rates of approximately 25–50% [98, 101–103]. Kemeny et al., for instance, achieved a liver metastases conversion rate of 47% (and noted an even higher percentage, 57%, in chemotherapy-naïve patients) in metastatic colorectal cancer patients treated with HAI-FUDR plus systemic oxaliplatin and irinotecan [104]. Ninety-two percent of the total 49 patients had either complete (8%) or partial response (84%) leading to a median overall survival from the commencement of HAI therapy of 50.8 and 35 months for chemotherapy-naïve and previously treated patients, respectively. Ammori et al. also shared their 10-year experience at the Memorial Sloan-Kettering Cancer Center using HAI and systemic chemotherapy for treating unresectable colorectal liver metastases, focusing on conversion to complete hepatic resection (noted ablation was also permitted) [105]. A total of 373 patients were retrospectively analyzed; 93 of them (25%) subsequently underwent complete liver resection/ablation. Median overall survival for the patients who converted to complete resection was 59 months against 16 months among those who did not undergo surgery (p < 0.001).

The literature also reveals several small studies which have combined HAI with systemic chemotherapy and monoclonal antibodies in attempts to further increase the liver metastases conversion rates mentioned above. Although the results of these studies are promising, there is not enough evidence to recommend this approach in current practice. In one such case, D'Angelica et al. found that 47% of their 49 patients treated with HAI-FUDR and systemic therapy (irinotecan, bevacizumab and either oxaliplatin or 5FU/LV depending on existing baseline residual neuropathy) were able to undergo complete resection [106]. Malka et al. investigated the efficacy and tolerability of HAI-oxaliplatin and 5-FU/LV and cetuximab in patients with unresectable colorectal liver metastases in a phase II trial [107]. Approximately one-third of the patients (11 out of 36) underwent subsequently complete liver resection and/or ablation. More recently, Lévi et al. also examined the role of HAI and systemic cetuximab in unresectable liver metastases from wild-type KRAS colorectal cancer in order to increase the conversion rate of curative liver resection [108]. Almost 30% of the patients in this phase II study were able to undergo R0/R1 resection achieving median overall survival of 35.2 months and survival rate at 4 years of 37.4%.

5.2. Post resection of liver metastases

The role of postoperative HAI following complete liver resection has also been tested in several randomized clinical trials comparing adjuvant HAI plus systemic chemotherapy versus chemotherapy alone [109, 110]. A Cochrane review of seven randomized controlled trials did not show significant long-term survival benefit for HAI (either FUDR or 5-FU) and systemic chemotherapy (5-FU/LV) versus 5-FU/LV alone as an adjuvant treatment [111]. Subsequently, the addition of newer (and improved) adjuvant chemotherapy regimens, such as FOLFOX, FOLFIRI or capecitabine–oxaliplatin (CapOx) to a HAI pump has been also examined with some promising results in early phase studies. Alberts et al., in a recent phase II study, investigated the combination of alternating HAI-FUDR and systemic CapOx following hepatic resection for colorectal liver metastases [112]. These authors reported a two-year overall survival rate of 85%. Similarly in another phase I/II study, Kemeny et al. found a 2-year survival rate of 89% among their 96 colon cancer patients treated with HAI-FUDR plus systemic irinotecan following complete hepatic resection [113]. We would like to mention two retrospective comparative studies looking at the efficacy of adjuvant HAI-FUDR and systemic oxaliplatin- or irinotecan-containing-regimens versus systemic chemotherapy alone. These studies suggest that patients who received HAI had better long-term outcomes compared with those patients treated without HAI. With a median follow-up of 43 months, House et al. found a higher 5-year survival among patients treated with HAI compared to patients treated with systemic chemotherapy alone (72 versus 52%, respectively; p = 0.004) [114]. The 5-year hepatic recurrence-free survival was also improved (79 versus 55%, respectively; $p < 0.001$). More recently, Koerkamp et al. reached the same conclusions after analyzing the outcomes of 1442 patients treated with adjuvant HAI in conjunction with oxaliplatin- or irinotecan-containing-regimens following liver resection [115]. With a median follow-up of 55 months, the median overall survival was 67 months with HAI versus 47 months without HAI ($p < .001$). It is important to underline that just as in the adjuvant chemotherapy setting, not all chemotherapeutic agents and targeted therapies have shown benefit following liver resection for hepatic metastatic disease. Kemeny et al. tested the adjuvant combination of HAI plus oxaliplatin-based therapy with/without bevacizumab [116]. In terms of efficacy, in this phase II study the results were disappointing. Moreover, this strategy was also associated with an increase in biliary toxicity leading to an early termination of the trial.

Several limitations exist on the use of HAI therapy for liver metastases. These include the lack of standardized systemic chemotherapeutic regimens, the requirement of specific technical expertise, and the potential for complications related either to the catheter (estimated at about 10% of cases in experienced centers) and extrahepatic infusion (5–10%) [117, 118] or to drug-related toxicity (biliary sclerosis 5% with FUDR alone, and 10–20% in polychemotherapy and gastritis and gastroduodenal ulcers in 15–20% of the patients according to some reported studies) [119, 120].

5.3. Summary

In summary, although there are prospective single arm studies showing promising results with the combination of HAI and systemic chemotherapy in both postoperative treatment after liver resection and conversion therapy for liver metastases, randomized phase III trials are needed before HAI can feasibly become standard practice in the treatment of colorectal liver metastases. At present, HAI therapy should only be considered as an option for rigorously selected patients and only under the care of physicians and institutions with extensive experience using this technique.

6. Conclusion

All treatment modalities have shown activity in different lines of treatment in CRLM. Consistent across all treatments is the heterogenous nature of trials and the relative lack of randomized, controlled trials with control arms which reflect current standard of care. SIRT and DEB-TACE currently only have evidence that would support their use in patients with progression after systemic therapy, with no survival benefit seen in first-line trials. RFA has shown evidence of survival benefit in one RCT, however this has been criticized for imbalances in treatment groups potentially confounding results. HAI has shown evidence of high response rates and conversion of liver metastases to resection, however it lacks comparison to highly active triplet chemotherapy which is current standard of care in this setting. All modalities are also lacking in data on their effects on quality of life, which should always remain a consideration in a mostly palliative population with not insignificant rates of serious toxicities observed for all of these treatments. While further trials are developed to fill these gaps in knowledge, the use of local therapies needs to continue to be assessed on a case by case basis, weighing up potential efficacy with costs, toxicity and quality of life of the patient.

Author details

Mark McGregor[1], Gonzalo Tapia Rico[2], Amanda Townsend[2,3] and Tim Price[2,3]*

*Address all correspondence to: timothy.price@sa.gov.au

1 Adelaide Oncology and Haematology, North Adelaide, Australia

2 Medical Oncology, The Queen Elizabeth Hospital, Adelaide, Australia

3 University of Adelaide, Adelaide, Australia

References

[1] World Health Organization International Agency for Research on Cancer. GLOBOCAN 2012: Estimated Cancer Incidence, Mortality and Prevalence Worldwide in 2012. [Updated: 2017]. Available from: http://globocan.iarc.fr/Pages/fact_sheets_population. aspx [Accessed: Aug 25, 2017]

[2] National Cancer Institute Surveillance, Epidemiology and End Results Program. Cancer Stat Facts: Colon and Rectum Cancer [Internet]. 2017. Available from: https://seer.cancer. gov/statfacts/html/colorect.html [Accessed: Aug 25, 2017]

[3] Cancer Research UK. Bowel Cancer Incidence Statistics [Internet]. Feb 15, 2017. Available from: http://www.cancerresearchuk.org/health-professional/cancer-statistics/statistics-by-cancer-type/bowel-cancer/incidence [Accessed: Aug 25, 2017]

[4] Heinemann V, von Weikersthal LF, Decker T, et al. FOLFIRI plus cetuximab versus FOLFIRI plus bevacizumab as first-line treatment for patients with metastatic colorectal cancer (FIRE-3): A randomised, open-label, phase 3 trial. Lancet Oncology. 2014;**15**(10):1065-1075. DOI: 10.1016/S1470-2045(14)70330-4

[5] Van Cutsem E, Nordlinger B, Adam R, et al. Towards a pan-European consensus on the treatment of patients with colorectal liver metastases. European Journal of Cancer. 2006;**42**(14):2212-2221. DOI: 10.1016/j.ejca.2006.04.012

[6] Helling TS, Martin M. Cause of death from liver metastases in colorectal cancer. Annals of Surgical Oncology. 2014;**21**(2):501-506. DOI: 10.1245/s10434-013-3297-7

[7] Padman S, Padbury R, Beeke C, et al. Liver only metastatic disease in patients with metastatic colorectal cancer: Impact of surgery and chemotherapy. Acta Oncologica. 2013;**52**(8):1699-1706. DOI: 10.3109/0284186X.2013.831473

[8] Morris EJ, Forman D, Thomas JD, et al. Surgical management and outcomes of colorectal cancer liver metastases. British Journal of Surgery. 2010;**97**(7):1110-1118. DOI: 10.1002/bjs.7032

[9] Kanas GP, Taylor A, Primrose JN, et al. Survival after liver resection in metastatic colorectal cancer: Review and meta-analysis of prognostic factors. Clinical Epidemiology. 2012;**4**(1):283-301. DOI: 10.2147/CLEP.S34285

[10] Delaunoit T, Alberts SR, Sargent DJ, et al. Chemotherapy permits resection of metastatic colorectal cancer: Experience from intergroup N9741. Annals of Oncology. 2005;**16**(3): 425-429. DOI: 10.1093/annonc/mdi092

[11] Jones RP, Poston GJ. Resection of liver metastases in colorectal cancer in the era of expanding systemic therapy. Annual Review of Medicine. 2017;**68**:183-196. DOI: 10.1146/annurev-med-062415-093510

[12] Grothey A, Sargent D, Goldberg RM, Schmoll H-J. Survival of patients with advanced colorectal cancer improves with the availability of fluorouracil-leucovorin, irinotecan and oxaliplatin in the course of treatment. Journal of Clinical Oncology. 2004;**22**(7):1209-1214. DOI: 10.1200/JCO.2004.11.037

[13] Tournigand C, Andre T, Achille E, et al. FOLFIRI followed by FOLFOX6 or the reverse sequence in advanced colorectal cancer: A randomized GERCOR study. Journal of Clinical Oncology. 2004;**22**(2):229-237. DOI: 10.1200/JCO.2004.05.113

[14] Saltz LB, Clarke S, Diaz-Rubio E, et al. Bevacizumab in combination with oxaliplatin-based chemotherapy as first-line therapy in metastatic colorectal cancer: A randomized phase III study. Journal of Clinical Oncology. 2008;**26**(12):2013-2019. DOI: 10.1200/JCO.2007.14.9930

[15] Arnold D, Lueza B, Douillard J-Y, et al. Prognostic and predictive value of primary tumour side in patients with RAS wild-type metastatic colorectal cancer treated with chemotherapy and EGFR directed antibodies in six randomized trials. Annals of Oncology. 2017;**28**(8):1713-1729. DOI: 10.1093/annonc/mdx175

[16] Adam R, Delvart V, Pascal G, et al. Rescue surgery for unresectable colorectal liver metastases downstaged by chemotherapy: A model to predict long-term survival. Annals of Surgery. 2004;**240**(4):644-658. DOI: 10.1097/01.sla.0000141198.92114.16

[17] Adam R, Wicherts DA, de Haas RJ, et al. Patients with initially unresectable colorectal liver metastases: Is there a possibility of cure? Journal of Clinical Oncology. 2009;**27**(11):1829-1835. DOI: 10.1200/JCO.2008.19.9273

[18] Pozzo C, Basso M, Cassano M, et al. Neoadjuvant treatment of unresectable liver disease with irinotecan and 5-fluorouracil plus folinic acid in colorectal cancer patients. Annals of Oncology. 2004;**15**(6):933-939. DOI: 10.1093/annonc/mdh217

[19] Alberts SR, Horvath WL, Sternfeld WC, et al. Oxaliplatin, fluouracil and leucovorin for patients with unresectable liver only metastases from colorectal cancer: A north central

cancer treatment group phase II study. Journal of Clinical Oncology. 2005;23(36):9243-9249. DOI: 10.1200/JCO.2005.07.740

[20] Emami B, Lyman J, Brown A, et al. Tolerance of normal tissue to therapeutic irradiation. International Journal of Radiation, Biology, Physics. 1991;21(1):102-122. DOI: 10.1016/0360-3016(91)90171-Y

[21] Gray BN, Buron MA, Kelleher D, et al. Tolerance of the liver to the effects of Yttrium-90 radiation. International Journal of Radiation Oncology, Biology, Physics. 1990;18(3):619-623. DOI: 10.1016/0360-3016(90)90069-V

[22] Welch JS, Kennedy AS, Thomadsen B, et al. Selective internal radiation therapy for liver metastases secondary to colorectal adenocarcinoma. International Journal of Radiation Oncology, Biology, Physics. 2006;66(2):S62-S73. DOI: 10.1016/j.ijrobp.2005.09.011

[23] Campbell AM, Bailey IH, Burton MA. Analysis of the distribution of intra-arterial microspheres in human liver following hepatic yttrium-90 microsphere therapy. Physics in Medicine & Biology. 2000;45(4):1023-1033. DOI: 10.1088/0031-9155/45/4/316

[24] Salem R, Thurston KG. Radioemoblization with 90 yttrium microspheres: A state-of-the-art brachytherapy treatment for primary and secondary liver malignancies. Journal of Vascular & Interventional Radiology. 2006;17(8):1251-1278. DOI: 10.1097/01.RVI.0000233785.75257.9A

[25] Gulec SA, Fong Y, et al. Yttrium 90 microsphere selective internal radiation treatment of hepatic colorectal metastases. Archives of Surgery. 2007;142(7):675-682. DOI: 10.1001/archsurg.142.7.675

[26] Gianmarile F, Bodei L, Chiesa C, et al. EANM procedure guideline for the treatment of liver cancer and liver metastases with intra-arterial radioactive compounds. European Journal of Nuclear Medicine and Molecular Imaging. 2011;38(7):1393-1406. DOI: 10.1007/s00259-011-1812-2

[27] Gray B, Van Hazel G, Hope M, et al. Randomised trial of SIR-spheres plus chemotherapy vs. chemotherapy alone for treating patients with liver metastases from primary large bowel cancer. Annals of Oncology. 2001;12(12):1711-1720. DOI: 10.1023/A:1013569329846

[28] Kennedy A, Douglas C, Nutting C, et al. Resin 90Y-microsphere brachytherapy for unresectable colorectal liver metastases: Modern USA experience. International Journal of Radiation Oncology, Biology, Physics. 2007;65(2):412-425. DOI: 10.1016/j.ijrobp.2005.12.051

[29] Mulcahy M, Lewandowski R, Ibrahim S, et al. Radioembolisation of colorectal hepatic metastases using yttrium-90 microspheres. Cancer. 2009;115(9):1849-1858. DOI: 10.1002/cncr.24224

[30] Cosimelli M, Golfieri R, Cagol PP, et al. Multicentre phase II clinical trial of yttrium-90 resin microshperes alone in unresectable, chemotherapy refractory colorectal liver metastases. British Journal of Cancer. 2010;103(3):324-331. DOI: 10.1038/sj.bjc.6605770

[31] Jakobs TF, Hoffmann R-T, Dehm K, et al. Hepatic yttrium-90 radioembolization of che-
      motherapy refractory colorectal cancer liver metastases. Journal of Vascular & Inter-
      ventional Radiology. 2008;19(8):1187-1195. DOI: 10.1016/j.jvir.2008.05.013

[32] Lim L, Gibbs P, Yip D, Shapiro J, et al. Prospective study of treatment with selective
      internal radiation therapy spheres in patients with unresectable primary or second-
      ary hepatic malignancies. Internal Medicine Journal. 2005;35(4):222-227. DOI: 10.1111/j.
      1445-5994.2005.00789.x

[33] Chua T, Bester L, Saxena A, et al. Radioembolization and systemic chemotherapy
      improves response and survival for unresectable colorectal liver metastases. Journal
      of Cancer Research and Clinical Oncology. 2011;137(5):865-873. DOI: 10.1007/s00432-
      010-0948-y

[34] Hendlisz A, Van den Eynde M, Peeters M, et al. Phase III trial comparing protracted
      intravenous fluorouracil infusion alone or with yttrium-90 resin microspheres radioem-
      bolisation for liver-limited metastatic colorectal cancer refractory to standard chemother-
      apy. Journal of Clinical Oncology. 2010;28(23):3687-3694. DOI: 10.1200/JCO.2010.28.5643

[35] Saxena A, Bester L, Shan L, et al. A systematic review on the safety and efficacy of
      yttrium-90 radioembolization for unresectable, chemorefractory colorectal cancer liver
      metastases. Journal of Cancer Research in Clinical Oncolofgy. 2014;140(4):537-547. DOI:
      10.1007/s00432-013-1564-4

[36] Grothey A, Van Cutsem E, Sobrero A, et al. Regorafenib monotherapy for previously
      treated metastatic colorectal cancer (CORRECT): An international, multicentre, ran-
      domised, placebo-controlled, phase 3 trial. Lancet. 2013;381(9863):303-312. DOI: 10.1016/
      S0140-6736(12)61900-X

[37] Yoshino T, Mizunuma N, Yamazaki K, et al. TAS-102 monotherapy for pretreated meta-
      static colorectal cancer: A double-blind, randomised, placebo-controlled phase 2 trial.
      Lancet Oncology. 2012;13(10):993-1001. DOI: 10.1016/S1470-2045(12)70345-5

[38] Van Hazel G, Blackwell A, Anderson J, et al. Randomised phase 2 trial of SIR-spheres
      plus fluorouracil/leucovorin chemotherapy versus fluorouracil/leucovorin chemother-
      apy alone in advanced colorectal cancer. Journal of Surgical Oncology. 2004;88(2):78-85.
      DOI: 10.1002/jso.20141

[39] Sharma R, Van Hazel G, Morgan B, et al. Radioembolization of liver metastases from
      colorectal cancer using yttrium-90 microspheres with concomitant systemic oxalipla-
      tin, fluorouracil, and leucovorin chemotherapy. Journal of Clinical Oncology. 2007;
      25(9):1099-1106. DOI: 10.1200/JCO.2006.08.7916

[40] Van Hazel G, Heinemann V, Sharma N, et al. SIRFLOX: Randomised phase 3 trial com-
      paring first line mFOLFOX6 (plus or minus bevacizumab) versus mFOLFOX6 (plus or
      minus bevacizumab) plus selective internal radiation therapy in patients with metastatic
      colorectal cancer. Journal of Clinical Oncology. 2016;34(15):1723-1731. DOI: 10.1200/
      JCO.2015.66.1181

[41] Wasan HS, Gibbs P, Sharma NK, et al. First-line selective internal radiotherapy plus chemotherapy versus chemotherapy alone in patients with liver metastases from colorectal cancer (FOXFIRE, SIRFLOX, and FOXFIRE-global): A combined analysis of three multicentre, randomised, phase 3 trials. Lancet Oncology. 2017;**18**(9):1159-1171. DOI: 10.1016/S1470-2045(17)30457-6

[42] Khattak MA, Martin HL, Beeke C, et al. Survival differences in patients with metastatic colorectal cancer and with single site metastatic disease at initial presentation: Results from south Australian clinical registry for advanced colorectal cancer. Clinical Colorectal Cancer. 2012;**11**(4):247-254. DOI: 10.1016/j.clcc.2012.06.004

[43] Hwang M, Jayakrishnan TT, Green DE, et al. Systematic review of outcomes of patients undergoing resection for colorectal liver metastases in the setting of extra hepatic disease. European Journal of Cancer. 2014;**50**(10):1747-1757. DOI: 10.1016/j.ejca.2014.03.277

[44] Ruers T, Punt C, van Coevorden F, et al. Radiofrequency ablation (RFA) combined with chemotherapy for unresectable colorectal liver metastases (CRC LM): Long term survival results of a randomised phase II study of the EORTC-NCRI CCSG-ALM Intergroup 40004 (CLOCC). Journal of Clinical Oncology. 2015;**33**(suppl 15):3501-3501. DOI: 10.1200/jco.2015.33.15_suppl.3501

[45] Van Hazel G, Heinemann V, Sharma N, et al. Impact of primary tumour location on survival in patients with metastatic colorectal cancer receiving selective internal radiation therapy and chemotherapy as first-line therapy. Annals of Oncology. Poster presentation at ESMO congress 2017;**28**(Suppl 3). DOI: 10.1093/annonc/mdx302.005

[46] Riaz A, Lewandowski RJ, Kulik LM, et al. Complications following radioembolization with yttrium-90 microspheres: A comprehensive literature review. Journal of Vascular & Interventional Radiology. 2009;**20**(9):1121-1130. DOI: 10.1016/j.jvir.2009.05.030

[47] Xing M, Kooby DA, El-Rayes BF, et al. Locoregional therapies for metastatic colorectal carcinoma to the liver- an evidence based review. Journal of Surgical Oncology. 2014;**110**(2):182-196. DOI: 10.1002/jso.23619

[48] Lewandowski RJ, Thurston KG, Goin J, et al. 90Y microsphere (TheraSphere) treatment for unresectable colorectal cancer metastases of the liver: Response to treatment at trageted doses of 135-150Gy as measured by (18F) fluorodeoxyglucose positron emission tomography and computed tomographic imaging. Journal of Vascular & Interventional Radiology. 2005;**16**(12):1641-1651. DOI: 10.1097/01.RVI.0000179815.44868.66

[49] Cianni R, Urigo C, Notarianni E, et al. Selective internal radiation therapy with SIR spheres for the treatment of unresectable colorectal hepatic metastases. Cardiovascular & Interventional Radiology. 2009;**32**:1179-1186. DOI: 10.1007/s00270-009-9658-8

[50] Abdalla EK, Bauer TW, Chun YS, et al. Locoregional surgical and interventional therapies for advanced colorectal cancer liver metastases: Expert consensus statements. HPB Journal. 2013;**15**(2):119-130. DOI: 10.1111/j.1477-2574.2012.00597.x

[51] Clark ME, Smith RR. Liver-directed therapies in metastatic colorectal cancer. Journal of gastrointestinal oncology. 2014;5(4):374-387. DOI: 10.3978/j.issn.2078-6891.2014.064

[52] Nicholl MB, Bilchik AJ. Thermal ablation of hepatic malignancy: Useful but still not optimal. European Journal of Surgical Oncology. 2008;34(3):318-323. DOI: 10.1016/j.ejso.2007.07.203

[53] Goldberg SN, Gazelle GS, Mueller PR. Thermal ablation therapy for focal malignancy: A unified approach to underlying principles, techniques, and diagnostic imaging guidance. AJR. American Rournal of Roentgenology. 2000;174(2):323-331. DOI: 10.2214/ajr.174.2.1740323

[54] Hur H, Ko YT, Min BS, et al. Comparative study of resection and radiofrequency ablation in the treatment of solitary colorectal liver metastases. American Journal of Surgery. 2009;197(6):728-736. DOI: 10.1016/j.amjsurg.2008.04.013

[55] Kim KH, Yoon YS, Yu CS, et al. Comparative analysis of radiofrequency ablation and surgical resection for colorectal liver metastases. Journal of the Korean Surgical Society. 2011;81(1):25-34. DOI: 10.4174/jkss.2011.81.1.25

[56] Hammill CW, Billingsley KG, Cassera MA, et al. Outcome after laparoscopic radiofrequency ablation of technically resectable colorectal liver metastases. Annals of Surgical Oncology. 2011;18(7):1947-1954. DOI: 10.1245/s10434-010-1535-9

[57] Abitabile P, Hartl U, Lange J, Maurer CA. Radiofrequency ablation permits an effective treatment for colorectal liver metastasis. European Journal of Surgical Oncology. 2007;33(1):67-71. DOI: 10.1016/j.ejso.2006.10.040

[58] Weng M, Zhang Y, Zhou D, et al. Radiofrequency ablation versus resection for colorectal cancer liver metastases: A meta-analysis. PLoS One. 2012;7(9):e45493. DOI: 10.1371/journal.pone.0045493

[59] Aloia TA, Vauthey JN, Loyer EM, et al. Solitary colorectal liver metastasis: Resection determines outcome. Archives of Surgery. 2006;141(5):460-467. DOI: 10.1001/archsurg.141.5.460

[60] Reuter NP, Woodall CE, Scoggins CR, et al. Radiofrequency ablation vs. resection for hepatic colorectal metastasis: Therapeutically equivalent? Journal of Gastrointestinal Surgery. 2009;13(3):486-491. DOI: 10.1007/s11605-008-0727-0

[61] Abdalla EK, Vauthey JN, Ellis LM, et al. Recurrence and outcomes following hepatic resection, radiofrequency ablation, and combined resection/ablation for colorectal liver metastases. Annals of Surgery. 2004;239(6):818-825; discussion 825-7. DOI: 10.1097/01.sla.0000128305.90650.71

[62] Poston GJ. Radiofrequency ablation of colorectal liver metastases: Where are we really going? Journal of Clinical Oncology. 2005;23(7):1342-1344. DOI: 10.1200/JCO.2005.10.911

[63] Mulier S, Ruers T, Jamart J, et al. Radiofrequency ablation versus resection for resectable colorectal liver metastases: Time for a randomized trial? An update. Digestive Surgery. 2008;25(1):445-460. DOI: 10.1159/000184736

[64] Sucandy I, Cheek S, Golas BJ, et al. Longterm survival outcomes of patients undergoing treatment with radiofrequency ablation for hepatocellular carcinoma and metastatic colorectal cancer liver tumors. HPB. 2016;**18**(9):756-763. DOI: 10.1016/j.hpb.2016.06.010

[65] Siperstein AE, Berber E, Ballem N, Parikh RT. Survival after radiofrequency ablation of colorectal liver metastases: 10-year experience. Annals of Surgery. 2007;**246**(4):559-565; discussion 565-567. DOI: 10.1097/SLA.0b013e318155a7b6

[66] Otto G, Duber C, Hoppe-Lotichius M, et al. Radiofrequency ablation as first-line treatment in patients with early colorectal liver metastases amenable to surgery. Annals of Surgery. 2010;**251**(5):796-803. DOI: 10.1097/SLA.0b013e3181bc9fae

[67] McKay A, Fradette K, Lipschitz J. Long-term outcomes following hepatic resection and radiofrequency ablation of colorectal liver metastases. HPB Surgery. 2009;**2009**:346863. DOI: 10.1155/2009/346863

[68] Stang A, Oldhafer KJ, Weilert H, et al. Selection criteria for radiofrequency ablation for colorectal liver metastases in the era of effective systemic therapy: A clinical score based proposal. BMC Cancer. 2014;**14**:500. DOI: 10.1186/1471-2407-14-500

[69] Evrard S, Rivoire M, Arnaud J, et al. Unresectable colorectal cancer liver metastases treated by intraoperative radiofrequency ablation with or without resection. British Journal of Surgery. 2012;**99**(4):558-565. DOI: 10.1002/bjs.8724

[70] Karanicolas PJ, Jarnagin WR, Gonen M, et al. Long-term outcomes following tumor ablation for treatment of bilateral colorectal liver metastases. JAMA Surgery. 2013;**148**(7):597-601. DOI: 10.1001/jamasurg.2013.1431

[71] Ruers T, Punt C, Van Coevorden F, et al. Radiofrequency ablation combined with systemic treatment versus systemic treatment alone in patients with non-resectable colorectal liver metastases: A randomized EORTC intergroup phase II study (EORTC 40004). Annals of Oncology. 2012;**23**(10):2619-2626. DOI: 10.1093/annonc/mds053

[72] Solbiati L, Ahmed M, Cova L, et al. Small liver colorectal metastases treated with percutaneous radiofrequency ablation: Local response rate and long-term survival with up to 10-year follow-up. Radiology. 2012;**265**(3):958-968. DOI: 10.1148/radiol.12111851

[73] Solomon B, Soulen MC, Baum RA, et al. Chemoembolization of hepatocellular carcinoma with cisplatin, doxorubicin, mitomycin-C, ethiodol, and polyvinyl alcohol: Prospective evaluation of response and survival in a U.S. population. Journal of Vascular and Interventional Radiology. 1999;**10**(6):793-798. DOI: 10.1016/S1051-0443(99)70117-X

[74] Llovet JM, Real MI, Montaña X. Arterial embolization or chemoembolization versus systemic treatment in patients with unresectable hepatocellular carcinoma: A randomised controlled trial. The Lancet. 2002;**359**(9319):1734-1739. DOI: 10.1016/S0140-6736(02)08649-X

[75] Heimbach J, Kulik LM, Finn R, et al. AASLD guidelines for the treatment of hepatocellular carcinoma. Hepatology. 2017;**67**:358-380. DOI: 10.1002/hep.29086

[76] Lang EK, Brown CL. Colorectal metastases to the liver: Selective chemoembolization. Radiology. 1993;**189**(2):417-422. DOI: 10.1148/radiology.189.2.8210369

[77] Martinelli DJ, Wadler S, Bakal CW, et al. Utility of embolization or chemoembolization as second-line treatment in patients with advanced or recurrent colorectal carcinoma. Cancer. 1994;**74**(6):1706-1712. DOI: 10.1002/1097-0142(19940915)74:6<1706

[78] Vogl TJ, Gruber T, Balzer JO, et al. Repeated transarterial chemoembolization in the treatment of liver metastases of colorectal cancer: Prospective study. Radiology. 2009;**250**(1):281-289. DOI: 10.1148/radiol.2501080295

[79] Albert M, Kiefer MV, Sun W, et al. Chemoembolization of colorectal liver metastases with cisplatin, doxorubicin, mitomycin C, ethiodol, and polyvinyl alcohol. Cancer. 2011;**117**(2):343-352. DOI: 10.1002/cncr.25387

[80] Memon K, Lewandowski RJ, Riaz A, et al. Chemoembolization and radioembolization for metastatic disease to the liver: Available data and future studies. Current Treatment Options in Oncology. 2012;**13**(3):403-415. DOI: 10.1007/s11864-012-0200-x

[81] Kim HK, Chung YH, Song BC, et al. Ischemic bile duct injury as a serious complication after transarterial chemoembolization in patients with hepatocellular carcinoma. Journal of Clinical Gastroenterology. 2001;**32**(5):423-427. DOI: 10.1097/00004836-200105000-00013

[82] Taylor RR, Tang Y, Gonzalez MV, et al. Irinotecan drug eluting beads for use in che-moembolization: In vitro and in vivo evaluation of drug release properties. European Journal of Pharmaceutical Sciences. 2007;**30**(1):7-14. DOI: 10.1016/j.ejps.2006.09.002

[83] Bower M, Metzger T, Robbins K, et al. Surgical downstaging and neo-adjuvant therapy in metastatic colorectal carcinoma with irinotecan drug-eluting beads: A multi-institu-tional study. HPB Journal. 2010;**12**(1):31-36. DOI: 10.1111/j.1477-2574.2009.00117.x

[84] Martin RC, Joshi J, Robbins K, et al. Hepatic intra-arterial injection of drug-eluting bead, irinotecan (DEBIRI) in unresectable colorectal liver metastases refractory to sys-temic chemotherapy: Results of multi-institutional study. Annals of Surgical Oncology. 2011;**18**(1):192-198. DOI: 10.1245/s10434-010-1288-5

[85] Fiorentini G, Aliberti C, Tilli M, et al. Intra-arterial infusion of irinotecan-loaded drug-eluting beads (DEBIRI) versus intravenous therapy (FOLFIRI) for hepatic metastases from colorec-tal cancer: Final results of a phase III study. Anticancer Research. 2012;**32**(4):1387-1395

[86] Martin 2nd RCG, Scoggins CR, Schreeder M, et al. Randomized controlled trial of iri-notecan drug-eluting beads with simultaneous FOLFOX and bevacizumab for patients with unresectable colorectal liver-limited metastasis. Cancer 2015;**121**(20):3649-3658. DOI: 10.1002/cncr.29534

[87] Fiorentini G, Aliberti C, Sarti D, et al. Locoregional therapy and systemic cetuximab to treat colorectal liver metastases. World Journal of Gastrintestinal Oncology. 2015;**7**(6):47-54. DOI: 10.4251/wjgo.v7.i6.47

[88] Ensminger WD, Gyves JW. Clinical pharmacology of hepatic arterial chemotherapy. Seminars in Oncology. 1983;**10**(2):176-182

[89] Michels NA. Newer anatomy of the liver and its variant blood supply and collateral circula-tion. American Journal of Surgery. 1966;**112**(3):337-347. DOI: 10.1016/0002-9610(66)90201-7

[90] Zervoudakis A, Boucher T, Kemeny NE. Treatment options in colorectal liver metastases: Hepatic arterial infusion. Visceral Medicine. 2017;**33**:47-53. DOI: 10.1159/000454693

[91] Zampino MG, Magni E, Ravenda PS, et al. Treatments for colorectal liver metastases: A new focus on a familiar concept. Critical Reviews in Oncology/Hematology. 2016;**108**: 154-163. DOI: 10.1016/j.critrevonc.2016.11.005

[92] Mocellin S, Pilati P, Lise M, Nitti D. Meta-analysis of hepatic arterial infusion for unresectable liver metastases from colorectal cancer: The end of an era? Journal of Clinical Oncology. 2007;**25**(35):5649-5654. DOI: 10.1200/JCO.2007.12.1764

[93] Piedbois P, Buyse M, Kemeny N, et al. Reappraisal of hepatic arterial infusion in the treatment of nonresectable liver metastases from colorectal cancer. Journal of the National Cancer Institute. 1996;**88**(5):252-258. DOI: 10.1093/jnci/88.5.252

[94] Harmantas A, Rotstein LE, Langer B. Regional versus systemic chemotherapy in the treatment of colorectal carcinoma metastatic to the liver. Is there a survival difference? Meta-analysis of the published literature. Cancer. 1996;**78**(8):1639-1645. DOI: 10.1002/(SICI)1097-0142(19961015)78:8<1639::AID-CNCR1>3.0.CO;2-9

[95] Kemeny N, Gonen M, Sullivan D, et al. Phase I study of hepatic arterial infusion of floxuridine and dexamethasone with systemic irinotecan for unresectable hepatic metastases from colorectal cancer. Journal of Clinical Oncology. 2001;**19**(10):2687-2695. DOI: 10.1200/JCO.2001.19.10.2687

[96] Kemeny N, Jarnagin W, Paty P, et al. Phase I trial of systemic oxaliplatin combination chemotherapy with hepatic arterial infusion in patients with unresectable liver metastases from colorectal cancer. Journal of clinical Oncology. 2005;**23**(22):4888-4896. DOI: 10.1200/JCO.2005.07.100

[97] Fazio N, Orsi F, Grasso RF, et al. Hepatic intra-arterial chemotherapy using a percutaneous catheter in pretreated patients with metastatic colorectal carcinoma. Anticancer Research. 2003;**23**(6D):5023-5030

[98] Boige V, Malka D, Elias D, et al. Hepatic arterial infusion of oxaliplatin and intravenous LV5FU2 in unresectable liver metastases from colorectal cancer after systemic chemotherapy failure. Annals of Surgical Oncology. 2008;**15**(1):219-226. DOI: 10.1245/s10434-007-9581-7

[99] Neyns B, Aerts M, Van Nieuwenhove Y, et al. Cetuximab with hepatic arterial infusion of chemotherapy for the treatment of colorectal cancer liver metastases. Anticancer Research. 2008;**28**:2459-2468

[100] Fiorentini G, Cantore M, Rossi S, et al. Hepatic arterial chemotherapy in combination with systemic chemotherapy compared with hepatic arterial chemotherapy alone for liver metastases from colorectal cancer: Results of a multi-centric randomized study. In Vivo. 2006;**20**(6A):707-710

[101] Ducreux M, Ychou M, Laplanche A, et al. Hepatic arterial oxaliplatin infusion plus intravenous chemotherapy in colorectal cancer with inoperable hepatic metastases:

A trial of the gastrointestinal group of the federation nationale des centres de lutte contre le cancer. Journal of Clinical Oncology. 2005;23(22):4881-4887. DOI: 10.1200/JCO.2005.05.120

[102] Elias D, Goere D, Boige V, et al. Outcome of posthepatectomy-missing colorectal liver metastases after complete response to chemotherapy: Impact of adjuvant intra-arterial hepatic oxaliplatin. Annals of Surgical Oncology. 2007;14(11):3188-3194. DOI: 10.1245/s10434-007-9482-9

[103] Goere D, Deshaies I, de Baere T, et al. Prolonged survival of initially unresectable hepatic colorectal cancer patients treated with hepatic arterial infusion of oxaliplatin followed by radical surgery of metastases. Annals of Surgery. 2010;251(4):686-691. DOI: 10.1097/SLA.0b013e3181d35983

[104] Kemeny NE, Melendez FD, Capanu M, et al. Conversion to resectability using hepatic artery infusion plus systemic chemotherapy for the treatment of unresectable liver metastases from colorectal carcinoma. Journal of Clinical Oncology. 2009;27(21):3465-3471. DOI: 10.1200/JCO.2008.20.1301

[105] Ammori JB, Kemeny NE, Fong Y, et al. Conversion to complete resection and/or ablation using hepatic artery infusional chemotherapy in patients with unresectable liver metastases from colorectal cancer: A decade of experience at a single institution. Annals of Surgical Oncology. 2013;20(9):2901-2907. DOI: 10.1245/s10434-013-3009-3

[106] D'Angelica MI, Correa-Gallego C, Paty PB, et al. Phase II trial of hepatic artery infusional and systemic chemotherapy for patients with unresectable hepatic metastases from colorectal cancer: Conversion to resection and long-term outcomes. Annals of Surgery. 2015;261(2):353-360. DOI: 10.1097/SLA.0000000000000614

[107] Malka D, Paris E, Caramella C, et al. Hepatic arterial infusion (HAI) of oxaliplatin plus intravenous (IV) fluorouracil (FU), leucovorin (LV), and cetuximab for first-line treatment of unresectable colorectal liver metastases (CRLM) (CHOICE): A multicenter phase II study. Journal of Clinical Oncology. 2010;28(15_suppl):3558-3558. DOI: 10.1200/jco.2010.28.15_suppl.3558

[108] Levi FA, Boige V, Hebbar M, et al. Conversion to resection of liver metastases from colorectal cancer with hepatic artery infusion of combined chemotherapy and systemic cetuximab in multicenter trial OPTILIV. Annals of Oncology. 2016;27(2):267-274. DOI: 10.1093/annonc/mdv548

[109] Portier G, Elias D, Bouche O, et al. Multicenter randomized trial of adjuvant fluorouracil and folinic acid compared with surgery alone after resection of colorectal liver metastases: FFCD ACHBTH AURC 9002 trial. Journal of Clinical Oncology. 2006;24(31):4976-4982. DOI: 10.1200/JCO.2006.06.8353

[110] Parks R, Gonen M, Kemeny N, et al. Adjuvant chemotherapy improves survival after resection of hepatic colorectal metastases: Analysis of data from two continents. Journal of the American College of Surgeons. 2007;204(5):753-61; discussion 761-3. DOI: 10.1016/j.jamcollsurg.2006.12.036

[111] Nelson RL, Freels S. Hepatic artery adjuvant chemotherapy for patients having resection or ablation of colorectal cancer metastatic to the liver. Cochrane Database of Systematic Reviews (Online). 2006;(4):CD003770. DOI: 10.1002/14651858.CD003770.pub3

[112] Alberts SR, Mahoney MR, Donohue J, et al. Systemic capecitabine and oxaliplatin administered with hepatic arterial infusion (HAI) of floxuridine (FUDR) following complete resection of colorectal metastases (M-CRC) confined to the liver: A north central cancer treatment group (NCCTG) phase II intergroup trial. Journal of Clinical Oncology. 2006;24(18_Suppl):3525-3525. DOI: 10.1200/jco.2006.24.18_suppl.3525

[113] Kemeny N, Jarnagin W, Gonen M, et al. Phase I/II study of hepatic arterial therapy with floxuridine and dexamethasone in combination with intravenous irinotecan as adjuvant treatment after resection of hepatic metastases from colorectal cancer. Journal of Clinical Oncology. 2003;21(17):3303-3309. DOI: 10.1200/JCO.2003.03.142

[114] House MG, Kemeny NE, Gonen M, et al. Comparison of adjuvant systemic chemotherapy with or without hepatic arterial infusional chemotherapy after hepatic resection for metastatic colorectal cancer. Annals of Surgery. 2011;254(6):851-856. DOI: 10.1097/SLA.0b013e31822f4f88

[115] Koerkamp BG, Sadot E, Kemeny NE, et al. Perioperative hepatic arterial infusion pump chemotherapy is associated with longer survival after resection of colorectal liver metastases: A propensity score analysis. Journal of Clinical Oncology. 2017;35(17):1938-1944. DOI: 10.1200/JCO.2016.71.8346

[116] Kemeny NE, Jarnagin WR, Capanu M, et al. Randomized phase II trial of adjuvant hepatic arterial infusion and systemic chemotherapy with or without bevacizumab in patients with resected hepatic metastases from colorectal cancer. Journal of Clinical Oncology. 2011;29(7):884-889. DOI: 10.1200/JCO.2010.32.5977

[117] Kemeny N, Daly J, Oderman P, et al. Hepatic artery pump infusion: Toxicity and results in patients with metastatic colorectal carcinoma. Journal of Clinical Oncology. 1984;2(6):595-600. DOI: 10.1200/JCO.1984.2.6.595

[118] Deschamps F, Rao P, Teriitehau C, et al. Percutaneous femoral implantation of an arterial port catheter for intraarterial chemotherapy: Feasibility and predictive factors of long-term functionality. Journal of Vascular and Interventional Radiology. 2010;21(11):1681-1688. DOI: 10.1016/j.jvir.2010.08.003

[119] Kemeny MM, Battifora H, Blayney DW, et al. Sclerosing cholangitis after continuous hepatic artery infusion of FUDR. Annals of Surgery. 1985;202(2):176-181

[120] Ito K, Ito H, Kemeny NE, et al. Biliary sclerosis after hepatic arterial infusion pump chemotherapy for patients with colorectal cancer liver metastasis: Incidence, clinical features, and risk factors. Annals of Surgical Oncology. 2012;19(5):1609-1617. DOI: 10.1245/s10434-011-2102-8

Permissions

All chapters in this book were first published in CMT, by InTech Open; hereby published with permission under the Creative Commons Attribution License or equivalent. Every chapter published in this book has been scrutinized by our experts. Their significance has been extensively debated. The topics covered herein carry significant findings which will fuel the growth of the discipline. They may even be implemented as practical applications or may be referred to as a beginning point for another development.

The contributors of this book come from diverse backgrounds, making this book a truly international effort. This book will bring forth new frontiers with its revolutionizing research information and detailed analysis of the nascent developments around the world.

We would like to thank all the contributing authors for lending their expertise to make the book truly unique. They have played a crucial role in the development of this book. Without their invaluable contributions this book wouldn't have been possible. They have made vital efforts to compile up to date information on the varied aspects of this subject to make this book a valuable addition to the collection of many professionals and students.

This book was conceptualized with the vision of imparting up-to-date information and advanced data in this field. To ensure the same, a matchless editorial board was set up. Every individual on the board went through rigorous rounds of assessment to prove their worth. After which they invested a large part of their time researching and compiling the most relevant data for our readers.

The editorial board has been involved in producing this book since its inception. They have spent rigorous hours researching and exploring the diverse topics which have resulted in the successful publishing of this book. They have passed on their knowledge of decades through this book. To expedite this challenging task, the publisher supported the team at every step. A small team of assistant editors was also appointed to further simplify the editing procedure and attain best results for the readers.

Apart from the editorial board, the designing team has also invested a significant amount of their time in understanding the subject and creating the most relevant covers. They scrutinized every image to scout for the most suitable representation of the subject and create an appropriate cover for the book.

The publishing team has been an ardent support to the editorial, designing and production team. Their endless efforts to recruit the best for this project, has resulted in the accomplishment of this book. They are a veteran in the field of academics and their pool of knowledge is as vast as their experience in printing. Their expertise and guidance has proved useful at every step. Their uncompromising quality standards have made this book an exceptional effort. Their encouragement from time to time has been an inspiration for everyone.

The publisher and the editorial board hope that this book will prove to be a valuable piece of knowledge for researchers, students, practitioners and scholars across the globe.

List of Contributors

Santi Tofani
University of Turin and Ivrea Hospital, Piemonte, Italy

Hugo de Seabra Martins Nunes, Ana Opinião, António Guimarães and Fátima Vaz
Department of Medical Oncology, Portuguese Institute of Oncology Lisbon Francisco Gentil, Lisbon, Portugal

Alexandra Mayer
Southern Portugal Cancer Registry (ROR-Sul), Portuguese Institute of Oncology Lisbon Francisco Gentil, Lisbon, Portugal

Ana Francisca Jorge
Department of Gynaecology, Portuguese Institute of Oncology Lisbon Francisco Gentil, Lisbon, Portugal

Teresa Margarida Cunha
Department of Radiology, Portuguese Institute of Oncology Lisbon Francisco Gentil, Lisbon, Portugal

Arkene Levy and Patricia C. Rose
Nova Southeastern University, Florida, USA

Alejandro Santini Blasco, Cristian Valdez Cortes, Veronica Sepúlveda Arcuch, Ricardo Baeza Letelier and Sergio Bustos Caprio
Centro Oncologico Antofagasta, Antofagasta, Chile

Roman Liubota and Roman Vereshchako
Department of Oncology, National Medical University named after O.O Bogomolets, Kyiv, Ukraine

Mykola Anikusko and Iryna Liubota
Municipal City Clinical Oncological Centre, Kyiv, Ukraine

Ambrogio P. Londero
Unit of Obstetrics and Gynecology, S. Polo Hospital, Monfalcone, GO, Italy

Serena Bertozzi, Roberta Di Vora, Luca Seriau, Andrea Risaliti and Carla Cedolini
Clinic of Surgery, University of Udine, Italy

Fabrizio De Biasio and Pier Camillo Parodi
Clinic of Plastic Surgery, University of Udine, Italy

Lorenza Driul
Clinic of Obstetrics and Gynecology, University of Udine, Italy

Laura Mariuzzi
Institute of Pathologic Anatomy, University of Udine, Italy

Ajda Coker-Gurkan, Pinar Obakan-Yerlikaya and Elif-Damla Arisan
Science and Leters Faculty, Department of Molecular Biology and Genetics, Istanbul Kultur University, Istanbul, Turkey

Shinichiro Morishita and Atsuhiro Tsubaki
Institute for Human Movement, Medical Sciences, Niigata University of Health and Welfare, Niigata, Japan

Mark McGregor
Adelaide Oncology and Haematology, North Adelaide, Australia

Gonzalo Tapia Rico
Medical Oncology, The Queen Elizabeth Hospital, Adelaide, Australia

Amanda Townsend and Tim Price
Medical Oncology, The Queen Elizabeth Hospital, Adelaide, Australia University of Adelaide, Adelaide, Australia

Index